BIOMATERIALS - PROPERTIES, PRODUCTION AND DEVICES

TYPE I COLLAGEN

BIOLOGICAL FUNCTIONS, SYNTHESIS AND MEDICINAL APPLICATIONS

BIOMATERIALS - PROPERTIES, PRODUCTION AND DEVICES

Additional books in this series can be found on Nova's website under the Series tab.

Additional E-books in this series can be found on Nova's website under the e-book tab.

STEM CELLS AND REGENERATIVE MEDICINE

Additional books in this series can be found on Nova's website under the Series tab.

Additional E-books in this series can be found on Nova's website under the e-book tab.

BIOMATERIALS - PROPERTIES, PRODUCTION AND DEVICES

TYPE I COLLAGEN

BIOLOGICAL FUNCTIONS, SYNTHESIS AND MEDICINAL APPLICATIONS

MARIA EDUARDA HENRIQUES
AND
MARCIO PINTO
EDITORS

New York

For permission to use material from this book please contact us:
Telephone 631-231-7269; Fax 631-231-8175
Web Site: http://www.novapublishers.com

Library of Congress Cataloging-in-Publication Data

ISBN 978-1-62257-625-8

Library of Congress Control Number: 2012943798

Published by Nova Science Publishers, Inc. † New York

CONTENTS

PREFACE

Type I collagen is a popular biomaterial for use in tissue engineering and regenerative medicine applications owing to its abundance in natural tissues and its natural functions within the body as a scaffold material with favorable cell-interactive properties. In this book, the authors present current research in the study of the biological functions, synthesis and medicinal applications of Type I collagen. Topics discussed include collagen type I as a candidate for in vivo delivery systems for cells, proteins, and drugs; degradation of type I collagen and the pathogenesis of infectious diseases; Type I collagen's synthesis, biological functions and medical applications during systemic inflammation; using collagen-based scaffolds in tissue engineering and repair; type I collagens from marine sources; and the role of extracellular matrix in the wound repair process.

Chapter 1- It is now recognized that biological macromolecules such as components of the extracellular matrix (ECM) are important as instructive templates in Regenerative Medicine applications. They are now increasingly used in the development of a new generation of bio-mimetic materials that allow for restoration of function when the self-renewal capacity of a tissue or organ cannot overcome degeneration caused by disease, injury or age-related wear. For example, macromolecules derived from connective tissue have been isolated, chemically modified, and used in medical applications ranging from tissue repair and reconstruction to drug and cell delivery systems. Common ECM macromolecules of vertebrates include collagen, proteoglycans, elastin and other cell-interactive proteins such as fibronectin and laminin. Of these, type I collagen is the most abundant ECM macromolecule and is the primary scaffolding material that maintains the 3-dimensional structure of tissues and organs within the body. It also provides the micro-environmental milieu for cellular attachment, migration, and proliferation. Animal-derived collagen is frequently used in tissue engineering applications due to its biocompatibility, but there are significant concerns about the immunogenicity of xenogeneic material as well as the possibility of pathogen transmission. Most recently, synthetic collagens and recombinant human collagens have been produced for medical application. Regardless of the source, however, macromolecules require processing and chemical treatment in order to improve their stability both *in vitro* and *in vivo*. This is most commonly achieved by cross-linking using a variety of agents. Cross-linking also allows for the development of "tailor-made" collagen-based biomaterials that possess specific properties for tissue engineering. Chemical cross-linkers such as glutaraldehyde and epoxy compounds are frequently used but their cytotoxicities have limited their clinical application. This has led to the use of zero-length cross-linkers such as carbodiimides and naturally derived agents such as genipin. Enzymatic cross-linking is becoming an attractive method to induce *in situ* biomaterial formation due to the mildness of the reaction. Naturally occurring enzymes such as transglutaminase are now commonly used. Photosensitizers used in combination with ultra-violet light irradiation can be used as exogenous cross-linkers. For example, riboflavin in combination with ultra-violet light is used clinically to augment the properties of collagen-based tissues such as the sclera and the cornea. Collagen type I is a good candidate for tissue engineering and *in vivo* delivery systems for cells, proteins, and drugs. Important to its versatile and functional nature are its chemotactic properties, which promote cellular proliferation and differentiation, richness in cross-linking sites, and biodegradability. Collagen based delivery matrices have been reported to improve the results of cell delivery by improving cell viability.

Chapter 2 - Collagen constitutes one-third of the proteins present in the human body and the main component of the extracellular matrix. Its singular structure renders collagen degradation a hard task and only specialized peptidases, known as collagenases, are able to mediate its hydrolysis. Collagenases generally belong to the family of zinc dependent matrix metalloproteases (MMPs) or bacterial collagenases of the M9 family, which have the ability to catalyze not only collagens but also other extracellular matrix components (ECM). Other independent types of collagenases have been reported as members of the serine and cysteine-protease family. Collagenase-like activity is still poorly understood but it seems to be associated to partially unfolded states adopted by collagen that could be recognized and cleaved by these proteases. While collagen degradation is a natural process for tissue homeostasis, its unusual hydrolysis has been recognized as contributing factor to multiple pathologies, among them cancer, chronic and infectious diseases. The identification of collagenases as agents of the infection process was first described in *Clostridium hystolyticum* with the isolation of an extracellular enzyme responsible for tissue putrefaction. At present, there is a wealth of data regarding collagenases in many pathogenic species of bacteria, fungus, protozoa and worms, involved in the pathogen spread in different host tissues. For this reason, collagenases are being considered promising targets for the design of new therapeutic drugs. Strategies for the advancement in this field are the detailed structural characterizations of pathogen collagenases and collagenase-like to assist in achieving drug selectivity to prevent infection accomplishment.

Chapter 3 - Collagens are proteins centrally involved in the formation of fibrillar and microfibrillar networks of the extracellular matrix. The biosynthesis of collagens starting with gene transcription within the nucleus, to the aggregation of collagen heterotrimers into large fibrils is a complex multistep process. It is characterized by the presence of a large number of co- and post-translational modifications, many of them being unique to collagens or collagen-like proteins. The fibril-forming collagens are synthesized as procollagens which is released to the extracellular space where undergo several modifications: removal of large procollagen N- and C-terminal peptides, ordered aggregation, crosslink formation. Biochemically, collagen is composed of a triple helix which consists of three α-chains. The amino acid composition of collagen is atypical for proteins, particularly with respect to its high hydroxyproline (Hyp) content. However, their size, function and tissue distribution vary considerably among collagens. To date, more than twenty genetically distinct collagen types have been described; being type I collagen the most abundant and best studied collagen of the body. It forms more than 90% of the organic mass of bone and is the major collagen of tendons, skin, ligaments, cornea, and many interstitial connective tissues with the exception of very few tissues such as hyaline cartilage, brain, and vitreous body. The collagen type I triple helix is usually formed as a heterodimer by two identical α1(I)-chains and one α2(I)-chain. In most organs and notably in tendons and fascia, type I collagen gives tensile stiffness and in bone, it defines substantial biomechanical properties regarding load bearing, tensile strength, and torsional stiffness in particular after calcification. The post-translational modifications of the collagenous matrix are important for both its structural and mechanical properties, and disruption of the cross-linking can result in severe dysfunction of the tissue. Both, biosynthesis and breakdown products are used in medicine as specific and sensitive bone markers to evaluate bone remodelling. In this regard N-terminal procollagen type I (PICP) is used as a bone formation marker while the crosslinks and the N and C-telopeptides (NTX and CT, respectively) are used as bone resorption markes.

Chapter 4 - Adult stem cell based tissue engineering for repair and regenerative purposes, has been an emerging area of intense investigation. The current major challenge to these approaches has been the inability to vascularize and perfuse in vitro engineered tissue constructs. Attempts to provide oxygen and nutrients to cells contained in biomaterial constructs have met with varying degrees of success. Engineering a tissue of clinically relevant magnitude requires the formation of extensive and stable microvascular networks within the tissue. Since most in vitro engineered tissue constructs do not contain the intricate microvascular structures of native tissue, the cells contained in scaffolds heavily rely on simple diffusion for oxygenation and nutritional delivery. The majority of cells need to be within 100-200 μm of a blood supply to receive adequate oxygen and nutrients for survival. Otherwise, due to limitations of diffusional transport, the cells in the interior regions of the artificial scaffold can experience hypoxia or anoxia and undergo cellular degeneration and necrosis. Hence, this necessitates the formation of appropriate in vitro three-dimensional (3-D) plexuses of new blood vessels within the pre-implanted biomaterial constructs through the process of in situ de novo vasculogenesis/angiogenesis for organ tissue engineering. To this end, here the authors demonstrate the application of 3-D matrix scaffolds composed of type I collagen to address these concerns.

Chapter 5 - Type I collagen is an important component in the wound-healing process and large quantities is found in scar tissue associated with a variety of pathological conditions. The equilibrium between synthesis and degradation of collagen has been targeted as therapeutic goal in chronic diseases. However, acute inflammation activated both fibrogenesis and degradation, which causes the release of activated extracellular matrix components causing a vicious cycle that would in turn contribute to the progression of the inflammatory process. The functional compromising of the organ by the collagen accumulation could aggravate the systemic inflammation. Consequently, type I collagen deposition have been investigated as an attractive target for anti-fibrotic therapies, marker of disease severity, as hemostatic sponges and implants to repair wounds and tissue engineering applications as scaffolds. The studies of biogenesis of collagen and the extracellular matrix components are crucial to determinate new therapeutic alternatives as medical application.

Chapter 6 - Tissue engineering is an emerging field that includes the development of structures that replace, repair, and maintain tissue functions. Tissue engineering is an attractive and cost-effective strategy when compared to conventional or surgical therapies. The technique involves in vitro seeding and attachment of human cells onto a scaffold. These cells then proliferate, migrate, and differentiate, as well as secrete extracellular matrix components in order to form and repair tissues. The type of scaffold and its components are therefore crucial for controlling the behavior of the cells and for the success of the therapy. Among the many scaffold materials that have been developed, the collagen-based scaffolds offer many advantageous features, as well as some limitations. The aim of this chapter is to describe the use of collagen-based scaffolds in tissue engineering and repair.

Chapter 7 - Among all the collagens, Type I collagen plays an important role in the extracellular matrix (ECM) of skin, bone and other tissues. This protein is involved in many human and animal diseases, including fibrosis, osteoporosis, cancer, atherosclerosis etc. In spite of or because of the fact that it is widely distributed in the body, the different parts (degradation products) of type I collagen molecule are frequently utilized to monitor physiological changes in tissues as well as being used as diagnostic tools in various pathophysiological conditions. Collagens from marine sources are proved to be suitable for human applications as is metabolically compatible, non-toxic, low inflammatory and less immunogenic, however, type I collagen from marine sources has not yet been made available for extensive commercial medical uses. Hence, in the current book chapter, for the first time, the authors provide comprehensive information on the past explorations of type I collagens exclusively from marine sources; isolation and characterization, biomedical applications basing on the author's previous experiences. Further, the future prospects and perspectives are well covered in the present manuscript in order to bring the wide-ranging viewpoints that are useful for the next generation ECM researchers as well as marine medical biologists.

Chapter 8 - The extracellular matrix (ECM) serves as scaffolding to hold tissues together, its form and its composition help to determine tissue characteristics. Wound repair processes heal by progressing through distinct but overlapping phases: haemostasis, inflammation, proliferation and remodeling. Throughout these phases, components of the ECM play an important role in regulating and integrating many key processes of healing mechanisms. The components of the ECM provide strength, elasticity and compressibility in normal skin. In acute wounds the provisional wound matrix, containing fibrin and fibronectin, plays several key roles, including providing a scaffold to direct cells into the injury as well as stimulating them to proliferate, differentiate and synthesize new ECM. It has also been proposed that the prolonged inflammatory phase causes increased levels of proteases such as MMPs, elastase, plasmin and thrombin, which destroy components of the ECM, damaging the growth factors and their receptors that are essential for healing. This article reviews the multifaceted molecular roles of ECM in normal and abnormal wound-healing process, and touches on potential therapies based on recent acquisitions of tissue biology.

In: Type I Collagen
Editors: Maria Eduarda Henriques and Marcio Pinto
ISBN: 978-1-62257-625-8

Chapter I

COLLAGEN TYPE I: A PROMISING SCAFFOLD MATERIAL FOR TISSUE ENGINEERING AND REGENERATIVE MEDICINE

Kimberly Merrett[1,2], Monika Kozak Ljunggren[1], Debasish Mondal[1], May Griffith[1,2] and Mehrdad Rafat[1,*]

[1]Integrative Regenerative Medicine Centre, and Department of Clinical and Experimental Medicine, Linköping University, Linkoping, Sweden
[2]Department of Cellular and Molecular Medicine, University of Ottawa, Ottawa, Ontario, Canada

ABSTRACT

It is now recognized that biological macromolecules such as components of the extracellular matrix (ECM) are important as instructive templates in Regenerative Medicine applications. They are now increasingly used in the development of a new generation of bio-mimetic materials that allow for restoration of function when the self-renewal capacity of a tissue or organ cannot overcome degeneration caused by disease, injury or age-related wear. For example, macromolecules derived from connective tissue have been isolated, chemically modified, and used in medical applications ranging from tissue repair and reconstruction to drug and cell delivery systems. Common ECM macromolecules of vertebrates include collagen, proteoglycans, elastin and other cell-interactive proteins such as fibronectin and laminin. Of these, type I collagen is the most abundant ECM macromolecule and is the primary scaffolding material that maintains the 3-dimensional structure of tissues and organs within the body. It also provides the micro-environmental milieu for cellular attachment, migration, and proliferation.

Animal-derived collagen is frequently used in tissue engineering applications due to its biocompatibility, but there are significant concerns about the immunogenicity of xenogeneic material as well as the possibility of pathogen transmission. Most recently, synthetic collagens and recombinant human collagens have been produced for medical application. Regardless of the source, however, macromolecules require processing and

* Corresponding author: Mehrdad Rafat, Ph.D. Department of Clinical and Experimental Medicine, Linköping University, 581 85 Linkoping, Sweden. Tel: +46 (0)73 461 3166. E-mail: Mehrdad.rafat@liu.se.

chemical treatment in order to improve their stability both *in vitro* and *in vivo*. This is most commonly achieved by cross-linking using a variety of agents. Cross-linking also allows for the development of "tailor-made" collagen-based biomaterials that possess specific properties for tissue engineering. Chemical cross-linkers such as glutaraldehyde and epoxy compounds are frequently used but their cytotoxicities have limited their clinical application. This has led to the use of zero-length cross-linkers such as carbodiimides and naturally derived agents such as genipin. Enzymatic cross-linking is becoming an attractive method to induce *in situ* biomaterial formation due to the mildness of the reaction. Naturally occurring enzymes such as transglutaminase are now commonly used. Photosensitizers used in combination with ultra-violet light irradiation can be used as exogenous cross-linkers. For example, riboflavin in combination with ultra-violet light is used clinically to augment the properties of collagen-based tissues such as the sclera and the cornea.

Collagen type I is a good candidate for tissue engineering and *in vivo* delivery systems for cells, proteins, and drugs. Important to its versatile and functional nature are its chemotactic properties, which promote cellular proliferation and differentiation, richness in cross-linking sites, and biodegradability. Collagen based delivery matrices have been reported to improve the results of cell delivery by improving cell viability.

INTRODUCTION

The collagens are a family of extracellular matrix (ECM) macromolecules that are ubiquitous within the body, contributing to both mechanical properties and biological function of various types of tissues such as skin, bone, tendons, ligaments, blood vessels, and the cornea. Collagens are found in multi-cellular animals, accounting for approximately 30% of all body proteins and are the most abundant constituent of naturally occurring scaffolds (Nimni et al., 1987). Twenty-nine types of collagens have now been described, but types I, II and III are the most abundant and make up the majority of the extracellular matrix macromolecules and have several roles. In general, collagens act as: (i) supporting scaffolds to maintain tissue structure (e.g. stromal fibers in the cornea that are responsible for maintaining the cornea's structure are mainly comprised of collagen type I); (ii) anchoring devices to promote cellular adhesion to non-cellular areas (e.g. fibrils that anchor epithelial cells to the corneal stroma are mainly comprised of collagen type VII) (Whikehart, 2003).

The name collagen appeared in the 19th century and comes from the Greek words meaning "glue" and "birth", as the first discovered property of these proteins was their ability to yield gelatin. Type I collagen is a popular biomaterial for use in tissue engineering and regenerative medicine applications owing to its abundance in natural tissues and its natural functions within the body as a scaffold material with favourable cell-interactive properties.

All collagens are protein complexes whose basic units consist of triple helices (tropocollagen) in which three polypeptide chains are wound around each other like a piece of rope. Collagen molecules are self-assembled into micro-fibrils and then fibrils. The basic structure of all collagen molecules is a triple helix formed by three α chains that are approximately 1000 amino acids long, comprised of repeats of the basic triplet Gly-X-Y, where X and Y are often proline and hydroxyproline, respectively. The proline and 4-hydroxyproline residues are also important for the correct conformation and stability of the triple helix. Non-hydroxylated type I collagen is denatured at 24 °C while the hydroxylated molecules are stable in temperatures up to 39 °C (Berg & Prockop, 1973; Jimenez et al.,

1973). The presence of glycine in every third position is necessary for the assembly of a right-handed superhelix (van der Rest et al., 1991). In homotrimeric collagens all three α chains are identical (e.g. collagen type II and III consisting of three identical α1 chains) whereas heterotrimeric molecules consist of two or three different α chains (e.g. collagen type I consisting of two α1 chains and one α2 chain). The collagen types in vertebrates can be grouped into fibrillar and non-fibrillar collagens based on their structures. The fibril-forming collagens (e.g. types I, II, III, V, XI, etc.) These collagens tend to aggregate into fibrils that provide tensile strength to tissues and define the shape of the tissue in which they are present. The non-fibrilar collagens (e.g. types IX, XII, XIV, XVI, etc.) are not capable of forming fibrils themselves; instead they associate with the surface of collagen fibrils and interact with other extracellular matrix components.

Collagens as Raw Materials

Extracted Collagens

As alluded to, collagen have now been extracted from a range of body tissues, including connective tissue and skin (bovine and porcine hides and more recently, fish skin) for use as biomaterials. They are then purified and made available for use as raw materials both with and without their telopeptides.

The immunogenicity of collagens differs among the various types. Collagen type I is much less immunogenic when compared with type II. The injection of type II native molecules evokes polyarthritis in rats, whereas type I, even in the presence of an adjuvant causes no great effect (Stuart et al., 1985). The high level of homology among collagen type I sequences and low content of aromatic amino acids are possible explanations for this phenomenon. However, immune reactions, anaphylaxis included, develop in 3-5% of the human population (Cooperman et al., 1984). In case of bovine collagen, a pre-sensitization mechanism has been suggested, probably the result of beef consumption (Soo et al., 1993). Most immunogenic epitopes are located on the α2(I) chains with the major histocompatibility complex involvement in the immune response (Sakaguchi et al., 1999). Fortunately, most of these adverse reactions are lenient and only rarely they necessitate the removal of a collagen implant of animal origin (Olsen et al., 2003).

There is current debate as to whether the telopeptides are the regions primarily responsible for the immunogenic properties of collagens. (Lynn et al., 2004) These nonhelical fragments exhibit a much lower degree of conservation and higher degree of intra-species variation (Furthmayr et al., 1976) that may evoke immune responses (Michaeli et al. 1969; Furthmayr et al., 1971). However, there are contradicting studies that suggest that the helical regions are the main antigenic determinants (Beil et al., 1973; Nowack et al., 1975). Furthermore, some of these epitopes may be hidden and become exposed as the helix unwinds, which might cause a problem while the implanted collagen degrades (Dodge et al., 1989). The immunogenicity issue becomes more evident when comparing various species as the donor-recipient pairs. In addition to the collagen type, the presence or absence of an immune response, as well as the location of antigenic determinants are also dependent on the interacting species. Therefore, the results of biocompatibility testing of a given animal collagen in a given host species cannot be directly extrapolated to all other species and humans. (Lynn et al., 2004). The belief that it is the telopeptides that are responsible for collagen immunogenicity lead to the production of atelocollagen, where the telopeptide regions have been removed by proteolytic enzymes (Vizarova et al., 1994). The lack of both the C and N terminus leads to impaired fibril assembly and consequently, the banding pattern is lost (Kadler et al. 1996). Atelocollagen is also characterised by an improved solubility, which along with its amorphous character may be beneficial for production purposes. However, the lack of immunogenicity postulated for atelocollagen has only been demonstrated in certain cases (Davison et al., 1967; Pontz et al., 1970) The benefits of using animal-extracted atellocollagen for human implantation are to be further investigated from a immunological point of view (Lynn et al., 2004) although porcine collagen products have been safely used in human for cosmetic applications such as dermal fillers.

From our own work on type I collagen, when carbodiimide crosslinked porcine atelocollagen hydrogels were implanted into pigs as partial thickness implants by lamellar keratoplasty (LKP), they were well-accepted with no adverse immune response (Rafat et al., 2008; Liu et al., 2006; Liu et al., 2009). We also implanted bovine collagen-polyNIPAAM copolymers in dogs (Li et al., 2003) and in pigs' corneas (Bentley et al., 2010) using LKP that were well-tolerated *in vivo*. However, when porcine collagen was implanted into mouse corneas as full-thickness corneal substitutes, the implants generated a low-grade anti-porcine collagen Type-1 antibody response two weeks post-operative while did not induce a significant T cell response. The antibody level continued to rise over several weeks. Overall, porcine collagen-EDC/NHS cross-linked corneas were tolerated well in murine recipients (Liu et al., 2007). Retro-corneal membrane formation was the main complication and barrier to clarity. Whether the antibody response and the retrograde membrane formation were due to full thickness implantation or due to an immune response will need to be further investigated.

Collagen Biosynthesis

The biosynthesis of fibril-forming collagens (mainly type I) has been extensively studied. Collagen fibrils ranging from simple ones containing Gly-X-Y repeats that have been stitched together to more sophisticated self-assembly triple helical fibres have been synthetically produced. Fibril-forming collagen genes are conserved among metazoans, which is an indication of the importance of this group of proteins. Even though collagen type I molecules contain about 1014 amino acids, the genes encoding α1 and α2 chains are approximately 5000 base pairs (bp) long, containing 51 and 52 exons, respectively (Marini et al., 2007). These exons are multiples of a 54 bp unit equal to six repeats of the basic collagen triplet Gly-X-Y. It is believed that this 54 bp repeat comes from a common ancestral gene from which all modern collagen genes have evolved through duplications and recombinations (Ramirez et al., 1985). Collagen synthesis takes place both intra- and extra-cellularly. After splicing, 5' capping and 3' polyadenylation, mature mRNA is translated by ribosomes bound to the rough endoplasmic reticulum (RER). The resulting pre-procollagen molecule undergoes hydroxylation of proline and lysine inside the RER. An abundance of 4-hydroxyproline leads to greater thermal stability of the molecule, thus this type of hydroxylation is not extensive among species living in lower temperatures (Cohen-Solal et al., 1986). Hydroxylysine is the site of glycosylation by both glucosyl- and galactosyl- residues and participates in cross-linking of collagen molecules within fibrils. The folding of the collagen chains into the triple helix begins at the C-pro-peptide and is catalyzed by a series of enzymes, including chaperones such as HSP47 (Lang et al., 1987; Clarke et al., 1991). The assembled triple helices are secreted through the Golgi apparatus and further processing occurs in the extracellular compartment. Both C and N pro-peptides are cleaved by specific proteases and have been suggested to play a role in the regulation of collagen expression (Wu et al., 1991).

Recombinantly Produced Collagen

The understanding of the complex transcription and translation of collagen has allowed the production of recombinant human collagen. Recombinant collagen is the collagen derived from recombinant DNA (rDNA), which is a form of synthetic DNA made by combining two or more DNA sequences that would not normally occur together. The goal in recombinant protein technology is to introduce recombinant genes into a host cell along with expression factor, so that the host cell expresses the desired protein. The key steps in collagen biosynthesis using recombinant technology are the formation of the triple helix and the post-translational modification of proline residues to hydroxyproline for stability at body temperature. Prior to these two steps, the selection of the essential genes, enzymes, and cell types in which the collagen molecules are expressed play a crucial role for production of recombinant collagen. Mammalian, baculoviral, and transgenic systems have been used for expression of recombinant collagen (Toman et al., 2000). Recombinant collagen accumulation has been reported in mammalian cell culture, insects' cell culture, yeast, bacteria, mice and cow milk, tobacco cell culture, and tobacco plants. Among variuos systems only mammalian cells transfected with collagen genes expressed stable hydroxylated full-length collagens. There has been no report of production of stable hydroxylated collagen using the rest of these expression systems unless they were co-expressed with prolyl 4-hydroxylase (P4H). Non-hydroxylated collagen molecules are susceptible to degradation and so not suitable for tissue engineering applications The co-expression of P4H with collagen in yeast fermentations has generated thermally stable recombinant human collagen Type I (Yang et al., 2004). Hanan et al. have also reported the synthesis of recombinant heterotrimeric collagen type I co-expressed in tobacco plants with the human prolyl-4-hydroxylase (P4H) and lysyl hydroxylase 3 (LH3) enzymes. Plant-derived thermally stable triple helical collagens with bio-functionalities similar to human tissue-derived collagen were formed.

Recombinant technology is a challenging field that may hold great promise for the future in synthesizing biological macromolecules or preventing or treating genetic diseases. However, it poses serious ethical and economical questions: are we equipped to deal with the environmental impact of recombinantly produced molecules that replace their natural counterparts, and whether these molecules can be produced in an economically viable way making them readily available to everyone who needs them.

COLLAGEN AS A BIOMATERIAL

Based on *in vitro* experiments, it has been postulated that procollagen molecules assemble spontaneously into organized fibrils. It is the hydrophobic and electrostatic interactions of these molecules that drive this phenomenon (Silver et al., 1992). However, it is believed that *in vivo*, integrins and fibronectin participate in the extracellular assembly of collagen fibrils inducing conformational changes that facilitate the process, therefore exhibiting a regulatory function in fibrillogenesis. The final mechanical properties of the fibrils are dependent on the number of cross-links formed between collagen molecules, which is a function of lysine hydroxylation in the telopeptides and is tissue-specific. Cartilage is characterized by complete lysine hydroxylation, whereas in skin no such hydroxylation occurs. Cross-linking is initiated by an enzymatically catalyzed formation of aldehydes leading to the spontaneous creation of reducible Schiff bases (lysine) or ketoimine (hydroxylysine) bonds. Permanent cross-links (pyridinium, pyrrolic or histidine adducts) are formed in further steps of tissue maturation. The location of these cross-links is usually between the C- or N-telopeptide and a residue of the helical region of the neighboring molecule (Gelse et al., 2003).

In vitro, however, the pathway leading to covalent bond formation does not occur and consequently, in its purified form, type I collagen forms a weakly cross-linked thermogel lacking the sufficient physical properties and resistance to biodegradation to make it adequate for most *in vitro* and *in vivo* tissue engineering applications (Kew et al., 2011; Bailey 1991; Di & Heath, 2009).Hence there is a requirement for a synthetic cross-linking process that can confer purified collagen with suitable physical properties and resistance to biodegradation whilst retaining its biocompatibility. It has been demonstrated that exogenous covalent bonds can be added between individual collagen molecules in the triple helix (intrahelical cross-links), between adjacent helices (intermolecular cross-links) or between collagen and other molecular species using chemical and/or physical methods (Lee et al., 1994). It has been reported that the formation of inter- and intra- covalent bonds improves antigenicity (Williams, 1985), thermal stability (Sionkowska, 2011), mechanical properties (Cornwell et al., 2007), and the resistance of collagen-based materials to biodegradation (Stricklin et al., 1988) without impeding the ability of the material to integrate into the surrounding host tissue and to promote regeneration. Despite the fact that collagen types I and III are reported to be non-immunogenic, e.g. not inducing autoimmune reactions (Trentham et al., 1977; Courtenay et al., 1980), the changes in antigenicity and immunogenicity induced by cross-linking methods are yet to be understood, and thus comprehensive *in vivo* experimental evidence is needed to determine the immunological effects of a given cross-linking treatment (Lynn et al., 2004).

Cross-linking approaches are used to produce implant materials that possess the desired mechanical properties for specific applications (e.g. tendon, skin, and cornea), Although mechanical properties are typically representing required tensile strength and elasticity for implantation and how well a biomaterial replicates the structure and mechanical characteristics of the natural tissue it is replacing, they are also important for maintaining the 3D architecture essential to cell attachment and cell migration (Tierney et al., 2008). Thus, mechanical properties of any collagen-based material are important in order to facilitate applications such as *in vitro* cell culture, *in vivo* implantation, as well as mechanical functionalities once implanted (Tierney et al., 2008).

Yet despite extensive research and development, there is to date no accepted "standard" cross-linking method for the production of collagen-based materials (Kew et al., 2011). Numerous chemical and physical cross-linking methods have been developed; each method employing different mechanisms. These methods often rely on the addition of synthetic polymers or natural polysaccharides to modulate and improve upon the properties of purified collagen (Rafat et al., 2008; Sang et al., 2010). The most significant factor involved in the cross-linking process is the number and availability of specific functional groups that will participate in the cross-linking reaction. In the case of type I collagen the majority of cross linking methods require reaction of the amine groups of lysine and hydroxylysine as well as the carboxylic groups of glutamic or aspartic acid residues. Most of these reactions are rapid and occur in high yield to give stable amide or in some cases secondary amine bonds. Common chemical cross-linkers include aldehydes such as glutaraldehyde (Daamen et al., 2003; Gough et al., 2002; Zhang et al., 2005; Wang et al., 2008) and formaldehyde (Singh et al., 2006), epoxides (Di & Heath, 2009; Tu et al., 1994), carbodiimides such as N-(3-Dimethylaminopropyl) N'-ethylcarboddimide hydrochloride (EDC) (Colazzo et al., 2011, Angele et al., 2004; Kim et al., 2005; Merrett et al., 2008), imidoesters (Hassel & Hand, 1974) and isocyanates (Rault et al., 1996; Zhang, Wu et al., 2011). Effective alternatives to chemical cross-linkers include the naturally derived cross-linkers such as genepin (Daamen et al., 2003; Torres-Giner et al., 2009; Zhang et al., 2011) and schizophyllan (Jayakumar et al. 2012). Physical cross-linking methods include ultra-violet (UV) and gamma irradiation (Ibrahim et al., 2011), dehydrothermal (DHT) (Tierney et al. 2008) methods as well as a variety of photochemical approaches that require the use of photo-initiators such as Rose Bengal and riboflavin (Ibusuki et al., 2007; Kew et al., 2011).

Not all of these methods are completely satisfactory in terms of producing collagen-based materials for particular tissue engineering applications. In the case of chemical cross-linking approaches, the relationship between the molecular structure of cross-linking agents and the properties of the resultant material are not clearly defined (Di & Heath, 2009; Lee et al., 1994). Studies have also shown that chemical cross-linkers are potentially cytotoxic; for example glutaraldehyde and formaldehyde are known to be carcinogenic (Gendler et al., 1984). Physical cross-linking imparts partial denaturation to the collagen molecules (Weadock et al., 1995), which markedly reduces the strength and increases the rate of degradation by enzymes (Ohan et al., 2002). And while cross-linking strategies are intended to improve the strength and stiffness of the material, some approaches may impair biocompatibility by altering the scaffold surface biochemistry in a manner that impedes cellular infiltration and the rate of new tissue ingrowth and remodelling (Cornwell et al., 2007; Nishi et al., 1995; Speer et al., 1980). For example, DHT treatment of self-assembled collagen threads, while providing mechanical stability, has been reported to compromise the rate of cellular migration onto the collagen-based scaffolds as compared to the equivalent material cross-linked using a carbodiimide such as EDC (Cornwell et al., 2004).

COLLAGEN CROSSLINKING

Of the organic, bis-aldehyde, homobifunctional collagen cross-linkers, glutaraldehyde has the most widespread application because of its relative low cost and high efficiency (Ulrich et al., 2011; Tung et al., 2011; Di & Heath, 2009; Cockerman & Hsu, 2009 ; Bao et al., 2008) (Figure 1 (a)). A large variety of reaction pathways may be involved when using glutaraldehyde to cross-link collagen; for a more extensive review see Old Damink et al. 1995. It is generally accepted that glutaraldehyde produces inter- and intra- molecular cross-links through the reaction of the aldehyde groups with the ε-amine groups of lysine or hydroxylysine residues of collagen to form Schiff bases; these Schiff base intermediates are unstable and may lead to several different reactions (e.g. secondary amines, pyridinium-type cross-links). Glutaraldehyde can also form cross-links with the sulfydryl groups of cysteine, phenolic and imidazole rings of tyrosine and histidine (Olde Damink et al., 1995; Hassel &Hand, 1974). The final results are stable covalent inter- and intra- molecular bonds that produce a stable cross-linked collagen-based material (Simionescu et al., 1991). Although the cross-linking reaction is most efficient at basic pH values, it has been shown that glutaraldehyde cross-linking at acidic pH values is preferred because materials cross-linked at acidic pH values have less pendant glutaraldehyde molecules thus decreasing the potential for glutaraldehyde related cytotoxicity (Olde Damink et al., 1995).

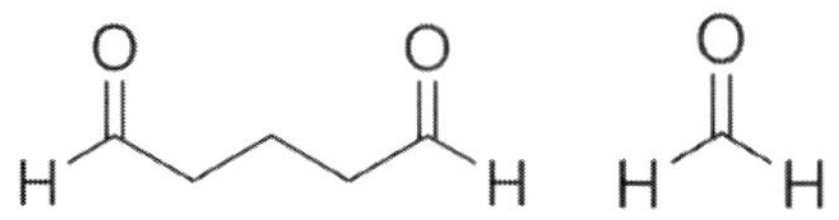

(a) (b)

Figure 1. Aldehyde-based cross-linkers: (a) Glutaraldehyde. (MW 100.12), (b) Formaldehyde (MW 30.03).

Glutaraldehyde has been widely used to cross-link a variety of collagen-based materials such as porcine aortic valve cusps and bovine pericardium for cardiac valve replacement (Duncan et al., 1996; Lyman et al., 1990). Glutaraldehyde is also a popular choice to cross-link chitosan and collagen blends to fabricate three dimensional carriers for the controlled drug release of ophthalmic drugs such as pilocarpine chlorohydrate (Flocea et al., 2010). The network structure and composition of these materials have been shown to be influenced by the nature and amount of chitosan used in the synthesis and the quantity of cross-linker used.

Glutaraldehyde in its vapour form has been reported to cross-link electro-spun collagen-chitosan nanofibers. Owing to the sensitivity of collagen-chitosan fiber to water, the conventional cross-linking approach of immersing samples into aqueous glutaraldehyde solution is not ideal. By placing the fibers into a dessicator filled with glutaraldehyde vapour, the collagen-chitosan fibers can be cross-linked. In this case, cross-linking of collagen and chitosan with glutaraldehyde involves the reaction of the free amino groups of chitosan and lysine or hydroxylysine amino acid residues of the polypeptide chains of collagen with the aldehyde groups of glutaraldehyde. After vapour cross-linking, the fiber matrix becomes yellowish and is slightly shrunk dimensionally. The color change is due to the establishment of CH=N linkages between the free amine groups of collagen-chitosan and aldehyde groups of glutaraldehyde (Chen et al., 2010).

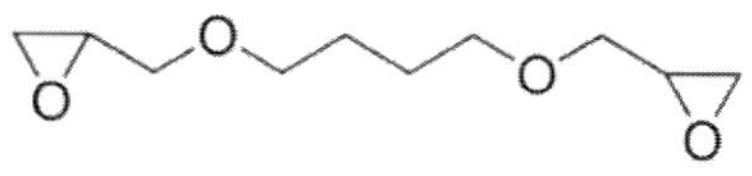

Figure 2. 1,4-(butanediol) diglycidyl ether (BDDGE) (MW 202.25).

Despite its popularity, glutaraldehyde cross-linking is associated with a number of concerns: (i) cytotoxicity due to post-implantation depolymerization and monomer release from the glutaraldehyde polymer (Gendler et al., 1984; Huang-Lee et al., 1990), (ii) impairment of endothelialisation over a certain cross-linking threshold (Titorencu et al., 2010; Nimni et al., 1987), and (iii) pre-disposition of implanted glutaraldehyde cross-linked material to calcification (Schoen et a., 1985; Golomb et al., 1987) The unstable Schiff bases formed as a result of glutaraldehyde cross-linking may lead to the leaching of residual glutaraldehyde with subsequent cytotoxic and inflammatory activity that can contribute to calcification (Nimni et al., 1987).

Formaldehyde, another aldehyde collagen cross-linker, is the smallest cross-linking reagent available that does not create a zero-length link between two molecules (Hermanson, 2008) (Figure 1(b)). Although technically not a bi-functional reagent, it undergoes cross-linking reactions as though it possessed two functional groups. It has seen less wide spread use as a collagen cross-linker in terms of fabricating collagen-based biomaterials as other commercial cross-linkers often result in superior products with respect to biocompatibility and mechanical properties (Madhaven et al., 2010). Its current primary use is that of a tissue fixative for the preservation of ultra-structural details for microscopy related studies (Kiernan, 2000).

Cross-linking by epoxides may afford another approach to cross-link collagen. The epoxide cross-linking reagents are homo-functional compounds containing epoxide groups on both ends and vary mainly in their chain length, ranging from 4-carbons to the popular 12-carbon 1,4-(butanediol) diglycidyl ether (BDDGE) (Sundberg & Porath, 1974; Zeeman et al., 2000) (Figure 2). Under basic conditions, an epoxide will react with the primary amines of the lysine and hydroxylysine residues of collagen in an oxirane ring opening process and by condensation or poly-addition reactions form stable covalent secondary amine bonds (Hermanson, 2008). Under acidic conditions, the epoxide group will be protonated and subsequently react through a nucleophilic attack of a carboxylate anion of glutamic or aspartic acid with the formation of an ester linkage (Zeeman et al., 2000). For a more extensive review on epoxide cross-linking mechanisms see Zeeman et al. (Zeeman et al., 2000).

The effect of pH conditions when using epoxides on the macroscopic appearance of the final collagen-based material is clearly demonstrated with BDDGE. BDDGE is the most commonly used homo-bifunctional epoxide compound used for cross-linking collagen. It is a viscous liquid, hygroscopic and corrosive; aqueous solutions usually possess a characteristic oily film on their surfaces, indicating limited solubility of the reagent (Hermanson, 2008). Cross-linking under basic conditions results in a stiff and compact material; the stiffness of the collagen material is enhanced with increasing pH and increasing BDDGE concentration. In contrast, cross-linking with BDDGE under acidic conditions results in a very soft and pliable material (Zeeman et al., 2000). To improve the resistance of collagen matrices cross-linked under acidic conditions to enzymes such as collagenase while retaining favourable tensile properties, epoxide cross-linked materials can be post-treated with 1-ethyl-3-(3-dimethyl aminopropyl) carbodiimide (EDC) in the presence of N-hydroxysuccinimide (NHS) (Figure 3) (Zeeman et al, 1999). In contrast, acylation of the residual amine groups of expoxide cross-linked materials with acetic acid N-hydroxysuccinimide ester (HAc-NHS) alone reduces the stability of the material towards enzymatic degradation.

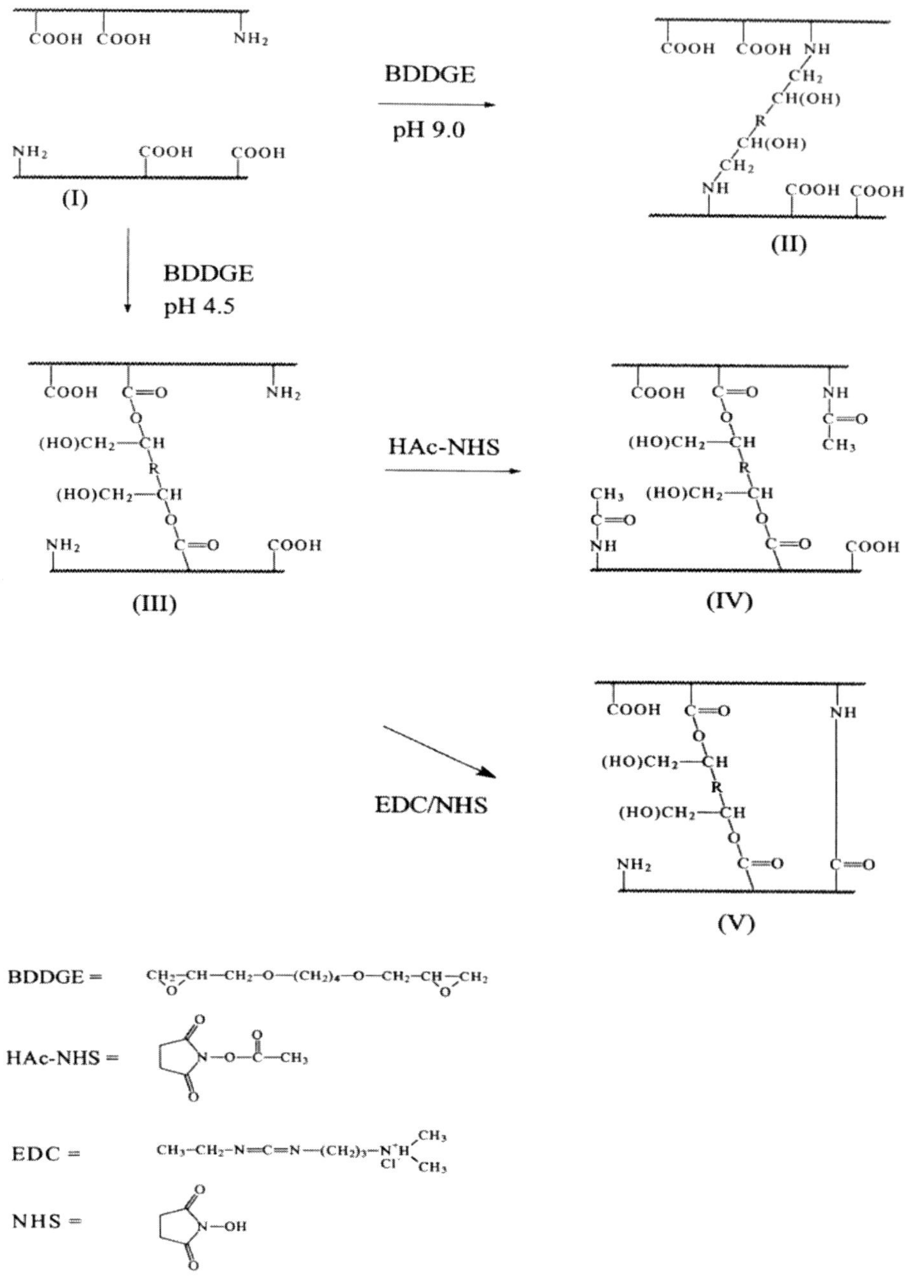

Figure 3. Successive epoxy and carbodiimide cross-linking of collagen type I (Zeeman et al., 1999).

Other common collagen epoxide cross-linkers include glycerol polyglycidyl ethers, and ethylene glycol polyglycidyl ethers (Lee et al., 1994). Studies have shown that these aliphatic glycidyl ether type epoxides can stabilize collagen but their efficiency has been found rather low in comparison to glutaraldehyde (Di & Heath, 2009). The ratio of epoxide to collagen used needs to be typically higher and the effective reaction period long, in many cases over three days to achieve a similar degree of cross-linking as achieved by glutaraldehyde. Some epoxide reagents previously studied to cross-link bio-prosthetic heart valves have shown poor results likely due to poor water solubility of the polyepoxides studied, chemical heterogeneity, and contamination with residual reactants such as organo-chlorides (Connolly et al., 2005). However, a significant benefit associated with epoxides can be seen in the work of Imamura et al.(Imamura et al., 1989) and Courtman et al. (Courtman et al., 1989) who have shown that over three months, there was no significant calcification of the epoxide cross-linked materials; by contrast the equivalent glutaraldehyde cross-linked materials showed calcification.

It has also been reported that triglycidylamine (TGA), a highly polar, water soluble, biocompatible polyepoxide cross-linking agent, confers calcification resistance because of its unique reactions with extra cellular matrix proteins (Connolly et al., 2005). TGA cross-linking, compared to glutaraldehyde cross-linking, can involve reactions with not only amine groups such as lysine amino side chains in collagen but also sulphur containing amino acids such as methionine and cysteine. Cross-linking of connective tissue with TGA is also postulated to result in a more complex structure involving collagen-collagen and collagen-protein bonds that would also hypothetically reduce collagenase digestibility (Connolly et al., 2005; Hunter et al., 2010).

A tri-functional polyepoxide triglycidyl isocyanurate (Tris (2, 3-epoxypropyl) isocyanurate (TEPIC) has been reported to have high reactivity for cross-linking collagen (Figure 4). TEPIC provides enhanced thermal stability due to the aromatic-like heterocyclic triazine nucleus in its molecular structure (Di&Heath, 2009). The poly-addition of the TEPIC epoxy rings to collagen takes place in basic conditions, optimally at pH 9. At lower pH values the reactivity of the epoxy group is reduced, while at higher pH values, side reactions such as hydrolysis of both the peptide and epoxy groups can occur.

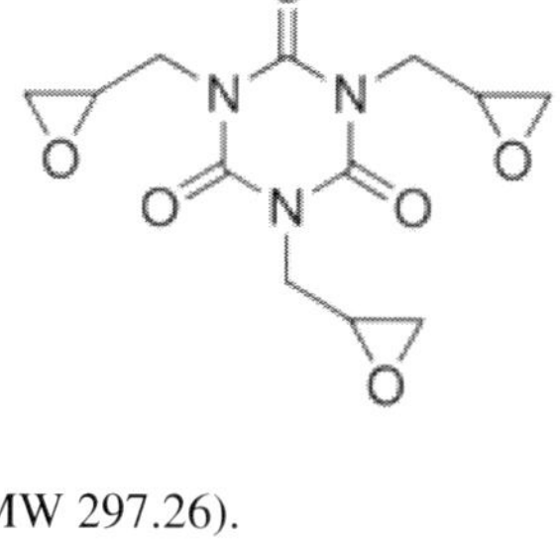

Figure 4. Tri-glycidyl isocyanurate (MW 297.26).

The carbodiimides are zero-length cross-linking agents used to mediate the formation of intra-molecular and inter-molecular amide linkages between a carboxylate group and a primary amine group of collagen, which are located within one nanometer from each other (Zeeman et al., 1999). They are called zero-length reagents because in forming these bonds no additional chemical structure is introduced between the conjugating groups. The most popular carbodiimide is the water soluble N-(3-dimethylaminopropyl) N'-ethylcarbodiimide hydrochloride (EDC or EDAC) (Hermanson, 2008) (Figure 5(a)). N-substituted carbodiimides can react with carboxylic acids to form highly reactive o-acylyisourea derivatives that are extremely short-lived. This active species reacts with a primary amine to form a covalent amide bond. Amide bond formation occurs with the highest yield at pH 4-6 (Nakajima & Ikada, 1995; Gilles et al., 1990; Hermanson, 2008). When working with collagen, EDC mediated cross-linking effectively occurs between pH 4.5-5.5. N-hydroxysuccinimide (NHS), or its water soluble analog sulfo-NHS, is often included in EDC cross-linking protocols to improve efficiency or to create a more stable amine-reactive intermediate (Duncan et al., 2010) (Figure 5(b)).

EDC has been reported to prepare hyaluronic acid/collagen-based scaffolds for brain tissue engineering. The scaffold in this study was designed for use as a potential neuron stem cell-seeded construct for implantation into a defect in the brain resulting from trauma. In this case, these reagents form amide bonds between carboxyl groups and amino groups as well as ester bonds between hydroxyl and carboxyl groups, resulting in Col-Col, HA-Col and HA-HA cross-links (Wang & Spector, 2009). EDC has been successfully used to cross-link collagen to produce scaffolds for potential use as corneal implants (Merrett et al., 2008); aligned nanofibrous blends of poly (DL-lactide-co-glycolide) (PLGA) and collagen to produce promising new materials for bone tissue engineering (Moncy et al., 2009); and collagen/chitosan/heparin complexes for potential use as a scaffolding material for bioartificial livers (Yu et al., 2005). Collagen-polymer hybrids have been successfully produced by using ethanol as the reaction solvent to prevent EDC hydrolysis, providing a longer period of time for collagen to crosslink to the polymer (Nam et al., 2010).

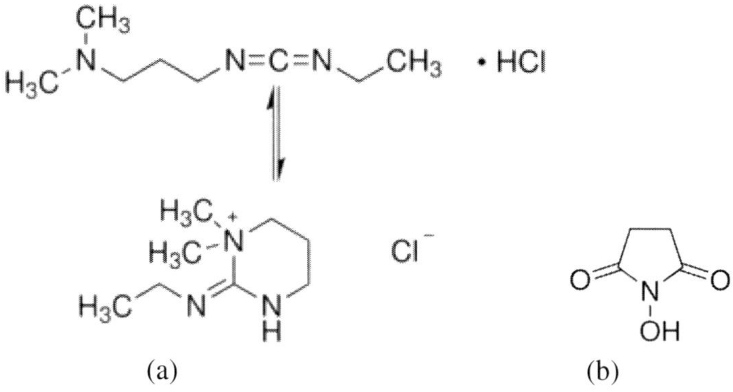

Figure 5. **(a)** N-(3-Dimethylaminopropyl) N'-ethylcarbodiimide hydrochloride (EDC) (MW 191.70), **(b)** *N*-Hydroxysuccinimide (NHS) (MW 115.09).

EDC is limited by the number of amine groups in collagen. A method of cross-linking collagen using multi-functional dendrimers was examined and compared with conventional cross-linking methods. In this study, cross-linking was affected by activating the carboxylic acid groups of glutamic and aspartic acid residues in collagen in the presence of EDC. It was hypothesized that the multi-terminal free amine groups of the polypropyleneimine octamine dendrimers can largely amplify the limited quantities of amine groups in collagen available for cross-linking, thus producing a highly cross-linked, stable collagen matrix (Duan & Sheardown, 2005).

NHS active esters have drawn attention mainly due to their cytocompatibility and biocompatibility. The use of a novel cross-linking agent, adipic acid activated NHS (NHS-AA) has been recently investigated (Zhang et al., 2011). This cross-linking agent has two active ester groups and is used to crosslink collagen by the reaction between ε-amino groups and active ester groups as shown in Figure 6.

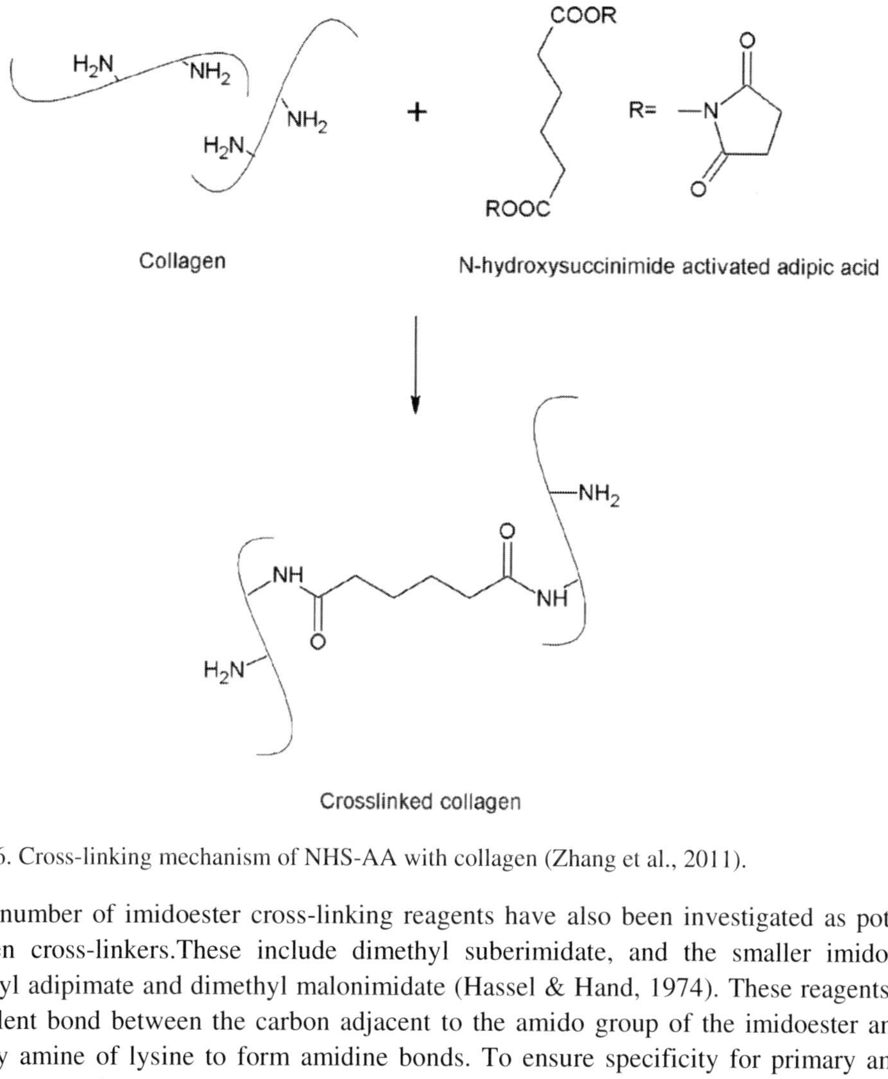

Figure 6. Cross-linking mechanism of NHS-AA with collagen (Zhang et al., 2011).

A number of imidoester cross-linking reagents have also been investigated as potential collagen cross-linkers.These include dimethyl suberimidate, and the smaller imidoesters dimethyl adipimate and dimethyl malonimidate (Hassel & Hand, 1974). These reagents form a covalent bond between the carbon adjacent to the amido group of the imidoester and the primary amine of lysine to form amidine bonds. To ensure specificity for primary amines, imidoester reactions are best done in amine-free, alkaline conditions. Imidoesters are unique in that they carry an amido group adjacent to the functional groups on the molecule and as a result do not alter the net charge on collagen after reaction (i.e. the resulting the amidine bond is protonated, therefore the cross-link has a positive charge at physiological pH, much like the primary amine that it replaced (Hassel & Hand, 1974). For this reason, imidoester cross-linkers were found to best used primarily to study protein structure and molecular associations in membranes and to immobilize proteins onto solid-phase supports while preserving the isoelectric point (pI) of the native protein rather than as cross-linkers for collagen-based materials. Although imidoesters are still used in certain procedures, the amidine bonds formed are reversible at high pH. Therefore, other more stable and efficient collagen cross-linkers have steadily replaced them in most applications.

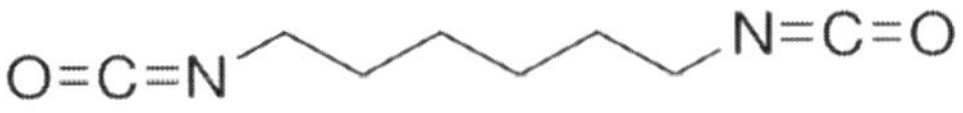

Figure 7. Hexamethylene diisocyanate (HMDC) (MW 168.19).

Diisocyanates, such as hexamethylene diisocyanate (HMDC) (Figure 7), react with the free amine groups of collagen to form stable isourea linkages and have been used to successfully to cross-link collagen to produce collagen sponges with high thermal stabilities (Rault et al., 1996). However, it has been recently predicted that isocyanate reagents will see limited use as collagen cross-linkers primarily due to toxicity concerns (Zhang et al., 2011). In addition, many commercial suppliers of chemical reagents have found isocyanate compounds too unstable to offer them for sale, since moisture rapidly decomposes them, releasing CO_2, and leaving an aromatic amine (Hermanson, 2008).

Concerns related to chemical toxicity have led to the development of naturally derived cross-linkers as alternatives to chemical reagents used to cross-link collagen. Recent studies have shown that naturally derived cross-linkers can stabilize collagen-based scaffolds and can bring about properties similar to native extracellular matrix assemblies while not compromising cell attachment, proliferation, and growth (Zeugolis et al., 2010). Naturally derived cross-linking reagents range from genipin (Figure 8), an aglycone derivative from an iridoid glycoside called geniposide found in gardenia fruit(Kosaraju et al., 2010) to transglutaminases, a family of enzymes that catalyze several post-translational modifications by forming inter- and intra-molecular bonds (Zeugolis et al., 2010).

Naturally derived genipin was first isolated from Genipa Americana during an extensive investigation of extracts from Mexican and South American plants (Djerassi et al., 1960). While it is difficult to extract genipin from gardenia fruits directly by common chemical methods (Yao et al., 2004) it can be isolated in large quantity by microbiological process involving *Penicillum nigricans* that produces B-glucosidase that in turn hydrolyzes the geniposidase into the aglycone genipin (Muzzarelli, 2009).

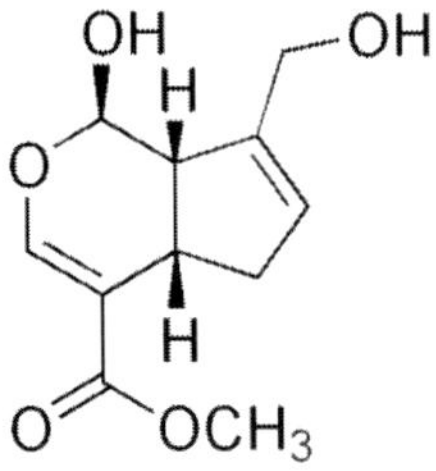

Figure 8. Genipin (MW 226.23).

Genipin, which behaves like a dialdehyde, reacts with the free amino groups in lysine and hydroxylysine (Sung et al., 2000). After cross-linking it has been observed that genipin imparts a dark-blue coloration to collagen-based materials. This coloration is associated with the oxygen radical-induced polymerization of genipin as well as its reaction with amino groups (Muzarelli, 2009). The results of studies investigating the structures of the intermediates leading to the blue pigment suggest that genipin may form intramolecular and intermolecular cross-links with cyclic structure within collagen fibrils in biological tissue (Touyama et al., 1994; Fukikawa et al., 1987). Genipin has been compared to formaldehyde and EDC in the development of collagen-based vascular constructs and has been shown to improve elongation and endothelial coverage (Madhaven et al., 2010). In orthopaedic applications, Fessel et al. have recently shown that cross-linking of collagenous tissue (e.g. tendons) with genipin improves tissue fatigue and tear resistance (Fessel et al., 2012).

A less known naturally derived cross-linker is derived from schizophyllan, a natural polysaccharide, produced by the fungi of the genus Schizophyllum. Periodate oxidation specifically cleaves the vicinal glycols in schizophyllan to form their dialdehyde derivatives referred to as scleraldehydes) (Jayakumar et al., 2012). Scleraldehyde cross-linking has been shown to impart high thermal and enzymatic stability to collagen based materials without any associated cytotoxicity concerns (Jayakumar et al., 2012).

The use of a novel extract from myrica rubra (*M.rubra*), a subtropical tree native to Eastern Asia, as a collagen cross-linker has recently been reported by Zeugolis et al., *M. rubra* cross-linked collagen fibres have been shown to possess thermal, structural, physical and mechanical properties comparable to native tissues such as tendon and anterior cruciate ligament. Therefore, stabilisation using *M . rubra* may be an alternative to aldehyde cross-linking approaches for the construction of three-dimensional scaffolds that would imitate native extracellular matrix assemblies(Zeugolis et al., 2010).

In a second study, Zeugolis et al. investigated transglutaminase as a potential collagen cross-linker for tissue engineering applications. This study reported that although transglutaminase cross-linked the collagen, the mechanical properties were found to be inferior to those produced using more conventional chemical cross-linking strategies (Zeugolis et al., 2010).

Tannic acid, a natural polyphenol, possessing antibacterial, and anti-enzymatic properties has seen considerable use in restorative dentistry to cross-link dentin (i.e. type I collagen) (Bedran-Russo et al., 2009) (Figure 9). It has also been reported as an effective alternative to the aldehydes for cross-linking purified collagen to produce matrices suitable for drug delivery applications (Albu et al., 2010).

Cross-linking techniques that do not incorporate new molecules into collagen such as the physical methods are the most appealing as they do not introduce potentially cytotoxic reagents into the collagen. Physical approaches include ultra-violet (UV) and gamma irradiation (Ibrahim et al., 2011), photochemical methods requiring the use of photo-sensitizers such as Rose Bengal and riboflavin (Ibusuki et al., 2007; Kew et al., 2011), as well as dehydrothermal techniques (DHT) (Tierney et al., 2008).

UV is a non-ionizing form of energy that can be absorbed by the aromatic ring residues of tyrosine and phenylalanine, creating free radical sites that can propagate reactions that cross-link collagen (Miyata et al., 1971). When compared to traditional chemical cross-linking techniques, cross-linkers such as EDC have been reported to be more effective than UV for stabilizing collagen scaffolds (Walters et al., 2012; Caruso et al., 2004). It is important to note that the UV generated free radicals that lead to collagen cross-linking also propagate reactions that cause excessive molecular fragmentation and denaturation. Limited exposure of collagen to UV results in an intermediate state consisting of molecules that are cross-linked but partially denatured because of multi-chain scissions along the helix (Miles et al., 2000). Similarly, gamma irradiation used primarily as a sterilization technique for collagen-based implants results in molecular fragmentation via chain scission of the collagen peptide chains (Ohan et al., 2003).

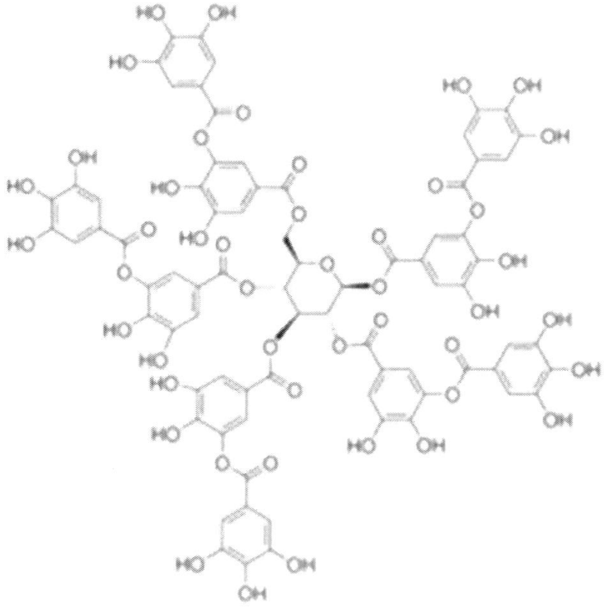

Figure 9. Tannic Acid (MW 1701.20).

The use of glucose as a protective agent when used in combination with UV and gamma irradiation has been investigated (Ohan et al., 2002; Ohan et al., 2003). The results of these studies have shown that the incorporation of glucose into collagen stabilizes the material via glucose-derived cross-link formation during irradiation consequently providing protection from the damaging effects of irradiation induced fragmentation (Ohan et al., 2003). Although glucose (in the absence of irradiation) has been reported as a method for cross-linking collagen biomaterials and cell seeded tissue-engineered products (Girton et al., 1999) glucose alone is a relatively ineffective cross-linker as collagen requires prolonged incubation (several days to months) in solutions containing high glucose concentrations under physiological conditions to generate cross-links (Ohan et al., 2002).

Photochemical cross-linking is a relatively new technique that is able to modify the physicochemical properties of collagen. In photochemical cross-linking, photochemical reactions are produced when the photosensitizers such as Rose Bengal (Chan et al., 2008) and riboflavin (Ibusuki et al., 2007), which are bound to or introduced to the collagen are activated by absorbing photons from a light source such as an argon laser or a UV/visible light source of a specific wavelength. The activated states of the photosensitizers and the photoproducts such as reactive oxygen species react with the amino acid residues in collagen, forming the cross-links. Rose Bengal (Figure 10(a)) and riboflavin (Figure 10(b)) initiate collagen cross-linking using 532- and 458 nm-light wavelengths, respectively (Ibushki et al., 2007). With respect to riboflavin, it has been reported that photodynamic modification of tyrosine probably contributes to the riboflavin-sensitized cross-linking of collagen through the formation of diotyrosine (Kato et al., 1994). Photochemical techniques do not involve organic solvents, and avoid the harsh conditions such as the extreme temperatures and pressures often associated with DHT, and therefore present a particularly suitable technique for cross-linking collagen-based materials (Chan et al., 2008).

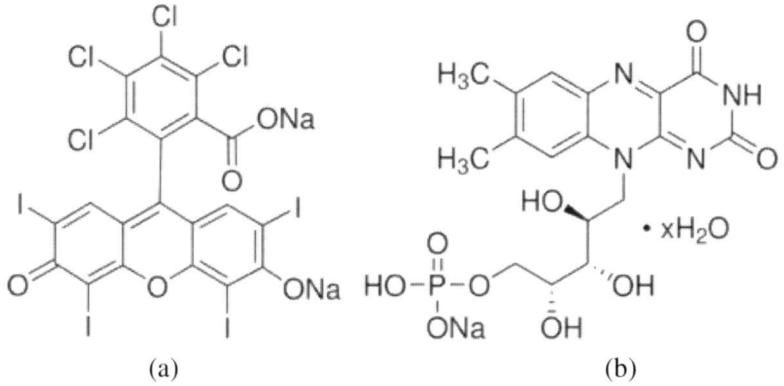

Figure 10. (a) Rose Bengal (MW 1017.64), (b) Riboflavin (MW 478.33 (anhydrous basis)).

A study comparing the use of Rose Bengal to riboflavin found that although both photosensitizers in combination with visible light cross-linked collagen, Rose Bengal was found to be toxic to cells even without irradiation. By contrast, the collagen photo-cross-linked with riboflavin and visible light permitted high levels of cell survival (Ibusuki et al., 2007). UVA-riboflavin cross-linking of collagen is currently used in the clinic to increase the mechanical and biochemical stability of the cornea damaged by corneal thinning disorders such as keratoconus, and iatrogenic keratectasia after laser in situ keratomileusis (LASIK) (Spoerl et al., 2007).

DHT cross-linking is a widespread technique for stiffening and stabilizing collagen-based materials. It involves subjecting the material to temperatures above 90 °C while under vacuum, creating bonds between the chains of amino acids present in the collagen molecule. It has been shown that reconstituted collagen fibers cross-linked with dehydrothermal treatment and cyanamide vapour achieved improvements to mechanical properties; most significantly to break strengths and low strain modulus (Kato et al., 1989). A further study by Wang et al. (1994) has reported that the use of high temperature and reduced pressure alone also results in high breaking strengths (Wang et al., 1994). However it is reported that DHT, like UV cross-linking results in lower mechanical strength when compared to chemical cross-linking techniques (Tierney et al., 2009). DHT cross-linking may also alter the surface wettability and protein conformations critical for cellular interaction and cause denaturation (Weadock et al., 1995).

Physical and chemical cross-linking techniques have been compared to determine the degree to which these methodologies could improve the mechanical properties and resistance to enzymatic degradation without negatively affecting cell migration rates on collagen based scaffolds (Weadock et al., 1996). In this study, UV, DHT and EDC methods were used. The results showed that all three methods significantly increased the mechanical properties and significantly decreased their respective enzymatic degradation rates. Analysis of cell migration rates showed that all three techniques decreased the rate of cell migration on the scaffold surface, although cell migration was faster on the EDC cross-linked material (Weadock et al., 1996). Furthermore, EDC cross-linked collagen was reported to swell to more than four times their dry cross-sectional area and to a significantly greater extent than physically cross-linked collagen upon rehydration. It has been postulated that that the increased swelling suggests that EDC cross-linked collagen has a lower cross-link density and more hydrophilic properties than the physically cross-linked collagen in this study (Weadock et al., 1996).

The presence and extent of collagen cross-linking in collagen-based materials can be assessed by several means, including (i) measurement of denaturation temperature by differential scanning calorimetry (DSC), (ii) measurement of resistance to enzymatic degradation, (iii) measurement of changes in mechanical properties, and (iv) measurement of unreacted lysyl and hydroxylysyl groups. The denaturation temperature is that temperature required to release the hydrogen bonding in the collagen triple helix producing a change to random coil configuration (Periara CA et al. 1990). The denaturation temperature is also an indicator of the cleavage of covalent bonds that stabilize the triple helices inter-molecularly and intra-molecularly. It is likely that intra-helical cross-linking, where it occurs, would be most effective in limiting uncoiling; however intermolecular cross-links may also contribute to some extent by coupling the non-helical terminal ends of collagen molecules to adjacent triple helix (Lee et al., 1994).

Measurement of resistance to enzymatic degradation involves exposure of the collagen-based material to proteolytic enzymes in optimized buffered solutions. In the case of collagen-based scaffolds the most popular enzyme of choice is collagenase (Merrett et al., 2008). This approach provides information related to the rate of degradation and thus may be of greater relevance to predicting the *in vivo* performance of the material than its denaturation temperature. However, it is unclear what type of cross-linking is being measured. If collagen chains are cleaved by the enzyme, either intra-helical or inter-molecular cross-linking could be expected to decrease solubility (Lee et al., 1994). For cross-linking methods that react with amino groups, chemical analysis for unreacted lysyl and hydroxylysyl residues should be an indicator of the completeness of reaction with collagen. The determination of free amino groups is commonly accomplished using a trinitrobenzenesulfonic acid (TNBS) assay, originally developed by Okuyama et al. to determine the free amino groups of amino acids and peptides in column eluates (Okuyama & Satake, 1960; Habeeb, 1966). However, this is not necessarily a direct measurement of cross-linking since an agent that reacted with these groups but did not cross-link would present similar results (Lee et al., 1994).

TISSUE ENGINEERING APPLICATIONS

The treatment of injured tissues or organs has focused traditionally on the use of autologous and allogenic grafts (Gomes et al., 2012). However, autologous grafts can cause donor site morbidity and loss of organ functionality. Allogenic grafts are associated with the risk of disease transmission and often require the use of immunosuppressants (Gomes et al., 2012). Tissue engineering of biomaterials offers an alternative approach by providing bio-resorbable scaffolds that promote the regeneration of the host tissue. These scaffolds may be derived from natural polymers such as fibrin, fibronectin, elastin, silk, keratin, alginate, amylase/amylopectin, hyaluronic acid and collagen (Gomes et al., 2012). Natural polymers are often used in combination with synthetic biodegradable polymers such as the polyesters containing glycolic (PLG) or lactic (PLL) acids and caprolactone (PCL) which have been approved for medical use by the US Food and Drug Administration (FDA) (Kohn et al., 2007).

Collagen, the focus of this chapter, is easy to process and modify; its abundance, non-antigenicity, biocompatibility and biodegradability make collagen an ideal choice (Lee et al., 2001). Collagen-based materials can be fabricated in a number of different forms such as tubes, sheets, sponges, hydrogels, powders, injectable solutions and dispersions for different biomedical applications (Gelse et al., 2003). A primary challenge associated with the use of collagen as a biomaterial is its rate of degradation in the presence of extracellular matrix collagenase. Collagen can be cross-linked to improve its resistance to biodegradation; however, there are some concerns associated with various cross-linking agents such as cytotoxicity, and calcification

Over the past 30 years, several collagen-based medical devices have been approved as a result of extensive safety profiling and an increased understanding of collagen-cell interactions (Kyle et al., 2009). Applications include haemostasis (Browder and Litwin, 1986) and soft tissue repair, artificial skin and bone, as well as cell and drug delivery (Pachence, 1996; Wachol-Drewek et al., 1996; Chan et al., 2010; Chan et al., 2008). Collagen from animal sources has long been used in the tissue engineering of heart valves, ligaments and tendons, nerves, cartilage, menisci, and blood vessels, yet the risks of pathogen transmission and immunogenicity make such sources clinically undesirable (Kyle et al., 2009). Research groups are therefore moving from animal source to human recombinant collagens to overcome these safety concerns (Merrett et al., 2008). Production of recombinant collagens has seen the greatest success to date using transgenic *Pichia pastoris* yeast, tobacco plant and *Escherichia coli* bacteria based approaches (Kyle et al., 2009).

Hemostasis

A femoral artery pseudoaneurysm (PSA) is a complication that may occur after arterial puncture for invasive cardiovascular procedures (Geutjes et al., 2010). Injectable collagen may be an attractive agent for the treatment of PSA. When collagen comes in contact with blood, platelets become activated, resulting in platelet adhesion, aggregation to the vessel wall, and the release of hemostasis-stimulating compounds, (Geutjes et al., 2010). In 2002, Hamraoui et al treated PSA patients with bovine fibrillar type I collagen demonstrating that the use of collagen is a safe and effective strategy (Hamraoui et al., 2002). Recently, Geutjes et al. (2010) have developed a well-characterized injectable collagen preparation that was evaluated in a porcine model for PSA treatment.

A primary concern with regards to the use of injectable collagen for medical applications is proper sterilization. In the above study, both ethylene oxide gas (EtO) and hydrogen peroxide gas plasma (H_2O_2) were compared. It was reported that the integrity of the collagen was not compromised by either approach however; EtO was selected for its tendency to have less of an effect on collagen-induced platelet aggregation. *In vivo*, the injectable collagen formed a dense network, which had partial hemostatic activity. Sterilized injectable collagen may be an effective therapeutic alternative for current femoral PSA treatment, but additional studies will be needed in the future to prove its efficacy (Geutjes et al., 2010).

Skin: Skin consists of an epidermis and a dermis layer. Damage to the epidermis often results in scar tissue lacking flexibility, elasticity, and strength (Clark et al., 2000). Thus, scar tissue limits movements, causes pain, and is cosmetically undesirable. Also, natural skin tissue grafts are not readily available. Therefore, artificial skin would be a viable alternative for wound dressings and regeneration of the dermis. Apligraf®, a composite bilayer of reconstructed skin consisting of a collagen gel populated with neonatal fibroblasts with an epidermis layer composed of neonatal keratinocytes, is commercialized as a temporary dressing for the treatment of ulcers (Edmonds 2008; and Karr, 2009). Commercial skin substitutes and dressing such as Integra® (an acellular collagen/GAG scaffold), Alloderm™ (human dermis), Amniograph™ (amniotic membrane), and OrCel® (Ortec International Inc.) are also commercially available.

Min et al. (2004) have developed nonwoven electrospun silk fibroin nanofibers for skin tissue engineering applications. This study reported that collagen type I coated fibrin nanofibers promote keratinocytes/fibroblast adhesion and spreading due to the high porosity and high surface area to volume ratio of the nanofibers, suggesting the potential use of these collagen coated nanofibers as scaffold materials (Min et al., 2004).

Rho et al. have reported on the fabrication of wound dressing comprised of electrospun nanofibrous matrices made of collagen type I that were functionally active in response to normal human keratinocytes (Rho et al., 2006).

An asymmetric chitosan matrix with nanosized collagen particles for skin tissue engineering applications has been designed (Chen et al., 2006). *In vivo* results have indicated that the scaffold promoted efficient re-epithelialization of the wound (Chen et al., 2006). Recently, a three-dimensional (3D) collagen scaffold with controlled pore structure was developed using a 3D dispensing system supplemented with a cryogenic and freeze drying process. In this study, the fabricated scaffold promoted cell migration and differentiation, but had poor mechanical stability due to its highly porous structure (Kim et al., 2009). As an alternative approach, a hybrid scaffold composed of an outer collagen shell and an inner alginate core was designed to overcome the limitations of the first design. The collagen/alginate hybrid scaffolds demonstrated good structural stability and good cell viability, and were shown to be a successful dermal substitute (Kim et al., 2009).

Large scale evaluation of potential skin tissue engineering biomaterials is time-consuming and limited by ethical considerations. In order to address this limitation, Lammers et al. (2009) have developed an array of 48 different, molecularly-defined films based on native fibrillar collagen (Lammers et al., 2009). These films differed in the type and amount of ECM components, method of preparation, and method and extent of cross-linking. The array was evaluated using cultured primary keratinocytes/fibroblasts and may be generally applicable and instrumental in the future for the selection of the appropriate set of matrix molecules for use as biomaterials for skin applications.

Bone

A large variety of synthetic and natural materials have been explored for bone tissue engineering applications. The physical properties of bone tissue such as mechanical strength, porosity, hardness, and overall 3D architecture are important factors to consider in the design of scaffolds for bone regeneration and/or replacement. Scaffolds with a pore size in the range of 100–350 μm and porosity greater than 90% are preferred for better cell/tissue in-growth and thus enhanced bone regeneration (Bruder and Caplan., 2000; Hutmacher et al., 2000). In order to increase the scaffolds' mechanical strength composites of collagen and other synthetic polymers such as polycaprolactone (PCL) (Venugopal et al., 2007), and poly-(3-hydroxybutyrate–cohydroxyvalerate) (PHBV) (Meng et al., 2007) have been used. The presence of collagen type I in hybrid materials has been reported to enhance cell adhesion, proliferation and differention (Vengopal et al., 2007; Salaszyk et al., 2004; Kundu et al., 2006; Meng et al., 2007). Collagen type I has also been used in combination with calcium phosphate (Du et al., 2000; Harley et al., 2010) and with hydroxyapatite (Dubey and Tomar, 2009; Liao et al., 2009) to form mineralized scaffolds for bone tissue engineering. Cai et al. (2010) have developed an electrospun poly(l-lactic acid) (PLLA)-collagen bilayer composite scaffold (Cai et al., 2010). After six weeks of implantation, a higher percentage of cortical bone formed on the bilayer composite compared to collagen only, suggesting a benefit of collagen composites for bone tissue engineering applications.

Wang et al. (2010) have developed a chitosan/collagen type I composite embedded with adult human bone marrow-derived stem cells (hBMSC). The group reported that the presence of collagen in a chitosan-collagen composite was associated with increased cell spreading and proliferation, as well as increased gel compaction resulting in a stiffer matrix (Wang et al., 2010). In a later study, they found that glyoxal, a dialdehyde with relatively low toxicity, could be used to cross-link matrices resulting in stiffer and less compact materials than the uncross-linked controls. These materials supported osteogenic differentiation in response to stimulation, suggesting that glyoxal-crosslinked chitosan/collagen composite materials have the potential to be used as cell delivery vehicles for enhancing bone damage repair (Wang et al., 2011).

An alternative to collagen composites to deliver cells is to coat traditional materials with collagen. For example, titanium (Ti) is often the material of choice for load-bearing, bone-contacting devices. However, because titanium cannot form a chemical bond with natural bone, the loosening of implant-bone interface has become a critical problem in clinical applications (Chen et al., 2009). Self-assembled monolayers (SAMs) and layer by layer (LBL) techniques have been proven to be effective surface modification methods to improve the biocompatibility of titanium. Ni et al. (2011) have reported on the use of decyl bis phosphonate (DBP) and collagen type I to modify titanium using a LBL technique. The stability of the DBP-collagen layer on titanium was reported to be very good; osteoblasts evaluated by a metabolic assay and alkaline phosphatase (ALP) activity showed that osteoblasts had improved activity, proliferation, and differentiation on collagen terminated samples. These results, along with good biomineralization and protein adsorption abilities of the Ti/DBP/collagen surface suggest titanium modified by this LBL technique has the potential to improve the bone-implant interface of titanium based medical implants (Ni et al., 2010).

Cartilage

Cartilage, composed of a collagen fiber network, has a limited self-regeneration potential, due to the absence of vascular supplies, limited proliferation of highly differentiated chondrocytes, low supply of progenitor cells, and low matrix turnover (Wu et al., 2002; Chung et al., 2008; Vasita et al., 2006; Lu et al., 2010).

Various types of scaffolds have been investigated as cartilage substitutes. However, a common problem encountered with porous scaffolds is the rapid formation of a thin layer of tissue on the outer edge of the material. This is likely caused by uneven cell seeding that leads the development of a necrotic core due to the limitations of cell penetration and nutrient exchange (Silva et al., 2006). A method has been recently developed using ice particulate templates to prepare collagen type I scaffolds with open surface and interconnected pores (Lu et al., 2010). The scaffolds facilitated cell penetration leading to spatially homogenous cell distribution (Figure 11). These porous scaffolds are potentially useful for future cartilage engineering applications.

Autologous chondrocyte-based tissue engineering may also provide a promising therapy for cartilage damage (Lu et al., 2010). Collagen-coated microspheres have been successfully used as cell carriers for chondrocytes and could potentially be used to fabricate injectable constructs for cartilage tissue regeneration (Hong et al., 2005).

Cornea

Recombinant human collagen Type I (RHC I) and Type III (RHC III) have been evaluated as corneal stromal matrix substitutes in pigs (Merrett et al., 2008). After 12 months post-transplantation, implants were well-integrated and optically clear. Implants were stably anchored with a stratified epithelium and ingrowth of stromal cells and corneal sensory nerves were observed. Recently, artificial corneas were developed to replace partial or full thickness of damaged or diseased corneas. Corneal implants fabricated from recombinant collagen type III were implanted in a phase 1 clinical trial. All implants were stably integrated and remained avascular. A morphologically-normal epithelium with normal tear film was regenerated and nerve growth was observed. This study has demonstrated that collagen based implants promote tissue regeneration and are a potential alternative to corneal allografting (Fagerholm et al., 2010). Collagen type I hydrogels have been similarly developed using various chemical cross-linkers to mimic the corneal stroma. These hydrogels have been successfully implanted into pigs with stable host-graft integration and optical clarity (Rafat et al., 2008; Liu et al., 2006; Liu et al., 2009)(Figure 12).

We have also employed surface modification techniques to modulate cell interaction properties of porcine collagen type I. One potential complication with full-thickness corneal implants is formation of post-operative retro-corneal membranes likely due to the attachment of remaining endothelial cells to the implant's posterior surface. We developed a method to prevent endothelialisation of full thickness corneal grafts including ammonia plasma functionalization followed by grafting with alginate macromolecules to the implant posterior surface (Rafat et al., 2009).

Collagen scaffolds have also been used for the delivery of limbal epithelial stem cells to damaged cornea (Dravida et al., 2008; Builles et al., 2010; De Miguel et al., 2010). Borene et al. (2004) have developed a collagen-based stromal scaffold cultured with human corneal stromal fibroblasts, however they found that the cell-scaffold interactions resulted in changes in mechanical properties and permeability of the hydrogels (Borene et al., 2004).

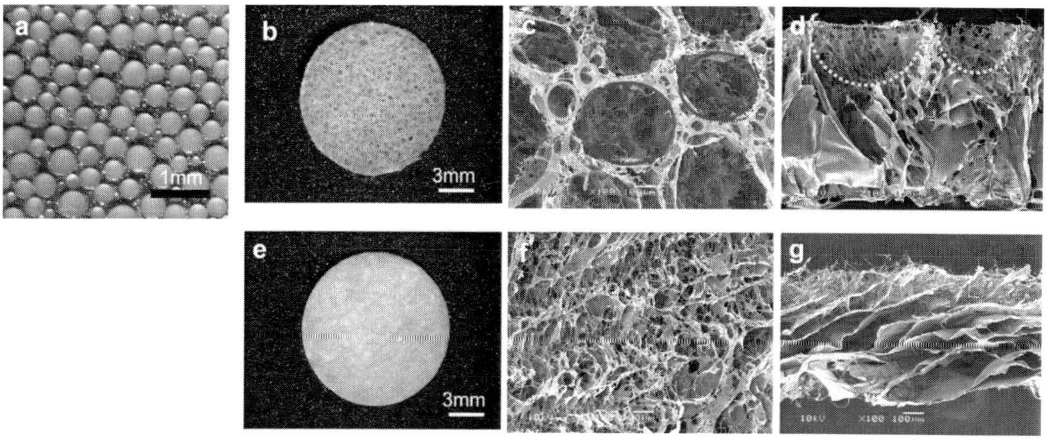

Figure 11. Photomicrograph of ice particulates with a mean diameter of about 400 μm (a) gross appearances (b,e), top surfaces SEM images (c,f) and cross section SEM images (d,g) of 400 μm, - 3ºC funnel-like collagen sponges (b-d) and control collagen sponge (e-g). Red circles, green circles and blue circles indicate large surface pores, small surface pores and inner bulk pores respectively (Lu et al., 2010).

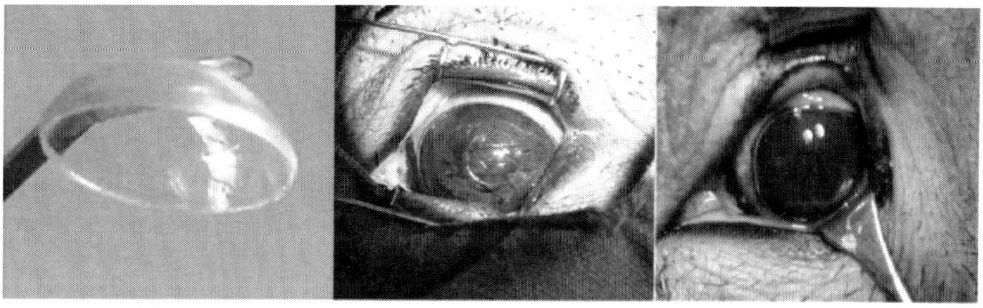

(a) (b) (c)

Figure 12. Corneal implants made from type I porcine collagen cross-linked with EDC/NHS/PEG-dibutyraldehyde: (a) before implantation, (b) right after implantation in mini pigs using overlaying sutures, and (c) 2-months post-implantation in pigs with stable host-graft integration (Rafat et al., 2008).

Cardiovascular

The formation of vascular tissue equivalents *in vitro* has been reported using natural proteins such as collagen, gelatin, alginate or synthetic polymers such as polyglycolic acid, and polyurethanes. The use of collagen-based materials for cardiovascular applications has been somehow limited by concerns associated with platelet adhesion that leads to platelet activation and thrombus growth (Hansen et al., 2011; van der Loo et al., 2011). However, development of new techniques for preventing platelet adhesion, e.g. endothelial cell seeding onto the surface of a graft (James et al., 1990) and heparin surface modifications are considered to be potential routes to further explore the use of collagen for blood contacting applications. Collagen based scaffold that could support the attachment, proliferation, and phenotypic maintenance of endothelial cells have shown potential for vascular tissue engineering applications (Wang et al., 2007; James et al., 1990).

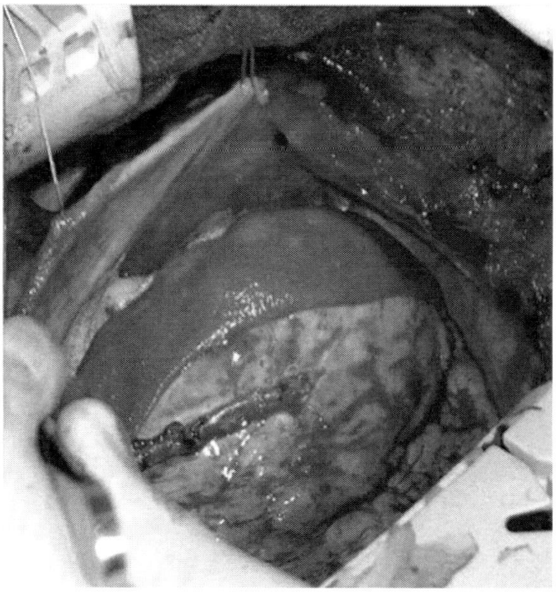

Figure 13. A human heart treated with a bone marrow cell-seeded collagen matrix patch after coronary artery bypass graft and cell injection (MAGNUM clinical trial) (Chachques et al., 2008).

In 1986, Weinberg and Bell reported on the construction of functional biological vascular grafts from collagen. Their model established the proof of concept for the fabrication of tubular structures with layers that match the intima, media, and adventia in natural blood vessels. However, in order to withstand physiological pressures, these constructs required the support of non-degradable Dacron sleeves. The properties of scaffolds for vascular applications have since improved using a variety of techniques ranging from glycation (Girton et al., 1999) to electrospinning collagen composite materials (Buttafoco et al., 2006; Boland et al., 2004; Mo et al. 2007). Electrospun polycaprolactone-collagen scaffolds for vascular tissue engineering were evaluated *in vivo* in a rabbit aorta-iliac bypass model (Tillman et al., 2009). This study demonstrated that electrospun scaffolds supported adherence and growth of vascular cells under physiologic conditions and that the endothelialized grafts resisted platelet adhesion. At retrieval, these scaffolds continued to maintain biomechanical strength that was comparable to the native artery suggesting that electrospun nanofibrous scaffolds combined with vascular cells may become an alternative to vascular grafts for vascular reconstruction (Tillman et al., 2009).

Recent developments in stem cell biology and bioactive collagen-based scaffolds have led to the development of engineered cardiac tissue *in vitro*. Collagen type I, a component of native cardiac muscle extracellular matrix (ECM), plays an important role in structural integrity and contractility in the myocardium (Fomovsky et al., 2010). Callegari et al. investigated the role of a collagen sponge for the repair of a cryo-injured left ventricles of rats for up to 60 days *in vivo* (Callegari et al., 2007). They found that the patches made of porous collagen scaffolds were able to promote angiogenesis immediately after injury. Collagen scaffolds have also been used to deliver cells such as human bone marrow-derived $CD133^+$ cells (Pozzobon et al., 2010), human mesenchymal stem cells (MSCs) (Simpson et al., 2007) and intra-myocardial cells (Hamdi et al., 2009). Collagen type I patch was also investigated for the MAGNUM (Myocardial Assistance by Grafting a New Bioartificial Upgraded

Myocardium) phase 1 clinical trial (Chachques et al., 2008). The collagen type I patch cultured with bone marrow cells was applied on 10 patients that had received a coronary artery bypass graft and intra-infarct implantation of autologous bone marrow cells (Figure 13). Left ventricular end diastolic (LVED) volume and scar thickness were improved in the patients that were treated with cell-seeded collagen patch combined with cellular injection compared with to those treated with cell injection alone (Chachques et al., 2008). A clinically approved cross-linked collagen I/III sponge (Avetine Ultrafoam) modified to present the RGD domain, has also been reported to support neonatal cardiomyocytes contractility and improved the viability of cardiomyocytes (Schussler et al., 2009).

Nerve Tissue

Neural tissue repair is a major objective in tissue engineering as neural injuries often lead to an irreversible loss of function. Disease, peripheral nerve injury, and tumour surgery require grafts to bridge the proximal and distal nerve ends. Autografts are the current available treatments, however, autografts are limited in supply, require a prolonged surgical time, and can cause donor site morbidity. As an alternative, a variety of conduit materials both natural and synthetic have been used as a nerve graft. Collagen can be used to align the reparative tissue with the long axis of the spinal cord and serve as a delivery vehicle for neural stem cells and the gene for glial cell line-derived neurotropic factor (GDNF) (Spilker et al., 2001; Cholas et al., 2012). Recently researchers have reported various compositions of collagen based materials for nerve conduit applications such as collagen/PCL blends that have shown to significantly enhance cell proliferation and axonal regeneration compared to PCL alone (Schnell et al., 2007).

Most collagen nerve guides, such as NeuraGen® from Integra™ are engineered from cross-linked collagen as tubular constructs. Although type I collagen is not a main component of the ECM of the central nervous system, it has been widely demonstrated to support the growth and differentiation of neurons *in vitro* and has been utilized as a scaffold *in vivo* (Ma et al., 2008; Watanabe et al., 2007; Willits et al., 2004). Collagen inhibits glial proliferation and therefore may decrease glial scar post-spinal cord injury (SCI) (Eccleston et al., 1989). The highest quality of peripheral nerve regeneration comparable to that of the nerve autografts has been demonstrated for collagen conduits implanted together with a collagen matrix with axially oriented pores (Chamberlain et al., 1998). The coupling of such collagen based devices has also been reported to facilitate the regeneration of peripheral nerves over long gaps e.g. greater than 10 mm). The pore structure of the collagen matrices can be controlled by properly tailoring the freeze drying process (O'Brien et al., 2004; Sannino & Madaghiele, 2009) and the degradation rate can be properly tuned by subjecting the collagen to different crosslinking treatments (Harley et al., 2004).

In a recent study by Volkenstein et al. (2012), spiral ganglion nerves were shown to survive on collagen-coated culture dishes with neurite growth oriented in the direction of the collagen fibrils. The ability to control directed neuronal growth is a significant contribution to neural tissue engineering, especially with respect to cochlear implant technology (Volkenstein et al., 2012). The coating of cochlear implant electrodes with oriented collagen could be used to promote a closer bioelectrical interface between the electrode array and the target tissue. Specifically, collagen could be used to attach neurotrophins such as brain derived neurotrophic factor, either in slow-release formulation, or covalently to promote spiral ganglion survival and neurite outgrowth toward the cochlear implant and further along the device, which would improve hearing results for affected patients (Volkenstein et al., 2012).

Therapeutic Agents Delivery

Collagen matrices have been widely used as delivery platforms for various therapeutic molecules including growth factors such as platelet-derived growth factor (PDGF), transforming growth factor-beta (TGF-beta) and fibroblast growth factor (FGF), as well as a variety of drugs (McPherson et al., 1992; Okafuji et al., 2006; Bareiss et al., 2010). Therapeutic agents can be incorporated into the matrix by direct absorption (Friedlaender et al., 2001; Armander et al., 2006), via nano- and microparticles containing the agent, or by covalent attachment of the agent to the scaffold (Li et al., 2012). For example, the Infuse Bone Graft (from Medtronic Inc.) is a collagen sponge delivery system used to deliver absorbed recombinant human bone morphogenetic protein-2 (hrBMP-2) to treat degenerative disc disease and cartilage defects (Sellers et al., 2000). Recently, Li et al. have developed a double-layer collagen membrane incorporating growth factor (bFGF) loaded chitosan-heparin nanoparticles for tissue repair (Li et al., 2012). Bareiss et al. (2010) have modelled the efficacy of delivery of an anti-viral drug, acyclovir, by using nanoparticles incorporated into collagen-based corneal implants demonstrating the feasibility of using collagen-based constructs as a drug release system in infected corneas (Bareiss et al., 2010)

Collagen scaffolds have been used for cell therapeutics *in vivo,* however, stem cell usage is limited by concerns caused by unwanted progenitors localizing at non-target sites, and causing unwanted tissue formation (Kuraitis et al, 2012). Collagen-based biomaterials have also been used for the delivery of mesenchymal stem cells to promote regeneration of damaged tissue (Trottier et al., 2008; Altman et al., 2008; Altman et al., 2008; Nie et al., 2009; Pabbruwe et al., 2010). The therapeutic potential of these types of implants requires future *in vivo* studies to access their long term effects.

Molecular and cellular therapy approaches have been studied for many years; however, the application of molecular delivery to support cell-based therapy has only recently been tested. Jay et al. (2010) have demonstrated the delivery of multiple therapeutic proteins – each with independent release kinetics and doses that facilitate their distinct biological functions to enhance the efficacy of cell-based therapeutic vascularization. Specifically, microparticles containing monocyte chemotactic protein-1 (MCP-1) and vascular endothelial growth factor (VEGF) were integrated into a collagen based gel to support endothelial cell transplantation. Their data suggests a potential benefit of combined delivery of MCP-1 and VEGF from endothelial cell-containing hydrogels as an alternative strategy.

Conclusion

Collagen type I, the most abundant collagen in the body, has been widely explored as a biomedical material regardless of its source whether extracted from natural tissues or recombinantly synthesized. In regenerative medicine, the applications range from biocompatible tissue-engineered scaffolds that promote endogenous progenitor cells, to matrices, hydrogels, and encapsulation systems that facilitate the delivery of therapeutic cells, drugs, and bioactive agents (e.g. growth factors, peptides) to encourage regeneration of the host tissue.

REFERENCES

Albu, M.G.; Ghica, M.V.; Leca, M.; Popa, L.; Borlescu, C.; Cremenescu, E.; Giurginca, M.; Trandafir, V. (2010). Doxcycyline delivery from collagen matrices cross-linked with tannic acid. *Molecular Crystals and Liquid Crystals*, 52391, 97-105.

Altman, A.M.; Chiu, E.S.; Bai, X.; Yan, Y.; Song, Y.H.; Newsome, R.E.; Alt, E.U. (2008). Human adipose-derived stem cells adhere to acellular dermal matrix. *Aesthetic Plast. Surg., 32*, 698-699.

Altman, A. M., Matthias, N., Yan, Y., Song, Y. H., Bai, X., Chiu, E. S., Slakey, D. P. & Alt, E. U. (2008). Dermal matrix as a carrier for *in vivo* delivery of human adipose-derived stem cells. *Biomaterials, 29*, 1431–1442.

Angele, P.; Abke, J.; Kujat, R.; Faltermeier, H.; Schumann, D.; Nerlich, M.; Kinner, B.; Englert, C.; Ruszczak, Z.; Mehrl, R.; Mueller, R. (2004). Influence of different collagen species on physico-chemical properties of cross-linked collagen matrices. *Biomaterials*, 25(14), 2831-2841.

Arnander, C., Westermark, A., Veltheim, R., Docherty-Skogh, A. C., Hilborn, J. & Engstrand, T. (2006). Three-dimensional technology and bone morphogenetic protein in frontal bone reconstruction. *J. Craniofac Surg., 17,* 275-279.

Bailey A.J. (1991).The chemistry of natural enzyme-induced crosslinks of proteins. *Amino Acids*, 1, 293-306.

Bao, L.; Yang, W.; Mao, X.; Mou, S.; Tang, S. (2008). Agar/collagen membrane as skin dressing for wounds. *Biomedical Materials*, 3(4), 1-7.

Bareiss, B., Ghorbani, M., Li, F., Blake, J. A., Scaiano, J. C., Zhang, J., Deng, C., Merrett, K., Harden, J. L., Diaz-Mitoma, F. & Griffith M. (2010). Controlled Release of Acyclovir Through Bioengineered Corneal Implants with Silica Nanoparticle Carrier. *The Open Tissue Engineering and Regenerative Medicine Journal, 3*, 10-17.

Barnes, M. J. and R. W. Farndale (1999). "Collagens and atherosclerosis. *Exp Gerontol* 34(4): 513-525.

Basel, D. & R. D. Steiner (2009). Osteogenesis imperfecta: recent findings shed new light on this once well-understood condition. *Genet Med* 11(6): 375-385.

Bedran-Russo, A.K.B.; Yoo, K.J.; Ema, K.C.; Pashley, D.H. (2009). Mechanical properties of tannic-acid treated dentin matrix. *J Dent Res*, 88(9), 807-811.

Beil, W., Timpl R., Furthmayr H. (1973). Conformation dependence of antigenic determinants on the collagen molecule. *Immunology,* 24(1): 13-24.

Bentley, E.; Murphy, C.J.; Li, F.; Carlsson D.J., Griffith, M. (2010). Biosynthetic corneal substitute implantation in dogs. *Cornea*, 29(8), 910-916.

Berg R.A. & Prockop D.J. (1973). The thermal transition of a non-hydroxylated form of collagen.Evidence for a role for hydroxyproline in stabilizing the triple-helix of collagen. *Biochem Biophys Res Commun*, 52(1), 115-120.

Birk, D. E. (2001). Type V collagen: heterotypic type I/V collagen interactions in the regulation of fibril assembly. *Micron*, 32(3), 223-237.

Boland, E. D., Matthews, J. A., & Pawlowski, K. J., *et al.*, (2004). Electrospinning collagen and elastin: preliminary vascular tissue engineering. *Front Biosci.*, 9, 1422-1432.

Boot-Handford, R. P. & Tuckwell, D. S. (2003). Fibrillar collagen: the key to vertebrate evolution? A tale of molecular incest. *Bioessays* 25(2): 142-151.

Borene, M. L., Barocas, V. H. & Hubel, A. (2004). Mechanical and cellular changes during compaction of a collagen-sponge-based corneal stromal equivalent. *Annals of Biomedical Engineering*, 32, 274-283.

Browder, I.W.; Litwin, M.S. (1986). Use of absorbable collagen for hemostasis in general surgical patients. *Am Surg.*, 52(9), 492-494.

Bruder, S. P. & Caplan, A. I. (2000). Bone regeneration through cellular engineering. in R.P. Lanza, R. Langer, & J. Vacanti (Eds.), *Principles of tissue engineering*: Academic Press, San Diego, pp. 683–696.

Builles, N., Janin-Manificat, H., Malbouyres, M., Justin, V., Rovère, M. R., Pellegrini, G., Torbet, J., Hulmes, D. J., Burillon, C., Damour, O. & Ruggiero F. (2010). Use of magnetically oriented orthogonal collagen scaffolds for hemi-corneal reconstruction and regeneration. *Biomaterials*, 31, 8313-8322.

Buttafoco, L., Boks, N. P., Engbers-Buijtenhuijs. P., Grijpma, D. W., Poot, A. A., Dijkstra, P. J., Vermes, I. & Feijen, J. (2006). Porous hybrid structures based on P(DLLA-co-TMC) and collagen for tissue engineering of small-diameter blood vessels. *J Biomed. Mater. Res. Part B,* 79B, 425-434.

Cai, Y. Z., Wang, L. L., Cai, H. X., Qi, Y. Y., Zou, X. H. & Ouyang, H. W. (2010). Electrospun nanofibrous matrix improves the regeneration of dense cortical bone. *J. Biomed. Mater. Res. A*, *95*, 49-57.

Callegari, A., Bollini, S., Iop, L., Chiavegato, A., Torregrossa, G., Pozzobon, M., Gerosa, G., De Coppi, P., Elvassore, N. & Sartore S. (2007). Neovascularization induced by porous collagen scaffold implanted on intact and cryoinjured rat hearts. *Biomaterials, 28,* 5449-5461.

Caruso, A.B.; Dunn, M.G. (2004). Functional evaluation of collagen fiber scaffolds for ACL reconstruction: Cyclic loading in proteolytic enzyme solutions. *Journal of Biomedical Materials Research,* 69A (1), 164-171.

Cerruti-Mainardi, P., G. Venturi, M. Spunton, E. Favaron, M. Zignani, S. Provera and B. Dallapiccola (2011). Infantile cortical hyperostosis and COL1A1 mutation in four generations. *Eur J Pediatr* 170(11): 1385-1390.

Chachques, J. C., Trainini, J. C., Lago, N., Cortes-Morichetti, M., Schussler, O. & Carpentier A. (2008). Myocardial Assistance by Grafting a New Bioartificial Upgraded Myocardium (MAGNUM trial): clinical feasibility study. *Ann. Thorac. Surg., 85,* 901-908.

Chamberlain, L. J., Yannas, I. V., Hsu, H-P., Strichartz, G. & Spector, M. (1998). Collagen-GAG substrate enhances the quality of nerve regeneration through collagen tubes up to the level of autograft. *Exp. Neurol.*, 154, 315-329.

Chan, B.P.; Hui, T.Y.; Wong, M.Y.; Yip, K.H.K.; Chan, G.C.F. (2010). Mesenchymal stem cell encapsulated collagen microspheres for bone tissue engineering. *Tissue Eng Part C*, 16, 225-235.

Chan O.C.M.; So, K.F.; Chan, B.P. (2008) Fabrication of nano-fibrous collagen microspheres for protein delivery and effect of photochemical crosslinking on release kinetics. *J Control Release*, 129, 135-143.

Chan, B.P.; Chan, O.C.M.; So, K.F. (2008). Effects of photochemical crosslinking on the microstructure of collagen and a feasibility study on controlled protein release. Acta Biomaterialia, 4(6), 1627-1636.

Chen, R. N., Wang, G. M., Chen, C. H., Ho, H. O. and Sheu, M. T. (2006). Development of N,O-(carboxymethyl)chitosan/collagen matrixes as a wound dressing. *Biomacromolecules, 7,* 1058-1064.

Chen, S.; Hirota, N.; Okuda, M.; Takeguchi, M.; Kobayashi, H.; Hanagata, N.; Ikoma, T. (2011). Microstructures and rheological properties of tilapia fish-scale collagen hydrogels with aligned fibrils fabricated under magnetic fields. *Acta Biomaterials*, 7(2), 644-652.

Chen, Y.J.; Feng, B.; Zu, Y.P.; Weng, J.; Wang, J.X.; Lu, X. (2009). Fabrication of porous titanium implants with biomechanical compatability. Mater Lett 63, 2659-2661.

Chen, Z.G.; Wang, P.W., Wei, B.; Mo, X.M., Cui, F.Z. (2010). Electrospun collagen-chitosan nanofiber; A biomimetic extracellular matrix for endothelial cell and smooth muscle cell. *Acta Biomaterialia*, 6920, 372-382.

Cholas, R. H., Hsu, H. P. & Spector, M. (2012). The reparative response to cross-linked collagen-based scaffolds in a rat spinal cord gap model. *Biomaterials,* 33, 2050-2059.

Chung, C. & Burdick, J. A. (2008). Engineering cartilage tissue. *Adv. Drug Delivery ReV., 60*, 243-262.

Clark, R. A. F. & Singer, A. J. (2000). Wound repair: basic biology to tissue engineering: In R. P. Lanza, R. Langer, & J. Vacanti (Eds.), *Principles of tissue engineering*: (855–78). Academic Press, San Diego.

Clarke, E. P., G. A. Cates, E. H. Ball and B. D. Sanwal (1991). A collagen-binding protein in the endoplasmic reticulum of myoblasts exhibits relationship with serine protease inhibitors. *J Biol Chem* 266(26), 17230-17235.

Cleutjens, J. P., Verluyten, M. J., Smiths J. F., and Daemen M. J. (1995). Collagen remodeling after myocardial infarction in the rat heart. *Am J Pathol* 147(2): 325-338.

Cockerman, K.; Hsu, V.J. (2009). Collagen-based dermal fillers: past, present, future. *Facial Plast Surg*, 25(2), 106-113.

Cohen-Solal, L., Castanet, J., Meunier, F. J., and Glimcher, M. J. (1986). Proline hydroxylation of collagens synthesized at different temperatures in vivo by two poikilothermic species. *Comp Biochem Physiol B*, 83(2), 483-486.

Colazzo, F.; Sarathchandra, P.; Smolenski, R.T.; Chester, A.H.; Tseng, Y.T.; Czernuszka, J.T.; Yacoub, M.H.; Taylor, P.M. (2011). Extracellular matrix production by adipose-derived stem cells: Implications for heart valve tissue engineering. *Biomaterials,* 3291, 119-127.

Connolly, J.M.; Alferiev, I.; Eidelman, N.; Sacks, M.; Palmatory, E.; Kronsteiner, A.; DeFelice, S.; Xu, J.; Ohri, R.; Narula, N.; Vyavahare, N.; Levy, R.J. (2005). Triglycidylamine crosslinking of porcine aortic valve cusps or bovine pericardium results in improved biocompatibility, biomechanics, and calcification resistance: Chemical and biologicial mechanisms. *The American Journal of Pathology*, 166(1), 1-13.

Cooperman, L. & Michaeli, D. (1984). The immunogenicity of injectable collagen. I. A 1-year prospective study. *J Am Acad Dermatol,* 10(4), 638-646.

Cornwell, K.; Downing, B.R.; Pins, G.D. (2004). Characterizing fibroblast migration on discrete collagen threads for applications in tissue regeneration. *J Biomed Mater Res A,* 71, 55-62.

Cornwell, K.G.; Lei, P.; Andreadis, T.; Pin, G.D. (2007). Crosslinking of discrete self-assembled collagen threads: Effects on mechanical strength and cell matrix interactions. *Journal of Biomedical Materials Research Part A,* 80A(2), 362-371.

Courtenay J.S., Dallman M.J., Dayan A.D., Martin A., Mosedale B. (1980). Immunisation against heterologous type II collagen induces arthritis in mice. *Nature,* 283, 666-668.

Courtman, D.W.; Wilson, G.J.; Lee, J.M.; Yeger, C.A.; Pereira, C.A.; Shearing, A.; Klement P. (1989). Mechanical characterization of an acellular matrix vascular graft: Comparison with natural arteries and effects of crosslinking. *Trans Soc Biomater* 15, 64-74.

Daamen, W.F.; Nillesen, S.T.M.: Wismans, RG; Reinhardt, DP; Hafmans, T; Veerkamp, JH et al. (2003). Preparation and evaluation of molecularly defined collagen-elastin-glycosaminoglycan scaffolds for tissue engineering. *Biomaterials* 24, 4001-4009.

Davison, P. F., L. Levine, M. P. Drake, A. Rubin and S. Bump (1967). The serologic specificity of tropocollagen telopeptides. *J Exp Med* 126(2): 331-346.

De Miguel, M. P., Alio, J. L., Arnalich-Montiel, F., Fuentes-Julian, S., de Benito-Llopis, L., Amparo, F. & Bataille, L. (2010). Cornea and ocular surface treatment. *Current Stem Cell Research Therapy, 5,* 195-204.

Di Y.; Heath R.J. (2009). Collagen stabilization and modification using a polyepoxide triglycidyl isocyanurate. *Polymer Degradation and Stability,* 94, 1684-1692.

Djerassi, C.; Gray, J.D.; Kincl, F. (1960). Naturally occurring oxygen heterocyclics. IX. Isolation and characterizationof genepin. *J Org Chem* 25, 2174-2177.

Dodge, G. R. Poole A. R. (1989). Immunohistochemical detection and immunochemical analysis of type II collagen degradation in human normal, rheumatoid, and osteoarthritic articular cartilages and in explants of bovine articular cartilage cultured with interleukin 1. *J Clin Invest* 83(2), 647-661.

Dravida, S., Gaddipati, S., Griffith, M., Merrett, K., Lakshmi Madhira, S. & Sangwan, V. S. (2008). A biomimetic scaffold for culturing limbal stem cells: a promising alternative for clinical transplantation. *Journal of Tissue Engineering Regenerative Medicine, 2,* 263-271.

Du, C, Cui, F. Z., Zhang, W., Feng, Q. L., Zhu, X. D. & de Groot, K. (2000). Formation of calcium phosphate/collagen composites through mineralization of collagen matrix. *Journal of Biomedical Materials Research Part A, 50,* 518-527.

Duan, X; & Sheardown, H. (2005). Crosslinking of collagen with dendrimers. *Journal of Biomedical Materials Research Part A,* 75A, 510-518.

Dubey, D. K. & Tomar V. (2009). Role of the nanoscale interfacial arrangement in mechanical strength of tropocollagen-hydroxyapatite-based hard biomaterials. *Acta Biomaterialia,* 5, 2704–2716.

Duncan, A.C.; Boughner, D.; Vesley, I. (1996). Dynamic glutaraldehyde fixation of a porcine aorticvalve xenograft: I. Effect of fixation conditions on the final tissue viscoelastic properties. *Biomaterials* 17(19), 1849-1856.

Dunn M.G., Avasarala N.P., Zawadsky J.P. (1993). Optimization of extruded collagen fibers for ACL reconstruction. *J Biomed Mater Res.*, (27),1545-1552.

Eccleston, P., Mirsky, R. & Jessen, K. (1889). Type I collagen preparations inhibit DNA synthesis in glial cells of the peripheral nervous system. *Exp. Cell Res.,* 182, 173-185.

Edmonds, M. (2009). Apligraf in the treatment of neuropathic diabetic foot ulcers. *Int. J. Low Extrem. Wounds, 28,* 11–18.

Fagerholm, P., Lagali, N.S., Merrett, K., Jackson, W.B., Munger, R., Liu, Y., Polarek J.W., Söderqvist, M. and Griffith, M. (2010) A biosynthetic alternative to human donor tissue for inducing corneal regeneration: 24 month follow-up of a Phase I clinical study. *Science Translational Medicine,* 2, 46ra61.

Fahenstock, S.R.; Steinbüchel A., (2003), editors. 2nd edn. Collagens and gelatins, Biopolymers, Polyamide and Complex Proteinaceous Materials, Vol. 8, Wiley-VCH.

Fessel, G.; Gerber, C.; Snedeker, J.G. (2012). Potential of collagen cross-linking therapies to mediate tendon mechanical properties. *Journal of Shoulder and Elbow Surgery* 21 (2), 209-217.

Fleischmajer, R., MacDonald E. D., Perlish J. S., R. E. Burgeson and L. W. Fisher (1990). Dermal collagen fibrils are hybrids of type I and type III collagen molecules." J Struct Biol 105(1-3), 162-169.

Flocea, P.; Verestiuc, L.; Popa, M.; Sunel, V.; Lungu, A. (2010). Crosslinked networks based on polysaccharides and collagen pilocarpine sustained release. *Journal of Macromolecular Science Part A: Pure and Applied Chemistry*, 47, 616-625.

Fomovsky, G.M., Thomopoulos, S. & Holmes, J. W. (2010). Contribution of extracellular matrix to the mechanical properties of the heart. *J. Mol. Cell. Cardiol., 48,* 490-496.

Franchi, M., A. Trire, M. Quaranta, E. Orsini and V. Ottani (2007). Collagen structure of tendon relates to function. *Scientific World Journal,* 7, 404-420.

Freiss, W. (1998). Collagen- biomaterial for drug delivery. *European Journal of Pharmaceutics and Biopharmaceutics,* 45, 113-136.

Friedlaender, G. E., Perry, C. R., Cole, J. D., Cook, S. D., Cierny, G., Muschler, G. F., Zych, G. A., Calhoun, J. H., LaForte, A. J. & Yin, S. (2001). Osteogenic protein-1 (bone morphogenetic protein-7) in the treatment of tibial nonunions. *J. Bone Joint Surg. Am.* 83-A Suppl 1 (Pt 2), 151-158.

Frisch, S. M. and H. Francis (1994). Disruption of epithelial cell-matrix interactions induces apoptosis. *J Cell Biol*, 124(4), 619-626.

Fujikawa, S.; Yokota, T.; Koga, K.; Kumada, J. (1987). The continuous hydrolysis of geniposide to genepin using immobilized ß-glucosidase on calcium alginate gel. *Biotechnol Lett* 9, 697-702.

Furthmayr, H., Beil, W. and Timpl R. (1971). Different antigenic determinants in the polypeptide chains of human collagen. FEBS Lett 12(6), 341-344.

Furthmayr, H. and Timpl, R. (1976). Immunochemistry of collagens and procollagens. *Int Rev Connect Tissue Res*, 7, 61-99.

Geiger, M., Li, R. H. & Friess,W. (2003). Collagen sponges for bone regeneration with rhBMP- 2. *Adv. Drug Deliv. Rev.* 55, 1613-29.

Gelse, K., Poschl, E. & Aigner, T. (2003). Collagens--structure, function, and biosynthesis. *Adv. Drug Deliv. Rev., 55,* 1531-1546.

Gendler, E.; Gendler, S.; Nimni, M.E. (1984). Toxic reactions evoked by glutaraldehyde-fixed pericardium and cardiac valve tissue bioprotheses. *J Biomed Mater Res,* 18(7), 727-736.

Gensure, R. C., Makitie, O., Barclay, C., Chan, C., Depalma, S. R., Bastepe, M., Abuzahra, H., Couper, R., Mundlos, S., Sillence, D., Ala Kokko, L., Seidman, J. G., Cole,W.G. and Juppner H. (2005). A novel COL1A1 mutation in infantile cortical hyperostosis (Caffey disease) expands the spectrum of collagen-related disorders. *J Clin Invest* 115(5), 1250-1257.

Gilles, M.A.; Hudson, A.Q.; Borders, C.l. (1990). Stability of water soluble carbodiimides in aqueous solution. *Anal Biochem,* 184, 244-248.

Girton T.S., Oegema T.R., Tranquillo R.T. (1999). Exploiting glycation to stiffen and strengthen tissue equivalents for tissue engineering. J Biomed Mater Res (46):87-92.

Girton, T. S., Oegema, T. R. & Tranquillo, R. T. (1999). Exploiting glycation to stiffen and strengthen tissue equivalents for tissue engineering, *J. Biomed. Mat. Res., 46,* 87–92.

Golomb, G.; Schoen, F.J.; Smith, M.S.; Linden, J.; Dixon, M.; Levy R.J. (1987). The role of glutaraldehyde induced crosslinks in calcification of bovine pericardium used in cardiac valve bioprostheses. *Am J Pathol,* 127, 122-130.

Gomes, S.; Leonor, I.; Mano, J.; Reis, L.; Kaplan, D. (2012). Natural and genetically engineered proteins for tissue engineering. *Progress in Polymer Science*, 37 (1), 1-17.

Gordon, M. K. and R. A. Hahn (2010). Collagens. *Cell Tissue Res* 339(1), 247-257.

Gough, J.E.;, Scotchford, C.A.; Downes, S. (2002). Cytotoxicity of glutaraldehyde crosslinked collagen/poly(vinyl alcohol) films is by the mechanism of apoptosis. *J Biomed Mater Res,* 61,121-125.

Grant, S. F., D. M. Reid, G. Blake, R. Herd, I. Fogelman and S. H. Ralston (1996). Reduced bone density and osteoporosis associated with a polymorphic Sp1 binding site in the collagen type I alpha 1 gene. *Nat Genet*, 14(2), 203-205.

Greilberger, J., O. Schmut and G. Jurgens (1997). In vitro interactions of oxidatively modified LDL with type I, II, III, IV, and V collagen, laminin, fibronectin, and poly-D-lysine. *Arterioscler Thromb Vasc Biol,* 17(11), 2721-2728.

Griffith, M.; Jackson, W.B.; Lagali, N.; Merrett, K.; Li, F. & Fagerholm, P. (2009). Artificial corneas: A regenerative medicine approach. *Eye,* 23, 1985-1989.

Habeeb, A.F.S. (2009). Determination of free amino groups in proteins by trinitrobenzenesulfonic acid. *Analytical Biochemistry* 1966 14,328-336.

Hamdi, H., Furuta, A., Bellamy, V., et al. (2009). Cell delivery: intramyocardial injections or epicardial deposition? A head-to-head comparison. *Ann. Thorac Surg., 87,* 1196-203.

Hamraoui, K.; Ernst, S.; van Desel, P.; Kelder, J.; Berg, J.; Suttorp, M.; Jaarsma, W.; Plokker, T. (2002). Efficacy and safety of percutaneoustreatment of iatrogenicfemoralarterypseudoaneurysm by biodegradablecollageninjection. *Journal of the American College of Cardiology*, 39(8), 1297-1304.

Hansen, A., McMillan, L., Morrison, A., Petrik, J. & Bradley, M. (2011). Polymers for the rapid and effective activation and aggregation of platelets, *Biomaterials, 32,* 7034-7041.

Harley, B. A., Lynn, A. K., Wissner-Gross, Z., Bonfield, W., Yannas, I. V. & Gibson, L. J. (2010). Design of a multiphase osteochondral scaffold. II. Fabrication of a mineralized collagen glycosaminoglycan scaffold. *Journal of Biomedical Materials Research Part A,* 92A, 1066–1077.

Harley, B.A.; Spilker, M.H.; Wu, J.W.; Asano, K.; Hsu, H.P.; Spector, M.; Yannas, V. (2004). Optimal degradation rate for collagen chambers used for regeneration of peripheral nerves over long gaps. *Cells, Tissues, Organs,* 176, 153-165.

Hassel J.; Hand A.R. (1974). Tissue fixation with diimidoesters as an alternative to aldehydes I. Comparison of crosslinking and ultrastructure obtained with dimethylsuberimidate and glutaraldehyde. *J Histochem. Cytochem*, 22, 223-239.

Hassell, J. R. & Birk D. E. (2010). The molecular basis of corneal transparency. *Exp Eye Res,* 91(3), 326-335.

Hassenkam, T., Fantner, G. E.,. Cutroni, J. A, Weaver, J. C., Morse D. E., and Hansma, P. K. (2004). High-resolution AFM imaging of intact and fractured trabecular bone. *Bone,* 35(1), 4-10.

Hay, E. D. (1981). Extracellular matrix. *J Cell Biol*, 91(3 Pt 2): 205s-223s.

Hermanson, G. T. (1996). Bioconjugate techniques. Academic Press, San Diego, CA.

Hermanson, GT. (2008). Bioconjugate Techniques. London, UK, Elsevier.

Hofmann, U., A. Bonz, S. Frantz, K. Hu, C. Waller, K. Roemer, J. Wolf, S. Gattenlohner, J. Bauersachs and G. Ertl (2012). A collagen alpha2(I) mutation impairs healing after experimental myocardial infarction. *Am J Pathol* 180(1), 113-122.

Hong, Y., Gao, C., Xie, Y., Gong, Y. & Shen, J. (2005). Collagen-coated polylactide microspheres as chondrocyte microcarriers. *Biomaterials. 26,* 6305-6313.

Huang-Lee, L.L.H.; Cheung, D.T.; Nimni, M.E. (2000). Biochemical changes and cytotoxicity associcated with degradation of polymeric glutaraldehyde derived crosslinks. *J Biomed Mater Res* 1990 24, 1185-1202.

Humphries, M. J. (2000). Integrin structure. *Biochem Soc Trans* 28(4), 311-339.

Hunter, S.A.; Rapopor, H.S.; Connolly, J.M.; Alferiev, I.; Fulmer, J.; Murti, B.H.; Herfat,M.; Noyes, F.R.; Butler, D.L.; Levy, R.J. (2010). Biomechanical and biologic effects of meniscus stabilization using triglycidyl amine. *Journal of Biomedical Materials Research Part A,* 93A (1), 235-242.

Hutmacher, D.W. (2000). Scaffolds in tissue engineering bone and cartilage. *Biomaterials,* 21, 2529-2543.

Hynes, R. O. (2002). Integrins: bidirectional, allosteric signaling machines. *Cel,l* 110(6), 673-687.

Ibrahim, S.; Kothapalli, C.R.; Kang, Q.K.; Ramamurthi, A. (2011). Characterization of glycidyl methacrylate- crosslinked hyaluronan hydrogel scaffolds incorporating elastogenic hyaluronan oligomers. *Acta Biomaterialia,* February 7(2), 653-665.

Ibusuki, S.; Halbesma, G.J.; Randolph, M.A.; Redmond, R.W.; Kochevar, I.E.; Gill, T.J. (2007). Photochemically crosslinked collagen gels as three-dimensional scaffolds for tissue engineering. *Tissue Engineering*, 13(8), 1995-2001.

Imamura, E.; Sawanti, H.; Koyanagi, Y.; Noishiki, Y.; Miyata T. (1989). Epoxy compounds as a new crosslinking agent for porcine aortic leaflets: Subcutaneous implant studies in rats. *J Cardiac Surg*, 4, 50-57.

Imamura. E.; Sawatani, O.; Koyanagi, H.; Noishiki, Y.; Miyata T. (1988). Anticalcification effects of expoxy compounds as crosslinking agent. *J Artif Organs*, 17, 1101-1103.

James, N. L., Schindhelm, K., Slowiaczek, P., Milthorpe, B. K., Dudman, N. P. B. & Johnson, G. *et al.* (1990). Endothelial Cell Seeding of Small Diameter Vascular Grafts. *Artif. Organs., 14,* 355-360.

Jay, S.M.; Shepherd, B.R.; Andrejecsk, J.W.; Kyriadkides, T.R.; Pober, J.S.; Saltzman, W.M. (20109. Dual delivery of VEGF and MCP-1 to support endothelial cell transplantation for therapeutic vascularization. *Biomaterials,* 31 (11), 3054-3062.

Jayakumar, G.C.; Kanth, S.V.; Sai, K.P.; Chandrasekaran, B.; Rao, J.R.; Nair, B.U. (2012). Scleraldehyde as a stabilizing agent for collagen scaffold preparation. *Carbohydrate Polymers,* 87(2), 1482-1489.

Jokinen, J., E. Dadu, P. Nykvist, J. Kapyla, D. J. White, J. Ivaska, P. Vehvilainen, H. Reunanen, H. Larjava, L. Hakkinen and J. Heino (2004). Integrin-mediated cell adhesion to type I collagen fibrils. *J Biol Chem* 279(30), 31956-31963.

Kadler, K. E., A. Hill and E. G. Canty-Laird (2008). Collagen fibrillogenesis: fibronectin, integrins, and minor collagens as organizers and nucleators. *Curr Opin Cell Biol*, 20(5), 495-501.

Kadler, K. E., D. F. Holmes, J. A. Trotter and J. A. Chapman (1996). Collagen fibril formation. *Biochem* J 316 (Pt 1), 1-11.

Karr, J. (2008). Utilization of living bilayered cell therapy (Apligraf) for heel ulcers. *Adv. Skin Wound Care, 21,* 270–274.

Kato Y.P., Christiansen D.L., Hahn R.A., Shieh S.J., Goldstein J.D., Silver F.H. (1989). Mechanical properties of collagen fibers: a comparison of reconstituted and rat tail tendon fibers. *Biomaterials*, 10(1), 38-42.

Kato, Y.; Uchida, K.; Kawakishi, S. (1994). Aggregation of collagen exposed to UVA in the presence of riboflavin; a plausible role of tyrosine modification. *Photochem Photobiol* 59, 343.

Kew, S.J.; Gwynne J.H.; Enea, D.; Abu-Rub, M.; Pandit, A.; Zeugolis, D.; Brooks, R.A.; Rushton, N.; Best, S.M.; Cameron, R.E. (2011). Regeneration and repair of tendon and ligament tissue using collagen-fibre biomaterials. Acta Biomaterialia, 7(9), 3237-3247.

Kiernan, J.A., (2000). Formaldehyde, formalin, paraformaldehyde and glutaraldehyde: What they are and what they do. *Microscopy Today* 00-1, 8-12.

Kim, G. H., Ahn, S. H., Yoon, H., Kim, Y. Y. & Chun, W. J. (2009). A cryogenic direct-plotting system for fabrication of 3D collagen scaffolds for tissue engineering. *Mater. Chem.,19,* 8817-8823.

Kim, H.W.; Li, L.H.; Lee, E.J.; Lee, S.H.; Kim, H.E. (2005). Fibrillar assembly and stability of collagen coating on titanium for improved osteoblast responses. Journal of Biomedical Materials Research Part A, 75A(3), 629-638.

Kodama, T., T. Doi, H. Suzuki, K. Takahashi, Y. Wada and S. Gordon (1996). "Collagenous macrophage scavenger receptors." Curr Opin Lipidol 7(5): 287-291.

Kohn J.; Welsh, W.J.; Knight, D.A. (2007). A new approach to the rationale discovery of polymeric biomaterials. Biomaterials 28, 4171-4177.

Kosaraju, S.L.; Puvanenthiran, A.; Lillford, P. (2010). Naturally crosslinked gelatin gels with modified material properties Food Research International 43 (10), 2385-2389.

Kundu, A. K. & Putnam, A. J. (2006). Vitronectin and collagen I differentially regulate osteogenesis in mesenchymal stem cells. *Biochem Biophys Res Commun., 347,* 347–357.

Kuraitis D.; Giordano, C.; Ruel, M; Musaro, A; Surronen, E.J. (2012). Exploiting extracellular matrix-stem cell interactions: A review of natural materials for therapeutic muscle regeneration. *Biomaterials* 33 (2), 428-443

Kurkinen, M., A. Vaheri, P. J. Roberts and S. Stenman (1980). Sequential appearance of fibronectin and collagen in experimental granulation tissue. *Lab Invest*, 43(1), 47-51.

Kyle, S.; Aggeli, A.; Ingham, E.; McPherson, M.J. (2009). Production of self-assembling biomaterials for tissue engineering. *Trends in Biotechnology*, 27 (7), 423-433.

Lammers, G.; Tjabringa, G.S.; Schalkwijk, J.; Daamen, W.F.; van Kuppevelt. (2009). *Biomaterials,* 30, 6213-6220.

Lang, K., Schmid F. X., and Fischer G. (1987). Catalysis of protein folding by prolyl isomerase. *Nature* 329(6136), 268-270.

Lee, C.H.; Singla, A.; Lee, Y. (2001). Biomedical Application of Collagen. *Int J Pharm*, 221, 1-22.

Lee, J.M.; Pereira, C.A.; Kan, L.W.K. (1994). Effect of moleculear structure of poly(glycidyl ether) reagents on crosslinking and mechanical properties of bovine pericardial xenograft materials. *J Biomed Mater Res*, 28, 981-992.

Li, F.; Carlsson, D.J.; Lohmann, C.; Suuronen, E.; Vascotto, S.; Kobuch, K.; Sheardown, H.; Munger, R.; Nakamura, M.; Griffith M. (2003). Cellular and nerve regeneration within a biosynthetic extracellular matrix for corneal transplantation, *PNAS*, 100 (26), 15346-5351.

Li, W., J. Fan, M. Chen, S. Guan, D. Sawcer, G. M. Bokoch and D. T. Woodley (2004). "Mechanism of human dermal fibroblast migration driven by type I collagen and platelet-derived growth factor-BB. *Mol Biol Cell,* 15(1), 294-309.

Li, X.; Wang, J.; Su, G.; Zhou, Z.; Shi, J.; Liu, L. (2012). Spatiotemporal control over growth factor delivery from collagen based membrane. *Journal of Biomedical Materials Research Part A*, 100 (2), 396-405.

Liao, S., Ngiam, M., Chan, C. K. & Ramakrishna, S. (2009). Fabrication of nanohydroxyapatite/collagen/osteonectin composites for bone graft applications. *Biomedical Materials, 4,* 025019.

Liu, L., Kuffova, L., Griffith, M., Dang, Z., Muckersie, E., Liu, Y., McLaughlin C and Forrester, J. (2007). Immunological responses in mice to full thickness corneal grafts engineered from porcine collagen. *Biomaterials*, 28, 3807-3814.

Liu, W., Deng, C., McLaughlin, C.R., Fagerholm, P., Watsky, M.A., Heyne, B., Scaiano, J.C., Lagali, N.S., Munger, R., Li, F. and Griffith, M. (2009). Collagen-phosphorylcholine interpenetrating network hydrogels as corneal substitutes. *Biomaterials,* 30, 1551-1559.

Liu, X., H. Wu, M. Byrne, S. Krane and R. Jaenisch (1997). Type III collagen is crucial for collagen I fibrillogenesis and for normal cardiovascular development. *Proc Natl Acad Sci U S A* 94(5), 1852-1856.

Lu, H.; Ko, Y.G.; Kawazoe, N.; Chen, G. (2010). Cartilage tissue engineering using funnel-like collagen sponges prepared with embossing ice particulate templates. *Biomaterials*, 31, 5825-5835.

Lyman, D.M.; Schwell, A.B., Factor, S.M.; Frater, R.W. (1990). Immunogenicity of glutaraldehyde tanned bovine pericardium. *J Thorac Cardiovasc Surg.* 99(6), 1082-90.

Lynn A.K., Yannas, I.V., Bonfield W. (2004). Antigenicity and Immunogenicity of Collagen. *J Biomed Mater Res Part B: Appl Biomater*, 71B, 343-354.

Ma, P. X. (2008). Biomimetic materials for tissue engineering. *Adv. Drug Deliv. Rev. 60,* 184-98.

Madhaven, K.; Belchenko, D.; Motta, A.; Tan W. (2010). Evaluation of composition and crosslinking effects on collagen-based composite constructs. *Acta Biomaterialia*, 6(4), 1413-1422.

Marini, J. C., A. Forlino, W. A. Cabral, A. M. Barnes, J. D. San Antonio, S. Milgrom, J. C. Hyland, J. Korkko, D. J. Prockop, A. De Paepe, P. Coucke, S. Symoens, F. H. Glorieux, P. J. Roughley, A. M. Lund, K. Kuurila-Svahn, H. Hartikka, D. H. Cohn, D. Krakow, M. Mottes, U. Schwarze, D. Chen, K. Yang, C. Kuslich, J. Troendle, R. Dalgleish and P. H. Byers (2007). Consortium for osteogenesis imperfecta mutations in the helical domain of type I collagen: regions rich in lethal mutations align with collagen binding sites for integrins and proteoglycans. *Hum Mutat* 28(3), 209-221.

McPherson, J. M. (1992). The utility of collagen-based vehicles in delivery of growth factors for hard and soft tissue wound repair. *Clin Mater.,* 9, 225-234.

Meng, W., Kim, S.Y., Yuan, J., Kim, J. C., Kwon, O. H., et al. (2007). Electrospun PHBV/collagen composite nanofibrous scaffolds for tissue engineering. *J Biomater Sci Polym Ed.,* 18, 81-94.

Merrett, K.; Fagerholm, P.; McLaughlin, C.R.; Dravida, S.; Lagali, N.; Shinozaki, N.; Watsky M.A.; Munger, R.; Kato, Y.; Li, F.; Marmo, C.J.; Griffith M. (2008). Tissue-engineered recombinant human collagen-based corneal substitutes for implantation: performance of type I versus type III collagen. *Invest Ophthalmol Vis Sci.*, 49(9), 3887-94.

Michaeli, D., G. R. Martin, J. Kettman, E. Benjamini, D. Y. Leung and B. A. Blatt (1969). Localization of antigenic determinants in the polypeptide chains of collagen. *Science*, 166(3912), 1522-1524.

Miles, C.; Sionkowska, A.; Hulin, S.; Sims, T.; Avery, N.; Bailey, A. (2000). Identification of an intermediate state in the helix-coil degradation of collagen by ultraviolet light. *J Biol Chem* (275), 33014-33020.

Min, B. M., Lee, G., Kim, S. H., Nam, Y. S., Lee, T. S. & Park, W. H. (2004). Electrospinning of silk fibroin nanofibers and its effect on the adhesion and spreading of normal human keratinocytes and fibroblasts in vitro. *Biomaterials*, 25, 1289-1297.

Miyata, T.; Sohde, T.; Rubin, A.L.; Stenzel, K.H. (1971). Effects of ultraviolet irradiation on native and telopeptide poor collagen. *Biochim Biophys Acta* 229, 672-680.

Mo, X., Chen, Z. & Weber, H. J. (2007). Electrospun nanofibers of collagen-chitosan and P(LLA-CL) for tissue engineering. *Front. Mater. Sci. China, 1,* 20-23

Moncy, J.V.; Vinoy, T.; Dean, D.R.; Nyairo E. (2009). Fabrication and characterization of aligned nanofibrous PLGA/Collagen blends as bone tissue scaffolds. *Polymer*, 50, 3778-3788.

Mosekilde, L. (2000). Age-related changes in bone mass, structure, and strength-effects of loading. *Z Rheumatol* 59 Suppl 1, 1-9.

Muzzarelli, R.A.A. (2009). Genepin-crosslinked chitosan hydrogels as biomedical and pharmaceutical aids. *Carbohydrate Polymers,* 77, 1-9.

Nakajima, N; Ikada, Y. Mechanism of amide formation by carbodiimide for bioconjugation in aqueous media. *Bioconjugate Chem*, 1995 6(1), 123-130.

Nam, K.; Kimuara, T.; Funamoto, S.; Kishida, A. (2010). Preparation of collagen/polymer hybrid gel designed for tissue membranes. Part I; Controlling the polymer-collagen cross-linking process using an ethanol/water co-solvent. *Acta Biomaterialia,* 6, 403-408.

Ni, Y.; Liu, Z.; Gao, W.; Qu, S.; Weng, J.; Feng, B. (2011). Characterization of self-assembled decyl bis phosphonate–Collagen layers on titanium by QCM-D and osteoblast-compatibility. *Applied Surface Science*, September 257 (22), 9287-9292

Nicholls, A. C., J. L. Sher, M. J. Wright, C. Oley, R. F. Mueller and F. M. Pope (2000). Clinical phenotypes and molecular characterisation of three patients with Ehlers-Danlos syndrome type VII. *J Med Genet,* 37(11), E33.

Nicolas, F. L. & Gagnieu, C. H. (1997). Denaturated thiolated collagen. *Biomaterials*, 18, 815-821.

Nie, C., Yang, D. & Morris, S. F. (2009). Local delivery of adipose-derived stem cells via acellular dermal matrix as a scaffold: A new promising strategy to accelerate wound healing. *Med. Hypotheses*, *72*, 679-682.

Nimni, M.E.; Cheung, D.; Strates, B.; Kodama, M.; Sheikh K. (1987). Chemically modified collagen: a natural biomaterial for tissue replacement. *J Biomed Mater Res* 21(6), 741-71.

Nishi, C.; Nakajima, N.; Ikada Y. (1995). In vivo evaluation of cytotoxicity of diepoxy compounts used for biomaterial modification. *Journal of Biomedical Material Research,* 29, 829-834.

Niyibizi, C. and D. R. Eyre (1989). Bone type V collagen: chain composition and location of a trypsin cleavage site. *Connect Tissue Res*, 20(1-4), 247-250.

Nowack, H., E. Hahn and R. Timpl (1975). Specificity of the antibody response in inbred mice to bovine type I and type II collagen. *Immunology* 29(4), 621-628.

O'Brien, F.J.; Harley, B.A.; Yannas, V.; Gibson L. (2004). Influence of freezing rate on pore structure of freeze dried collagen—GAG scaffolds Biomaterials 25(6), 1077-1086.

Ohan, M.P.; Dunn, M.G. (2003). Glucose stabilizes collagen sterilized with gamma irradiation. *J Biomed Mater Res*, 67A, 1188-1195.

Ohan, M.P.; Weadock, K.S.; Dunn, M.G. (2002). Synergistic effects of glucose and ultraviolet irradiation on the physical properties of collagen. *Journal of Biomedical Materials Research,* 60(3), 384-391.

Okafuji, N., Shimizu, T., Watanabe, T., Kimura, A., Kurihara, S., Furusawa, K., Hasegawa, H. & Kawakami, T. (2006). Tissue reaction to poly (lactic-co-glycolic acid) copolymer membrane in rhBMP used rabbit experimental mandibular reconstruction. *Eur. J. Med. Res. 11*, 394-396.

Okuyama, T.; Satake, K. (1960). *J Biochem,* 47, 454.

Olde Damink, L.H.H; Dijkstra, P.J.; Van Luyn, M.J.A.; Van Wachem, P.B.; Nieuwenhuis, P; Feijen, J. (1995). Glutaraldehyde as a crosslinking agent for collagen-based biomaterials. *J of Materials Science: Materials in Medicine,* 6, 460-472.

Olde Damink, L. H., Dijkstra, P. J., van Luyn, M. J., van Wachen, P. B., Nieuwenhuis, P. & Feijen, J. (1996). In vitro degradation of dermal sheep collagen cross linked using a water-soluble carbodiimide. *Biomaterials*, *17,* 679-684.

Olsen, D., C. Yang, M. Bodo, R. Chang, S. Leigh, J. Baez, D. Carmichael, M. Perala, E. R. Hamalainen, M. Jarvinen and J. Polarek (2003). Recombinant collagen and gelatin for drug delivery. *Adv Drug Deliv Rev* 55(12), 1547-1567.

Ottani, V., M. Raspanti and A. Ruggeri (2001). Collagen structure and functional implications. *Micron* 32(3), 251-260.

Pabbruwe, M.B.; Kafienah, W.; Tarlton, J.F.; Mistry, S.; Fox, D.J.; Hollander, A.P. (2010). Repair of meniscal cartilage white zone tears using a stem cell/collagen-scaffold implant. *Biomaterials,* 31(9), 2583-2591

Pachence, J.M. (1996). Collagen-based devices for soft tissue repair. *J. Biomed. Mater. Res.* 33, 35.

Pereira, C.A.; Lee, J.M.; Haberer, S.A. (1990). Effect of alternative crosslinking methods on low strain rate viscoelastic properties of bovine pericardial bioprosthetic material. *J Biomed Mater Res*, 24, 345-361.

Pickering, J. G., C. M. Ford, B. Tang and L. H. Chow (1997). Coordinated effects of fibroblast growth factor-2 on expression of fibrillar collagens, matrix metalloproteinases, and tissue inhibitors of matrix metalloproteinases by human vascular smooth muscle cells. Evidence for repressed collagen production and activated degradative capacity. *Arterioscler Thromb Vasc Biol* 17(3): 475-482.

Plant, A. L., K. Bhadriraju, T. A. Spurlin and J. T. Elliott (2009). Cell response to matrix mechanics: focus on collagen. *Biochim Biophys Acta* 1793(5), 893-902.

Plenz, G. A., M. C. Deng, H. Robenek and W. Volker (2003). Vascular collagens: spotlight on the role of type VIII collagen in atherogenesis. *Atherosclerosis* 166(1), 1-11.

Pontz, B., W. Meigel, J. Rauterberg and K. Kuhn (1970). Localization of two species specific antigenic determinants on the peptide chains of calf skin collagen. *Eur J Biochem* 16(1), 50-54.

Pozzobon, M., Bollini, S. & Iop, L., et al. (2010). Human bone marrow-derived CD133+ cells delivered to a collagen patch on cryoinjured rat heart promote angiogenesis and arteriogenesis. *Cell transplantation, 19,* 1247– 1260.

Radu, F. A., Bause, M., Knabner, P., Lee, G. W. & Friess, W. C. (2002). Modeling of drug release from collagen matrices. *J. Pharm. Sci. 91,* 964-972.

Rafat, M., Matsuura, T., Li, F. & Griffith, M. (2009). Surface modification of collagen-based artificial cornea for reduced endothelialization. *Journal of Biomedical Materials Research Part A, 88*, 755–768.

Rafat, M.; Li, F.; Lagali, N.S.; Watsky, M.A.; Munger, R.; Matsuura, T.; Griffith, M. (2008). PEG-stabilized carbodiimide crosslinked collagen-chitosan hydrogels for corneal tissue engineering. *Biomaterials*, 29(29), 3960-72.

Ramanujan, S., Pluen, A., McKee, T. D., Brown, E. B., Boucher, Y. & Jain, R. K. (2002). Diffusion and convection in collagen gels: implications for transport in the tumor interstitium. *Biophys J. 2002, 83,* 1650–60.

Ramirez, F., M. Bernard, M. L. Chu, L. Dickson, F. Sangiorgi, D. Weil, W. De Wet, C. Junien and M. Sobel (1985). Isolation and characterization of the human fibrillar collagen genes. *Ann N Y Acad Sci,* 460, 117-129.

Rault, I.; Frei, V.; Herbage, D.; Abdul-Marak, N.; Hue, A. (1996). Evaluation of different chemical methods for crosslinking collagen gels ,films and sponges. *J Mater Sci Med*, 7, 215-221.

Rauterberg, J., E. Jaeger and M. Althaus (1993). Collagens in atherosclerotic vessel wall lesions. *Curr Top Pathol,* 87, 163-192.

Rekhter, M. D. (1999). Collagen synthesis in atherosclerosis: too much and not enough. *Cardiovasc Res* 41(2), 376-384.

Rho, K. S., Jeong, L., Lee, G., Seo, B. M., Park, Y. J. & Hong, S. (2006). Electrospinning of collagen nanofibers: effects on the behavior of normal human keratinocytes and early-stage wound healing. *Biomaterials, 27,* 1452-1461.

Ricard-Blum, S. and F. Ruggiero (2005). The collagen superfamily: from the extracellular matrix to the cell membrane. *Pathol Biol (Paris),* 53(7), 430-442.

Robinson, T. F., L. Cohen-Gould and S. M. Factor (1983). Skeletal framework of mammalian heart muscle. Arrangement of inter- and pericellular connective tissue structures. *Lab Invest* 49(4), 482-498.

Sajithal, GB; Chithra, P; Chandrakasan, G. Advanced glycation end products induce cross-linking of collagen in vitro. *Biochimica Biophysica Acta (BBA)/Molecular Basis of Disease*, 1998 1407(3), 215-224.

Sakaguchi, M., H. Hori, S. Hattori, S. Irie, A. Imai, M. Yanagida, H. Miyazawa, M. Toda and S. Inouye (1999). IgE reactivity to alpha1 and alpha2 chains of bovine type 1 collagen in children with bovine gelatin allergy. *J Allergy Clin Immunol* 104(3 Pt 1), 695-699.

Salasznyk, R. M., Williams, W. A., Boskey, A., Batorsky, A. & Plopper. G. E. (2004). Adhesion to vitronectin and collagen I promotes osteogenic differentiation of human mesenchymal stem cells. *J Biomed Biotechnol*, 24–34.

Sang, L.; Luo, D.; Xu, S.; Wang, X.; Li, X. (2011). Fabrication and evaluation of biomimetic scaffolds by using collagen-alginate fibrillar gels for potential tissue engineering applications. *Materials Science and Engineering C,* 31(2), 262-271.

Sannino, A.; Madaghiele, M. (2009). Tuning the Porosity of Collagen-based Scaffolds for Use as Nerve Regenerative Templates. *Journal of Cellular Plastics*, 45 (2), 137-155.

Sasaki, N., A. Tagami, T. Goto, M. Taniguchi, M. Nakata and K. Hikichi (2002). Atomic force microscopic studies on the structure of bovine femoral cortical bone at the collagen fibril-mineral level. *J Mater Sci Mater Med*, 13(3), 333-337.

Schnell, E., Klinkhammer, K., Balzer, S., Brook, G., Klee, D., Dalton, P. & Mey, J. (2007). Guidance of glial cell migration and axonal growth on electrospun nanofibers of poly-epsilon-caprolactone and a collagen/poly-epsilon-caprolactone blend. *Biomaterials, 28,* 3012-3025.

Schoen, F.J.; Levy, R.J.; Nelson, A.C.; Bernard, W.F.; Nashef, A.; Hawley, M. (1985). Onset and progression of experimental bioprosthetic heart valve calcification of porcine aortic valve fibroblasts. *Lab Invest* 52, 523-532.

Schuppan, D., M. Schmid, R. Somasundaram, R. Ackermann, M. Ruehl, T. Nakamura and E. O. Riecken (1998). Collagens in the liver extracellular matrix bind hepatocyte growth factor. *Gastroenterology*, 114(1), 139-152.

Schussler, O., Coirault, C., Louis-Tisserand, M., Al-Chare, W., Oliviero, P., Menard, C., Michelot, R., Bochet, P., Salomon, D. R., Chachques, J. C., Carpentier, A. & Lecarpentier Y. (2009). Use of arginine-glycineaspartic acid adhesion peptides coupled with a new collagen scaffold to engineer a myocardium-like tissue graft. *Nat. Clin. Pract. Cardiovasc Med., 6,* 240-249.

Sellers, R. S., Zhang, R., Glasson, S. S., Kim, H. D., Peluso, D., D'Augusta, D. A., Beckwith, K. & Morris, E. A. (2000) Repair of articular cartilage defects one year after treatment with recombinant human bone morphogenetic protein-2 (rhBMP-2), *J Bone Joint Surg., 82,* 151-60.

Sheu, M. T., Huang, J. C., Yeh, G. C. & Ho, H. O. (2001). Characterization of collagen gel solution and collagen matrices for cell culture. *Biomaterials, 22,* 1713–1719.

Silva, M.M.C.G.; Cyster, L.A.; Barry, J.J.A., Yang, X.B., Oreffo, R.O.C., Grant, D.M., Scotchford' C.A.; Howdle, S.M.; Shakescheff; K.M.; Rose, R.F.A.J. (2006). The effect of anistropic architecture on cell and tissue infiltration into tissue engineering scaffolds. *Biomaterials,* 27, 5909-5917.

Silver, D., J. Miller, R. Harrison and D. J. Prockop (1992). Helical model of nucleation and propagation to account for the growth of type I collagen fibrils from symmetrical pointed tips: a special example of self-assembly of rod-like monomers. *Proc Natl Acad Sci USA,* 89(20), 9860-9864.

Simionescu, A.; Simionescu, D.; Deac, R. (1991). Lysine-enhanced glutaraldehyde crosslinking of collagenous biomaterials. *Journal of Biomedical Materials Research,* 25, 1495-1505.

Simpson, D., Liu, H., Fan, T. M., Nerem, R. & Dudley, S. C. (2007). A tissue engineering approach to progenitor cell delivery results in significant cell engraftment and improved myocardial remodeling. *Stem Cells, 25. 2350* –2357.

Singh, A.; Narvi, S.; Dutta, P.; Pandey, N. (2006). External stimuli response on a novel chitosan hydrogel crosslinked with formaldehyde. *Bull Mater Sci,* 29, 233-238.

Sionkowska, A. (2011). Current Research on the blends of natural and synthetic polymers as new biomaterials:Review. *Progress in Polymer Science*, 36, 1254-1276.

Skinner, M. P., E. W. Raines and R. Ross (1994). Dynamic expression of alpha 1 beta 1 and alpha 2 beta 1 integrin receptors by human vascular smooth muscle cells. Alpha 2 beta 1 integrin is required for chemotaxis across type I collagen-coated membranes. *Am J Pathol*, 145(5), 1070-1081.

Soderhall, C., I. Marenholz, T. Kerscher, F. Ruschendorf, J. Esparza-Gordillo, M. Worm, C. Gruber, G. Mayr, M. Albrecht, K. Rohde, H. Schulz, U. Wahn, N. Hubner and Y. A. Lee (2007). Variants in a novel epidermal collagen gene (COL29A1) are associated with atopic dermatitis. *PLoS Biol* 5(9), e242.

Somasundaram, R., M. Ruehl, B. Schaefer, M. Schmid, R. Ackermann, E. O. Riecken, M. Zeitz and D. Schuppan (2002). Interstitial collagens I, III, and VI sequester and modulate the multifunctional cytokine oncostatin M. *J Biol Chem*, 277(5), 3242-3246.

Somasundaram, R., M. Ruehl, N. Tiling, R. Ackermann, M. Schmid, E. O. Riecken and D. Schuppan (2000). Collagens serve as an extracellular store of bioactive interleukin 2. *J Biol Chem,* 275(49), 38170-38175.

Soo, C., G. Rahbar and R. L. Moy (1993). The immunogenicity of bovine collagen implants. *J Dermatol Surg Oncol* 19(5), 431-434.

Speer, D.P.; Chvapil, M.; Eskelson, C.D.; Ulrich J. (1980). Biological effects of glutaraldehyde in glutaraldehyde tanned collagen biomaterials. *Journal of Biomedical Material Research* 14, 753-764.

Spilker, M. H., Yannas, I. V., Kostyk, S. K., Norregaard, T. V., Hsu, H. P. & Spector, M. (2001). The effects of tubulation on healing and scar formation after transection of the adult rat spinal cord. *Restor Neurol Neurosci., 18,* 23-38.

Spoerl, E.; Mrochen, M.; Sliney, D.; Trokel, S.; Seiler, T. (2007). Safety of UVA-riboflavin cross-linking of the cornea. *Cornea* 26, 385-389.

Stein, H., Dgany O., Wilensky M., Tsafrir Y., Rosenthal M., Amir R., Avraham T., Ofir K., Yayon A. and Soseyov O. (2009) Production of bioactive, post-translationally modified, heterotrimeric, human recombinant type-I collagen in transgenic tobacco. *Biomacromolecules 10(9):2640-5.*

Stricklin G.P., Hibbs M.S., Nimmi M.E. (Eds) (1988). Collagen Boca Ratan: CRC Press;.

Stuart, J. M., A. S. Townes and A. H. Kang (1985). Type II collagen-induced arthritis. *Ann N Y Acad Sci*, 460, 355-362.

Sundberg, L.; Porath, J. (1974). Preparation of adsorbents for biospecific affinity chromatography. Attachment of group containing ligands to insoluble polymers by means of bifunctional oxiranes. *J Chromatogr,* 90, 87-98.

Sung, H.W.; Hsu, H.L.; Shih, C.C.; Lin, D.S. (1996). Crosslinking characteristics of biological tissues fixed with monofunctional or multifunctional epoxy compounds. *Biomaterials*, 17(4), 1405-1410.

Tierney, C.M.; Haugh, M.G.; Liedl, J.; Mulcahy, F.; Hayes, B.; O'Brien, F.J. (2009). The effects of collagen concentration and crosslink density on the biological, structural and mechanical properties of collagen-GAG scaffolds for bone tissue engineering. *Journal of the Mechanical Behaviour of Biomedical Materials*, 2, 202-209.

Tillman, B. W., Yazdani, S. K., Lee, S. J., Geary, R. L., Atala, A. & Yoo, J. J. (2009). The in vivo stability of electrospun polycaprolactone-collagen scaffolds in vascular reconstruction. *Biomaterials, 30,* 583-588.

Titorencu, I.; Albu, M.G.; Giurginca, M.; Jinga, V.; Antoniac, I.; Trandafir, V.; Cotrut, C.; Miculescu, F.; Simionescu, M. (2010). In vitro biocompatibility of human endothelial cells with collagen-doxycycline matrices. *Molecular crystals and liquid crystals,* 523(1), 82-96.

Torres-Giner, S.; Gimeno-Alcaniz, J.V., Ocio, M.J.; Lagaron, J.M. (2009). Comparative performance of electrospun collagen nanofibers cross-linked by means of different methods. *ACS Applied Materials Interfaces*, 1(1), 218-233.

Touyama, R.; Takeda, Y.; Inoue, K.; Kawamura, I.; Yatsuzuka, M.; Ikumoto, T.; Shingu, T.; Yokoi, T.; Inouye, H. (1994). Studies on the blue pigments produced from genepin and methylamine. I. Structures of the brownish-red pigments leading to the blue pigments. *Chem Pharm Bull,* 42, 668-673.

Trentham D.E., Townes AS, Kang A.H. (1977). Autoimmunity to Type II collagen: An experimental model of arthritis. *J Exp Med*, 146, 857-868.

Trottier. V., Marceau-Fortier, G., Germain, L., Vincent, C. & Fradette J. (2008). IFATS collection: Using human adipose-derived stem/stromal cells for the production of new skin substitutes. *Stem Cells, 26,* 2713–2723.

Tsipouras, P. and F. Ramirez (1987). Genetic disorders of collagen. *J Med Genet* 24(1), 2-8.

Tu, R.; Shen, S.H.; Lin, D.; Hata, C.; Thvagarajan, K.; Noishiki, Y.; et al. (1994). Fixation of bioprosthetic tissues with monofunctional and multifunctional polyepoxy compound. *J Biomed Mater Res,* 28(6), 677-84.

Tung, F.I.; Chiu, C.T.; Chang, Y.P.; Wang, Y.J. (2011). Collagen fibers constructed by gravity filament forming process. *Artificial Cells, Blood Substitutes and Biotechnology*, 39(5), 335-340.

Tzaphlidou, M. (2005). The role of collagen in bone structure: an image processing approach. *Micron* 36(7-8), 593-601.

Ulrich, T.A.; Lee, T.G.; Shon, H.K.; Moon, D.W.; Kumar, S. (2011). Microscale mechanisms of agarose-induced disruption of collagen remodeling. *Biomaterials*, 32(34), 5633-5642.

Van der Loo, B., Spring, S. & Koppensteiner, R. (2011). High-dose atorvastatin treatment in patients with peripheral arterial disease: Effects on platelet aggregation, blood rheology and plasma homocysteine, *Clin Hemorheol Microcirc.*, *47*, 241–251.

van der Rest, M. and R. Garrone (1991). Collagen family of proteins. *FASEB J*, 5(13), 2814-2823.

Vasita, R. & Katti, D. S. (2006). Nanofibers and their applications in tissue engineering. *Int. J. Nanomed.*, 1, 15-30.

Venugopal, J., Vadgama, P., Kumar, T. S. S. & Ramakrishna, S. (2007). Biocomposite nanofibres and osteoblasts for bone tissue engineering. *Nanotechnology*, *18,* 055101.

Vizarova, K., D. Bakos, M. Rehakova and V. Macho (1994). Modification of layered atelocollagen by ultraviolet irradiation and chemical cross-linking: structure stability and mechanical properties. *Biomaterials,* 15(13), 1082-1086.

Volkenstein, S.; Kirkwood, J.E.; Lai, E.; Dazert, A.; Fuller, G.G.; Heller, S. (2012). Oriented collagen as a potential cochlear implant electrode surface coating to achieve directed neurite outgrowth. *Eur Arch Otorhinolaryngol*, 269, 1111-1116.

Wachol-Drewek, Z.; Pfeiffer, M.; Scholl, E. (1996). Comparativeinvestigation of drugdelivery of collagenimplantssaturated in antibioticsolutions and aspongecontaininggentamicin. *Biomaterials* 17(7), 1733-1738.

Wallace, J. M., B. Erickson, C. M. Les, B. G. Orr and M. M. Banaszak Holl (2010). Distribution of type I collagen morphologies in bone: relation to estrogen depletion. *Bone* 46(5), 1349-1354.

Walters, V.I.; Kwansa, A.L.; Freeman, J.W. (2012). Design and Analysis of Braid-Twist Collagen Scaffolds, *Connective Tissue Research*, 53 (3), 255-266.

Wang M.C., Pins G.D., Silver F.H. (1994). Collagen fibers with improved strength for the repair of soft tissue injuries. *Biomaterials*, 15(7), 507-12.

Wang, L. & Stegemann, J. P. (2010). Thermogelling chitosan and collagen composite hydrogels initiated with b-glycerophosphate for bone tissue engineering. *Biomaterials. 31*, 3976–3985.

Wang, L. & Stegemann, J. P. (2011). Glyoxal crosslinking of cell-seeded chitosan/collagen hydrogels for bone regeneration. *Acta Biomater. 7,* 2410-2417.

Wang, T.W.; Spector, M. (2009). Development of hyaluronic acid-based scaffolds for brain tissue engineering. *Acta Biomaterialia* 5(7), 2371-2384.

Wang, X., Lin, P., Yao, Q. & Chen, C. (2007). Development of small-diameter vascular grafts. *World J. Surg.*, *31,* 682-689.

Wang, X.; Zhang, J.; Wang, Q. (2008). Surface modification of GTA crosslinkied collagen-based composite scaffolds with low temperature plasma technology. *Journal of Macromolecular Science Part A*, 45(7), 585-589.

Watanabe K., Nakamura M., Okano H., Toyama Y. (2007). Establishment of threedimensional culture of neural stem/progenitor cells in collagen type-1 gel. *Restor Neurol Neurosci*;25:109-17.

Weadock, K.S.; Miller, E.J.; Bellincampi, L.D.; Zawadsky, J.P.; Dunn, M.G. (1995). Physical crosslinking of fibers:comparison of ultraviolet radiation and dehydrothermal treatment. *J Biomed Mater Res*, 29, 1373-1379.

Weadock, K.S.; Miller, E.J.; Keuffel, E.L.; Dunn, M.G. (1996). Effect of physical crosslinking methods on collagen-fiber durability in proteolytic solutions, *Journal of Biomedical Materials Research*, 32 (2), 221-226.

Weinberg, C. B. & Bell, E. (1986). A blood vessel model constructed from collagen and cultured vascular cells, *Science, 231,* 397–400.

Whikehart, D,R. (2003). Biochemistry of the eye. Pennsylvania: Butterworth Heinemann, p.15.

Williams DF. Biocompatibility of Tissue Analogs. Vol 1. Boca Raton FL:CRC Press; 1985.

Willits, R. K. & Skornia, S. L. (2004). Effect of collagen gel stiffness on neurite extension. *J Biomater Sci Polym Ed.* 15, 1521-1531.

Wu, C. H., C. M. Walton and G. Y. Wu (1991). Propeptide-mediated regulation of procollagen synthesis in IMR-90 human lung fibroblast cell cultures. Evidence for transcriptional control. *J Biol Chem,* 266(5), 2983-2987.

Wu, J. Z. & Herzog, W. (2002). Elastic anisotropy of articular cartilage is associated with the microstructures of collagen fibers and chondrocytes. *J. Biomech., 35,* 931-942.

Yamaguchi, Y., D. M. Mann and E. Ruoslahti (1990). Negative regulation of transforming growth factor-beta by the proteoglycan decorin. *Nature,* 346(6281), 281-284.

Yang C., Hillas PJ, Báez JA, Nokelainen M, Balan J, Tang J, Spiro R, Polarek JW. The application of recombinant human collagen in tissue engineering. *BioDrugs,* 200418(2),103-19.

Yao, XS; Wu, L.J.; Wu, J.Z. (2004). Natural medicinal chemistry (4rth ed). Beijing, China People's Medicinal Publishing House.

Yu, X., Bichtelen, A.; Wang, X.; Yan, Y.; Lin, F.; Xiong, Z.; Wu, R.; Zhang, R.; Lu, Q. (2005). Collagen/chitosan/heparin complex with improved biocompatibility for hepatic tissue engineering. *Journal of Bioactive and Compatible Polymers,* 20(1), 15-28.

Zeeman R., Dijkstra P.J., Van Wachem P.B., Van Luyn M.J., Hendriks M., Cahalan P.T., (1999). Successive epoxy and carbodiimide cross-linking of dermal sheep collagen. *Biomaterials,* 20, 921–31.

Zeeman, R.; Dijkstra, P.J.; van Wachem, P.B.; van Luvn, M.J.; Hendricks, M.; Cahalan, P.T.; Feijen J. (2000). The kinetics of 1,4-butanediol glycidyl ether crosslinking of dermal sheep collagen. *J Biomed Mater Res,* 51(4), 541-548.

Zeugolis D.I., Paul R.G., (2010). Attenburrow G. The influence of a natural crosslinkcross-linking agent (myrica ruba) n the properties of extruded collagen fibers for tissue engineering applications. *Mater Sci Eng C,* 30(1), 190-5.

Zeugolis, D.I.; Panengad, P.P.; Yew, E.S.Y.; Sheppard, C.; Phan, T.T.; Raghunath, M. (2010). An in situ and in vitro investigation for the transglutaminase potential in tissue engineering. *Journal of Biomedical Materials Research Part A,* 92A (4), 1310-1320.

Zhang, L.; Hu, M.; Li, Y.; Jiang, H.; Chu, C.; Wang, M. (2005). Study on modification of collagen with chondroitin sulphate on the microcosmic level. *Artificial Cells, Blood Substitutes and Biotechnology,* 33(2), 215-226.

Zhang, L.; Li, K.; Xiao, W.; Zheng, L.; Xiao, Y.; Fan, H.; Zhang, X. (2011). Preparation of collagen-chondroitin sulphate-hyaluronic acid hybrid hydrogel scaffolds and cell compatibility in vitro. *Carbohydrate Polymers,* 84(1), 118-125.

Zhang, M.; Wu, K.; Li, G. (2011). Interactions of collagen molecules in the presence of N-hydroxysuccinimide activated adipic acid (NHS-AA) as a crosslinking agent. *International Journal of Biological Macromolecules,* 49 (4), 847-854.

In: Type I Collagen
Editors: Maria Eduarda Henriques and Marcio Pinto
ISBN: 978-1-62257-625-8

Chapter II

Degradation of Type I Collagen and Pathogenesis of Infectious Diseases

Flávia Nader Motta[1,2], Clênia Azevedo[1,2], Carla Nunes de Araújo[1,2], Jaime M. Santana[1] and Izabela M. D. Bastos[1*]

[1]Laboratory of Pathogen-Host Interface, Department of Cell Biology, The University of Brasília, Brazil
[2]Faculty of Ceilândia,The University of Brasília, Brazil

Abstract

Collagen constitutes one-third of the proteins present in the human body and the main component of the extracellular matrix. Its singular structure renders collagen degradation a hard task and only specialized peptidases, known as collagenases, are able to mediate its hydrolysis. Collagenases generally belong to the family of zinc dependent matrix metalloproteases (MMPs) or bacterial collagenases of the M9 family, which have the ability to catalyze not only collagens but also other extracellular matrix components (ECM). Other independent types of collagenases have been reported as members of the serine and cysteine-protease family. Collagenase-like activity is still poorly understood but it seems to be associated to partially unfolded states adopted by collagen that could be recognized and cleaved by these proteases. While collagen degradation is a natural process for tissue homeostasis, its unusual hydrolysis has been recognized as contributing factor to multiple pathologies, among them cancer, chronic and infectious diseases. The identification of collagenases as agents of the infection process was first described in *Clostridium hystolyticum* with the isolation of an extracellular enzyme responsible for tissue putrefaction. At present, there is a wealth of data regarding collagenases in many pathogenic species of bacteria, fungus, protozoa and worms, involved in the pathogen spread in different host tissues. For this reason, collagenases are being considered promising targets for the design of new therapeutic drugs. Strategies for the advancement in this field are the detailed structural characterizations of pathogen

*Corresponding to: The University of Brasília – UnB, Department of Cell Biology - IB, Laboratory of Pathogen-Host Interface, 70910-900, Brasília, D. F., Brazil. Tel.: 55 61 31073051; E-mail: *dourado@unb.br*.

collagenases and collagenase-like to assist in achieving drug selectivity to prevent infection accomplishment.

INTRODUCTION

Collagens are the most abundant proteins found in the different tissues of vertebrates. Around 28 different types of collagens are discribed and differ from each other according to their amino acid sequences that result in a variety of arrangements such as fibrils, network and transmembrane collagens.

In spite of these different forms, the collagens share a basic three-dimensional structure, a triple right-handed helix, as outcome of three polyproline-glycine rich chain assembly [Brodsky and Persikov, 2005]. This unique molecular structure confers to collagens, mainly the fibril-forming collagen, an extraordinary mechanical resistance, necessary to accomplish their crucial role as scaffold of tendon, cartilage, bone and skin [Kadler et al., 1996].

The type I collagen is the major fibril-forming collagen and the most abundant protein in human. Its ability to arrange into fibrils is due to the uninterrupted Gly-X-Y domain composed by ~1000 amino acid residues that allows the staking of triple-helix molecules in 67 nm periodic microfibrils [Chapman et al., 1990]. Their fibrils can range in narrow diameter from 12 nm to ~500 nm found in tendon and in indeterminate length [Di Lullo et al., 2002; Kadler et al., 1996].

The collagen fibrils fill the extracellular spaces forming not only a physical support for different tissues, but also a dynamic environment, since collagens present several binding sites to cell-associated molecules. These include the integrins, proteoglycan, discoidin domain receptors, molecules bridging cell surfaces and the extracellular matrix, such as fibronectin [Di Lullo et al., 2002].

Among these binding molecules, integrin is certainly the most crucial determinant in cell-collagen interactions [Sweeney et al., 2008]. Such interactions are a known route for cell signaling involved in many biological processes as angiogenesis, endothelial activation, osteoblast differentiation, and cell adhesion [Baronas-Lowell et al., 2004; Reyes and García, 2004; Sweeney et al., 2003].

The scaffold formed by collagen, in association with other components in ECM, is a natural key barrier against human pathogens infections [Lemichez et al., 2010]. However, invasive microorganisms possess an array of molecules able to directly degrade collagens counteracting their physical barrier and also, in many cases, inducing host inflammatory responses that amplify the tissue damage and facilitate the pathogen spreading in the body [Diacovich and Gorvel, 2010].

However, its tight bind triple helix structure render collagens resistant to hydrolysis by the most of proteases except specialized enzymes known as collagenases of the metalloprotease family, and a few others collagenases-like belonging to other protease families.

In this chapter we will present an overview of these proteases focusing in their structural and enzymatic features and soon afterwards, how the diverse human pathogens employ collagenases to counteract host barriers and thus to accomplish successful infection.

METALLOPROTEASE COLLAGENASES

Matrix Metalloproteases

Matrix metalloproteases (MMPs) are a major group of zinc-dependent proteolytic enzymes that regulate cell-matrix composition. The MMPs are known for their ability to catalyze the degradation of several ECM constituents, as well as non-matrix proteins [Armstrong and Jude, 2002; Das et al., 2003]. They comprise a large family of over 20 different secreted or membrane-bound proteases that share common structural and functional elements [Birkedal-Hansen et al., 1993; Nagase et al., 2006; Sternlicht and Werb, 2001].

MMPs are constituted by a modular combination of inserts and domains (Figure 1A). These may include, from N- to C-terminus, a signal peptide for secretion; a zymogenic pro-peptide (PRO) domain for latency until a signal for activation is given; a zinc- and calcium-dependent catalytic domain (CAT); a linker region that, theoretically, allows the C-terminal domain to fold back on the catalytic one and a hemopexin-like domain (HPX) for collagen binding, pro-MMP activation, and dimerization [Tallant et al., 2010]. Gelatinases (MMP-2 and MMP-9) have additional amino acid residues inserted between the catalytic and zinc binding domains comprising three fibronectin related type II modules involved in the binding of denatured collagens or gelatin. On a mechanistic level, little is known on how this last domain participates in the collagenolytic process [Bertini et al., 2012; Das et al., 2003]. Several of those domains and/or regions cited above have been implicated in collagenolysis.

Selected members of the MMP family catalyze the hydrolysis of collagen and exploit multiple domains to efficiently achieve this function. The collagenolytic MMPs consist of MMP-1, MMP-2, MMP-8, MMP-9, MMP-13 and membrane-bound MT1-MMP and MT2-MMP [Bertini et al., 2012]. These collagenolytic MMPs cleave type I collagen between Gly775-Ile776 of α1(I) chain and Gly775-Leu776 of the α2(I) chain generating characteristic ¾- and ¼-length parts [Nagase et al., 2006].

The PRO domain prevents MMPs to perform extensive non-controlled protein degradation and seems to function by a cysteine switch mechanism that links the unpaired propeptide Cys residue in the conserved sequence PRCGVPDV to the active site zinc ion thus blocking substrate entry [Docherty and Murphy, 1990; Springman et al., 1990; Van Wart and Birkedal-Hansen, 1990].

The CAT domain contains two zinc ions - a structural one, and another in the active site essential for the proteolytic activity of MMPs that interacts with the three histidine residues in the sequence AHEXGHXXGXXH– and at least one calcium ion coordinated to various residues [Das et al., 2003; Geurts et al., 2012].

The HPX domain is formed by a four bladed β- propeller. It has a critical role in collagenolysis, as removal of the MMP-1, MMP-8, MMP-13 or MT1-MMP HPX domain results in the loss of their characteristic capability to cleave triple helical collagen, but does not significantly affect hydrolytic activity toward small natural substrates [Clark and Cawston, 1989; Hurst et al., 2004; Knäuper et al., 1993; Murphy et al., 1992; Netzel-Arnett et al., 1994; Ohuchi et al., 1997; Sternlicht and Werb, 2001]. In general, the consensus function of HPX domain is its ability to bind and partially unwind the triple helical collagen substrate, allowing a single α-chain to enter the active site cleft of the CAT domain [Chung et al., 2004; Leikina et al., 2002]. Thus HPX domain is an "exosite" – region that, although it has no hydrolytic machinery, is required for recognition and cleavage of the natural substrate (reviewed by [Overall, 2002].

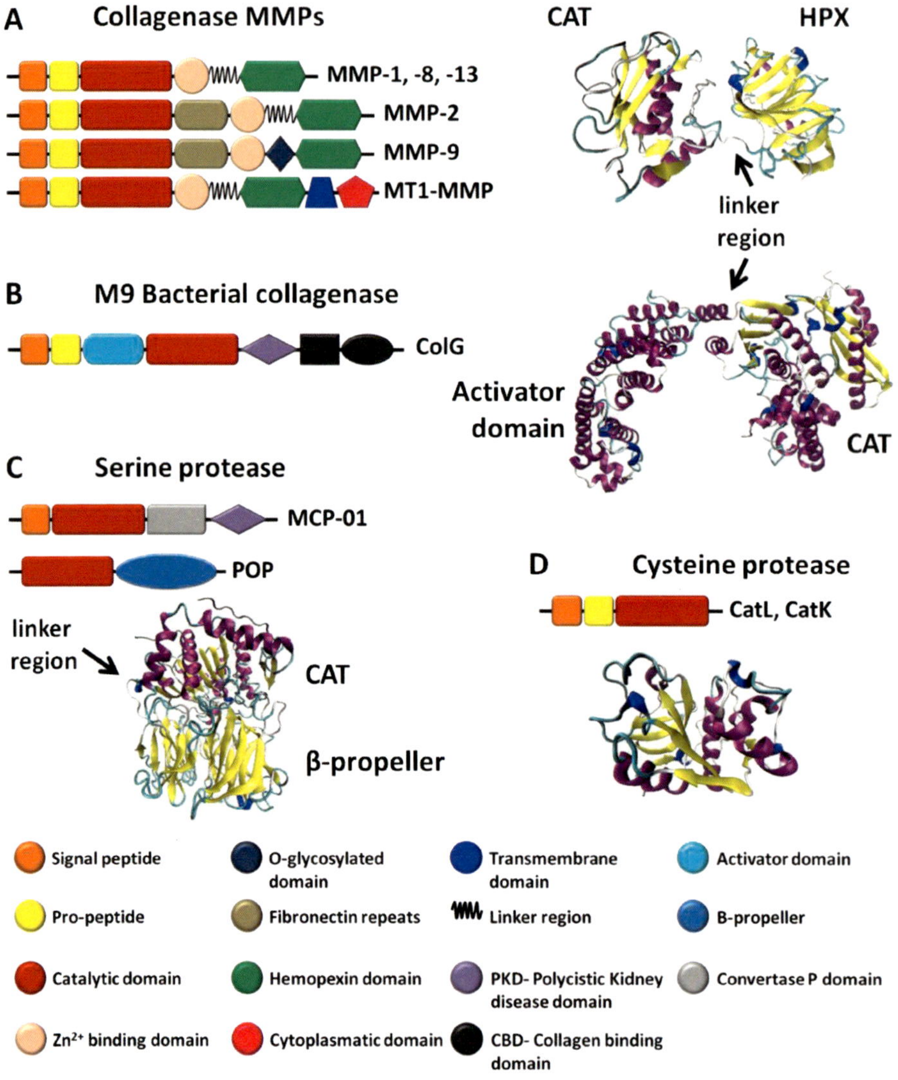

Figure 1. Schematic representation of domain organization and active tridimensional structure of collagenase MMPs, M9 bacterial collagenases and collagenolytic serine- and cysteine proteases. A. Collagenases MMPs are basically composed of a CAT domain and a HPX domain connected by a hinger of variable length. The HPX domain binds and partially unwinds the triple helical collagen. The prototype of this family is MMP-1 whose structure has been crystallized and solved (PDB 2CLT). B. ColG, the clostridial collagenase, has a CBD (PKD and CDB-a and CDB-b) domain responsible for the interaction and recruitment of triple helix collagen without unwinding it. The CBDs were not present in the crystallized structure of ColG (PDB 2Y50). C. The serine-protease deseasin MCP-01 has a PKD domain at its C-terminus that functions as a CBD improving the collagenolytic efficiency of its catalytic domain. The three-dimensional molecular model of POP Tc80 revealed a two-domain structure: α/β hydrolase catalytic domain and β-propeller domain associated by a linker region. D. Cathepsin L and K fold into a bi-lobed mature domain separated by a substrate-binding cleft (PDB 1ATK). Those cysteine-proteases do not present a CDB (hemopexin or PKD domain) and their biochemical approach to interact with and cleave collagen is unknown.

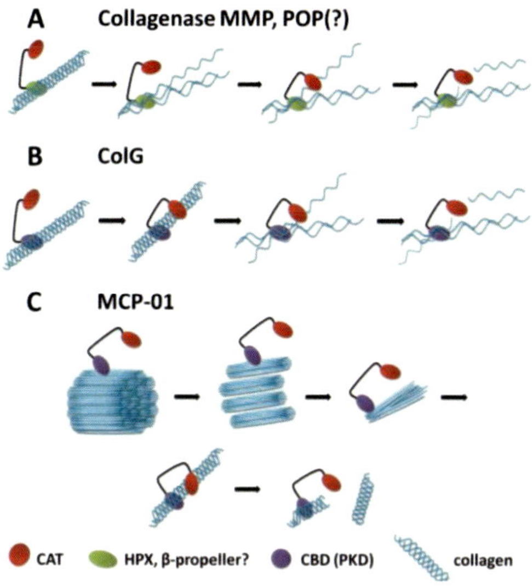

Figure 2. Presumed catalytic mechanisms of collagenases. A. Collagenases MMP expose their HPX domains which interact with triple helix collagen, unwinding it to be subsequently hydrolyzed by the enzyme CAT domains [Arnold et al., 2011; Bertini et al., 2012; Lauer-Fields et al., 2009]. B. ColG CBD recruits and partly swells triple helix collagen without unwinding it. Next, ColG CAT domain surrounds collagen until it is completely unwound and cleaved [Eckhard et al., 2011]. C. MCP-01 PKD domain binds collagen structures (fascicles, fibrils and microfibrils) and swell them until the exposition of collagen triple-helical monomers to their cleavage by CAT domain [Wang et al., 2010]. CAT – Catalytic Domain; HPX – Hemopexin Domain; CBD – Collagen-binding Domain; PKD – Polycystic Kidney Disease Domain.

Although biochemical approaches by which MMPs achieve the hydrolysis of collagen have been hypothesized, they are paradoxical and not validated on a molecular level [Bertini et al., 2012]. The catalytic mechanism of collagenase MMPs (Figure 2A), in overall view, is the binding of collagen to the HPX domain that will act as a helicase unwinding triple helical collagen, so a single chain can be hydrolyzed by CAT domain. All this process requires the flexibility of collagenase MMP domains that allows, so far, two known conformational states:

1. A dislocated conformation in which HPX will be completely exposed enabling its interaction with collagen; and
2. A compact conformation that allows the contact of the exosite and CAT domain to collagen triple helix leading to its catalysis [Arnold et al., 2011; Lauer-Fields et al., 2009].

M9 Bacterial Collagenases

Crystal structure and enzymatic properties of collagenase G (ColG) from *Clostridum histolyticum* have been recently elicited providing, for the first time, an integrated mechanistic model of collagen recognition and processing by exogenous bacterial collagenases [Eckhard et al., 2011]. ColG belongs to class I clostridial collagenases, a class of enzymes with a particular preference for degrading collagen substrates in a processive manner [Bond and Van Wart, 1984; Eckhard et al., 2009; Hesse et al., 1995]. Eckhard and co-workers (2011) were able to derive a conformational two-state model of bacterial collagenolysis that consists of an unified collagenase opening and closing steps that ensure recognition and unraveling of collagen microfibrils, and its subsequently hydrolysis.

The domain organization and architecture of ColG (Figure 1B) revealed an unexpected segmentation of the N-terminal collagenase module. The smaller N-terminal saddle flap acts as an activator domain (Tyr119–Asp388) followed by the peptidase catalytic subdomain (Asp398–Gln669) that resembles a thermolysin-like fold [Eckhard et al., 2011]. This segment represents the collagenase module of the ColG being imperative for its full collagenolytic activity. The activator domain and the catalytic subdomain constitute the "seat" of the saddle topology proposed by Eckhard and co-workers (2011), which is achieved by a solvent-exposed glycine-rich linker (Gly389–Tyr397) positioned at the twist of the saddle seat.

To complete its tridimensional arrangement, ColG presents an accessory domain composed of a PKD-like domain (Ala791–Asn880) positioned at the rear of the peptidase domain and two collagen-binding domains (CBDs) (Glu881–Gly1001/CBD-a, Leu1002–Lys1118/CBD-b) [Ducka et al., 2009; Eckhard et al., 2011]. The collagen-binding domains were not present in the crystal structure of ColG from *C. histolyticum* solved by Eckhard and co-workers (2011); nevertheless, the structural information of CBD of *C. histolyticum* ColG was available allowing its orientation and positioning into the final tridimensional display to satisfy biochemical data [Wilson et al., 2003].

The collagen-binding domains are also present in collagenases that belong to MMPs superfamily. In general, these enzymes have the same modular structure with an N-terminal domain - a catalytic domain belonging to M10, a linker peptide, and a C-terminal domain – a CBD called hemopexin-like domain with an unique four-bladed β-propeller structure as mentioned above. In these MMPs, CBDs deal with protein–substrate and protein–inhibitor interactions and in activation events. Bacterial CBDs are also known to promote protein-collagen interaction even thought they share no sequence or structural homology to any eukaryotic collagen-binding proteins [Wilson et al., 2003]. As for the PKD-like domain, it was first identified in human polycystin-1 gene [Bycroft et al., 1999], but it has been found in bacterial collagenases [Matsushita et al., 1994], proteases [Miyamoto et al., 2002; Oda et al., 1996], cellulases [Ahsan et al., 1996] and chitinases [Orikoshi et al., 2005; Perrakis et al., 1994]. The PKD domain has similar structure and function as the CBD of collagenase MMPs (hemopexin-like domain). It has a β-sandwich fold with 5 parallel β-sheets [Chen et al., 2007].

By combining the structural data with enzymatic and mutagenesis studies, Eckhard and collaborators (2011) concluded that ColG can adopt two preferred conformational states: a crystallized open state where the peptidase domain directly interacts with a collagen triple helix; still, at this state, the activator domain cannot interact with the substrate and there is no collagenolytic activity. The second conformation - a closed state – that allows the collagen triple helix to contact both the activator and peptidase domains, a prerequisite for collagen proteolysis, initiating the unwinding of the triple-helix α-chains and its subsequently hydrolysis [French et al., 1992; French et al., 1987]. Therefore, the structure of ColG revealed a chew-and-digest mechanism of bacterial collagenolysis (Figure 2B) based on the saddle topology of the N-terminal collagenase module. Contrasting with collagenase MMPs where CBD (hemopexin-like domain) is crucial for collagen binding, unwinding of the triple helix and catalytic turnover [Sanchez-Lopez et al., 1993], ColG accessory domains (PKD-like domain and CBD) serve to recruit and partly to swell insoluble collagen without unwinding its triple-helical structure [Wang et al., 2010; Wilson et al., 2003].

Finally, the knowledge of *C. hystoliticum* ColG structure associated with its enzymatic properties provide an integrated mechanistic model of collagen recognition and processing by bacterial collagenases allowing to explore the field of novel structure-based drug design that would avoid drug resistance problems typical of classical antibiotics.

NON-METALLOPROTEASE COLLAGENASES

Serine Proteases

There is a considerable example of serine proteases involved in hydrolysis of collagen, not only type I, but of other types, as well as other components of the ECM {reviewed by [Singh et al., 2012]}. But unlike MMPs, only certain details are known about the structural (Figure 1C) and enzymatic properties of collagenolytic serine proteases.

Zhao and colleagues [2008] and Wang and co-workers (2010) have well described the mechanism by which the serine protease deseasin MCP-01 (subtilase, Clan SB and S8 Subtilisin Family) [Rawlings et al., 2012] from the marine *Pseudoalteromona* ssp. is capable of digesting insoluble collagens (Figure 2C). Deseasin MCP-01 is implied in the degradation of deep-sea sediments [Zhao et al., 2008]. This multidomain protease has a PKD domain at its C-terminus that was proven by site directed mutagenesis combined with biochemical, biophysical, scanning electron and atomic force microscopy studies to function as a CBD. Moreover, PKD domain improves the collagenolytic efficiency of deseasin MCP-01 catalytic domain – capable of hydrolyzing collagen alone but in a less extended manner.

During collagenolysis by MCP-01, the C-terminal PKD domain binds collagen and swells collagen aggregate to the exposure of its monomers. Then, the N-terminal catalytic domain accommodates the triple-helical collagen monomer in its catalytic cavity and cleaves it. Therefore, the PKD domain of deseasin MCP-01 can destroy the aggregate structures of collagen but has no triple-helicase activity, different from the hemopexin-like domains of MMPs [Wang et al., 2010].

The prolyl oligopeptidases (POP, Clan SC and S9 Prolyl Oligopeptidase Family) [Rawlings et al., 2012] from *T. cruzi* (POP Tc80) and *T. brucei* (POP Tb) are examples of collagenolytic serine proteases. POP Tc80 and POP Tb have been proposed to participate in the ontogeny and/or maintenance of Chagas´ disease and sleeping sickness, respectively [Bastos et al., 2005; Grellier et al., 2001]. The three-dimensional molecular model of POP Tc80 was proposed based on the crystallized porcine POP [Fülöp et al., 1998] and revealed a two-domains structure: α/β hydrolase catalytic domain and β-propeller domain. To understand how a large molecule as collagen would interact with a protease that supposedly only cleaves substrates smaller than 30 amino acids [Camargo et al., 1979], docking calculations followed by molecular dynamics/minimization were performed. The result showed that collagen would access the catalytic pocket of POP Tc80 through a side opening situated in the interface between the α/β-hydrolase and β-propeller domain [Bastos et al., 2005]. Possibly, POP Tc80 β-propeller domain function as a CBD, facilitating collagenolytic efficiency, since its organization into a bladed β-propeller resembles the hemopexin domain of collagenase MMPs. Additionally, the collagen binding function of the β-propeller domain of collagenolytic POPs has already been suggested for dipeptidyl peptidase IV and FAPα, both POP family members [Beauvais et al., 1997a; Beauvais et al., 1997b; Cheng et al., 1998; Löster et al., 1995].

Cysteine Proteases

There are a few examples of collagenolytic cysteine proteases [Singh et al., 2012], and analogously to serine protease family, limited structural (Figure 1D) and enzymatic features of those proteases are known.

Accordingly to the literature, of all cysteine proteases capable of cleaving collagen, only two examples have their classification determined: human cathepsin K that has a highly restricted distribution in osteoclasts and seems to be involved in cartilage breakdown and bone remodeling [Atley et al., 2000; Kafienah et al., 1998] and *Fasciola hepatica* cathepsin L that adds sufficient proteolytic capacity for the parasite infection [Robinson et al., 2011; Robinson et al., 2008b; Stack et al., 2008].

Both enzymes belong to the papain family [Rawlings et al., 2012] of cysteine protease that folds into a bi-lobed mature domain separated by a substrate-binding cleft. The left-hand lobe is predominantly helical in composition and the right-hand one contains several elements of β-sheet [Stack et al., 2008; Zhao et al., 1997]. Distinctly from collagenase MMPs and serine proteases, collagenolytic cathepsin L and K do not present a CBD (hemopexin or PKD domain) that would help to understand in how these enzymes are able to interact with its target site in the intact triple helix collagen. Human cathepsin K cleaves type I collagen at the N-terminal end of its triple helix where, presumably, there is laxity of the helix to facilitate enzyme-substrate interaction [Atley et al., 2000; Kafienah et al., 1998].

By molecular simulations, Robinson and colleagues [2011] began to elucidate the unique collagenase-like activity of the three secreted cathepsins L (FhCL1, FhCL2 and FhCL3) present in *F. hepatica*. Their data suggest that FhCL3 has the greatest ability to digest type I collagen among these three proteases and Trp 67 residue in the S2 subsite is critical to accommodate either Gly or Pro residues at P2 of the substrate, such as type I collagen. In the case of FhCL2, Tyr 67 is the residue that enables the enzyme to cleave substrates with Pro in the P2 position. They also showed that FhCL1 does not readily accept Pro into the S2 subsite and thus its activity against type I collagens is restricted to the non-collagenous domains [Robinson et al., 2011].

Human Pathogens Versus Collagen Degradation

Clostridium spp.

Species of *Clostridium* cause various diseases resulting from the release of potent toxins responsible for severe clinical complications in botulism, tetanus and gas gangrene [Rood et al., 1997]. They are Gram-positive anaerobic recognized by the effective resistance acquired from the formation of spores [Rood et al., 1997]. Besides the toxins, it is believed that the virulence of pathogenic clostridia is also associated with the production of hydrolytic enzymes by the bacteria, serving as important virulence factors to facilitate the dispersion of both the bacteria (Figure 3) and their toxins, enhancing the harmful effect [Smith, 1979].

The initial studies that evidenced the proteolytic enzyme capable of degrading collagen arose from the observation that organisms, such as *C. perfringens* and *C. histolyticum*, were important in tissue putrefaction [MacLennan et al., 1953]. Decades after, this enzyme was called collagenase [Bidwell and Van Heyningen, 1948; Oakley et al., 1946] and since then, the clostridial collagenases became references in this class of enzymes.

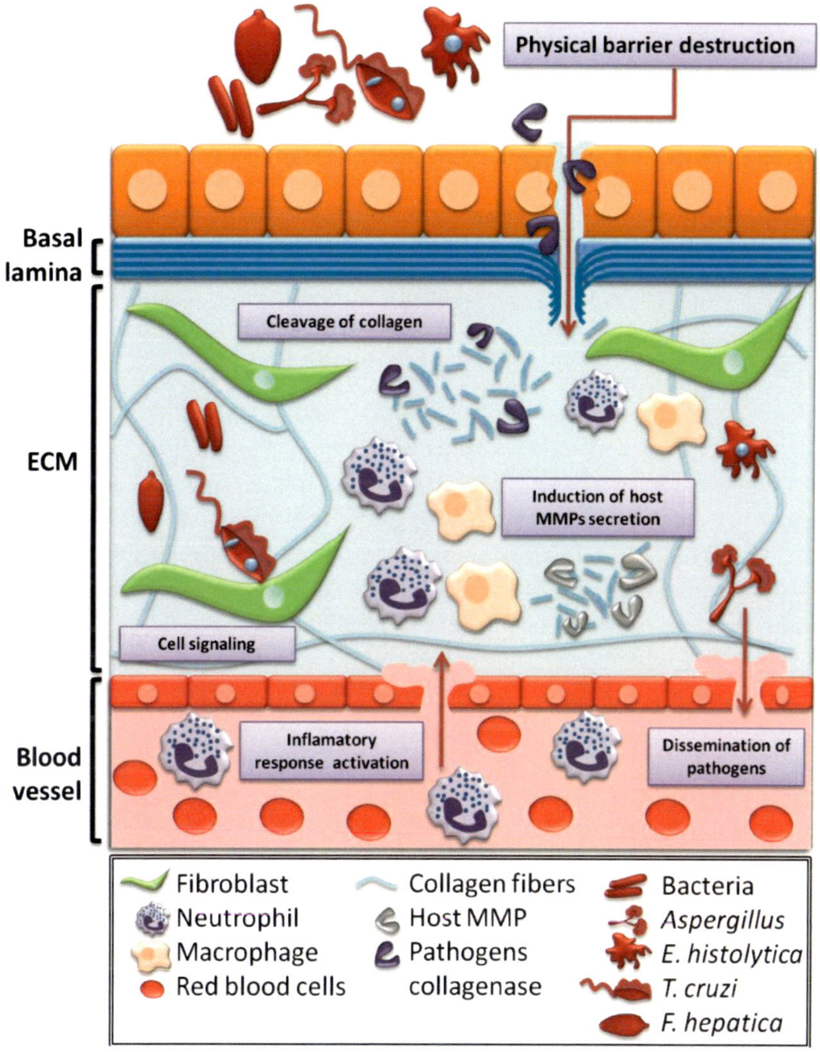

Figure 3. Roles of collagenolytic activity from several pathogens in host tissue invasion. The collagenases secreted by pathogens may act in different ways to achieve the establishment of the disease. They may: 1) destroy the physical barriers (basal lamina) allowing pathogens to enter the human body; 2) degrade extracellular matrix components, inducing an inflammatory response with recruitment of immune cells, 3) stimulate the release of host MMPs, giving rise to peptides that may enhance the immune response; and 4) interact with cells, such as fibroblasts, altering the cell signaling. These events facilitate systemic dissemination of the pathogen.

Myonecrosis is a disease primarily associated with infection by *C. perfringens* developed by the entering of their vegetative cells or sporulated forms in traumatic injury or surgical wound. Also known as gas gangrene, the disease is characterized by extracellular toxins production by these anaerobic bacteria, leading to production of gas and tissue damage, and if not controlled with antibiotics, there is risk of developing systemic toxemia and shock [MacLennan, 1962; Rood et al., 1997]. Among them, κ-toxin is a collagenase expressed by colA gene of *C. perfrigens*, as a preprocollagenase [Katayama et al., 1996].

C. histolyticum is the second of its genus associated with myonecrosis and also produces collagenases that degrade several types of collagen and gelatin. These collagenases have catalytic activity more potent than those of vertebrate collagenases [Peterkofsky, 1982] and various uses have been assigned to them, as their therapeutic use in Dupuytren's disease [Gelbard et al., 1993; Starkweather et al., 1996].

There are two collagenases that share similar molecular weights in *C. histolyticum*: ColG, the ColA orthologous from *C. perfringens*, and ColH. Shi and colleagues [2010] confirmed the collagenolytic activity of *Clostridium* collagenases on collagen types I, III and IV and also demonstrated that this enzyme acts on collagen type V.

Bacillus cereus

Bacillus cereus is an ubiquitous bacterium found in the natural environment, which inhabits the organic matter in soil, sea water and fresh water and is also part of the intestinal tract of invertebrates [Jensen et al., 2003]. It consists in a Gram-positive, aerobic facultative bacterium capable of forming spores in nature and acts as a vegetative cell when colonizes the human host. Because of the ability of spore adhesion to food products, *B. cereus* are easily disseminated [Stenfors Arnesen et al., 2008]. In addition to gastrointestinal infection, *B. cereus* is also involved in other pathogenic processes, such as endophthalmitis, periodontal disease, fulminate bacteremia, and pneumonia (reviewed in [Bottone, 2010].

B. cereus secretes toxins and enzymes important for the establishment of these infections that are powerful enough to destroy the host tissue. Among them there are the hemolysins, the phospholipases, emesis-inducing toxin, hemolysin BL, nonhemolytic enterotoxin and cytotoxin K [Granum, 1994; Granum and Lund, 1997; Lund et al., 2000]. Thus, probably these toxins play a decisive role in the severity of infection, determining its course [Beecher et al., 2000].

Well as in other bacteria, collagenases appear as promising virulence factors by their ability to cleave native collagen, opening a gateway to the spread of bacteria and their toxins [Peterkofsky, 1982]. A non-haemolytic enterotoxin is also suggested to be involved in this process, since it cleaves type I collagen [Lund and Granum, 1999]. It was found that the N-terminal of this toxin has high similarity with the ColA of *C. perfringens* and *C. histolyticum* [Matsushita et al., 1994; Yoshihara et al., 1994].

Another infection caused by *B. cereus* is posttraumatic and metastatic bacterial endophthalmitis, what turns this bacterium one of the most aggressive to the eye [Pflugfelder and Flynn, 1992], which can lead to blindness [Davey and Tauber, 1987; Vahey and Flynn, 1991]. The main characteristics of this infection are progressive corneal ring abscess, pain and retinal hemorrhage [Callegan et al., 1999; Martinez et al., 2007]. The phosphatidylcholine-preferring phospholipase C (PC-PLC) is a potent toxin because its hydrolytic capacity reaches phosphatidylcholine, phosphatidylethanolamine and phosphatidylserine, phospholipids components in retinal tissue [Beecher et al., 2000; Hergenrother and Martin, 1997]. Besides the influence of this toxin in tissue damage, collagenases were detected in the fluids of infected eyes, reinforcing the need for bacteria to break down the protective barrier of lens capsule composed primarily of type IV collagen. *B. cereus* collagenases allow its invasion by altering the permeability of the membrane and inducing the inflammatory response [Beecher et al., 2000; Berman, 1991].

Pseudomonas aeruginosa

Pseudomonas aeruginosa is a Gram-negative bacterium of critical clinical importance associated with various diseases such as cystic fibrosis and granulocytopenia. Its relation with the high incidence is worrisome because nosocomial infections by *P. aeruginosa* affects debilitated or immunosuppressed patients with clinical severity, leading to a necrotizing pneumonia. To effectively establish it is required that the bacteria invade host tissues, affecting the epithelial arrangement [Bodey et al., 1983; Pollack, 1985].

It is known that *P. aeruginosa* produces extracellular enzymes [Morjhara and Homma, 1985; Woods and Iglewski, 1983; Wretlind and Pavlovskis, 1983] capable of degrading collagen. Although this is just one of many factors that contribute to virulence mechanism, necrosis is, in part, attributed to *Pseudomonas* elastase and *P. aeruginosa* alkaline protease [Blackwood et al., 1983; Döring et al., 1987; Morjhara and Homma, 1985; Pollack, 1984]. *Pseudomonas* elastase is capable of degrading types IV and III collagens [Bejarano et al., 1989; Heck et al., 1986]. Type IV collagen is one of the major components that give mechanical strength to the basal lamina, ECM located in connective tissue and epithelial cells [Abrahamson, 1986; Bejarano et al., 1989]. Type III collagen is found in the composition of the dermis, lung and also blood vessel walls, being considered an interstitial collagen [Miller and Gay, 1982]. The capacity of this enzyme in cleaving type I collagen is limited to the cleavage of cross-linked beta chain monomer to the alpha chains [Heck et al., 1986]. *In vivo* studies observed that *P. aeruginosa* with elastase gene knocked-out produced a less severe pneumonia in rats compared with that one produced by wild type, probably due to the cleavage of type IV collagen as an important factor in the disruption of elastic lamina of arterioles and arteries [Heck et al., 1986; Woods et al., 1982].

Aspergillus

Aspergillus fumigatus is an opportunistic fungus responsible for pulmonary invasive aspergillosis [Balloy and Chignard, 2009], which mortality rates may reach 95% in certain situations [Abad et al., 2010; Maschmeyer et al., 2007]. This saprophytic fungus produces a great number of resistant spores, being abundant in soil and decaying organic matter. Humans inhale these spores daily, which are eliminated by pulmonary defense mechanisms in immunocompetent hosts, normally without causing harm [Balloy and Chignard, 2009]. The virulence of this mold depends on the combination of biological characteristics of the fungus and on the immune status of the patient. In this context, aspergillosis can be regarded as a broad spectrum of diseases [Park and Mehrad, 2009].

One of the key events involved in a successful invasion strategy by the fungus is proteolytic degradation of the lung tissue, counteracting its structural barriers, and necessary to acquire nutrients from mammalian tissues [Palmer et al., 2008]. Among *A. fumigatus* proteases, the serine alkaline proteases (ALPs) of the subtilisin family (S8) show high collagenolytic activity and ability to degrade elastin, collagen, fibrinogen and casein [Kolattukudy et al., 1993; Reichard et al., 1990]. Recently it was demonstrated that they degrade the complement components C3, C4, C5, and C1q as well as immunoglobulin G, thus controlling complement activation in *A. fumigatus* hyphaes [Behnsen et al., 2010]. ALPs are also major allergens of several prevalent *Aspergillus* species [Shen et al., 1999] and have been found to enhance immune, inflammatory, and airway remodeling responses, which may also apply for Aspergillus-induced allergy [Kurup and Grunig, 2002].

Another serine protease capable of hydrolyzing collagen, the dipeptidyl peptidase IV (DPP IV), was characterized in culture supernatants of *A. fumigatus*. DPP IV is a member of prolil oligopeptidase family (S9) known by hydrolyzing biological peptides such as chemokines and cytokines, activating or inactivating them [Bauvois et al., 1992; Mentlein et al., 1993]. *A. fumigatus* DPP IV bind to native collagen and releases N-terminal X-Pro and to lesser extent Xaa-Ala dipeptides. In addition, its role in pathogenesis is reinforced by the observation that DPP IV genes are strongly expressed when the fungus is cultivated on a medium containing ECM proteins [Vermout et al., 2008].

The possibility of *A. fumigatus* DPP IV modulation of the host immune responses (Figure 3) during the fungus infection has been evoked [Beauvais et al., 1997a; Beauvais et al, 1997b]. Landis and colleagues [2008] showed that the pre-treatment of rabbits with recombinant *A. fumigatus* DPP IV reduces inflammation caused by histamine, possibly by the inactivation of neuropeptides and other immuno-modulatory peptides [Landis et al., 2008].

Entamoeba histolytica

Entamoeba histolytica is an enteroprotozoan causative of amebiasis, a significant cause of morbidity and mortality in developing countries, responsible for up to 100.000 deaths worldwide each year [Haque et al., 2003]. This illness is due to the capability of *E. histolytica* trophozoites to settle in the human colon and actively penetrate into the mucosa, destroying the underlying tissues, thereby causing ulceration [Keene et al., 1986; Moncada et al., 2003]. Amebic penetration through ulcers facilitates subsequently spread to the liver [Ankri et al., 1999; Keene et al., 1986; Moncada et al., 2003], leading to abscesses development. *E. dispar* and *E. moshkovskii* infections, both morphologically indistinguishable from *E. histolytica*, are also common in humans [Beck et al., 2008; Fotedar et al., 2008; Khairnar et al., 2007], although their trophozoites are not invasive.

In order to invade the colonic mucosa, *E. histolytica* trophozoites combine cell shape deformation due to adopting 'amoeboid' migration mode [Arhets et al., 1998; Coudrier et al., 2005; Labruyère et al., 2003; Wolf et al., 2003], and protease activity. The mechanism of tissue damage is attributed to the latter and activity of various lytic factors synthesized by the parasite after interaction of *E. histolytica* trophozoites with ECM [Stanley and Reed, 2001]. As collagens are major components of the basal lamina and the ECM of the intestine, which are primarily damaged [Minor, 1980; Prockop et al., 1979; Rojkind, 1979], *E. histolytica* collagenase activity plays an important role in tissue invasion.

Preliminary data available for this peptidase suggested it was a membrane-bound protease capable of hydrolyzing native type I and type III collagen fibers, although it was shown to be more active against type I, and that its behavior in the presence of several enzyme inhibitors resembled that of collagenase MMPs [Muńoz et al., 1982].

The genome of this protozoa parasite encodes a variety of protease gene families, many of which may be associated with virulence. Nevertheless, no MMPs were predicted in *E. histolytica* genome (*http://merops.sanger.ac.uk/cgi-bin/speccards?sp=sp000377;type=peptidase*). The absence of genes encoding for the M9 and M10 MMPs families in *E. histolytica* reinforces the need of other protease families that possess collagenolytic activity.

Recently it was shown that *E. histolytica*'s collagenolytic activity is mainly performed by its cysteine proteinases. These enzymes are encoded by 50 *E. histolytica* genes [Clark et al., 2007; Tillack et al., 2007] and invasive trophozoites secrete 10-1.000-fold more cysteine proteinases than non-invasive *E. dispar* [Reed et al., 1989]. Several *E. histolytica* cysteine proteases (EhCPs) have been characterized; however, EhCP-A5 is the major enzyme responsible for *E. histolytica*'s collagenolytic activity and is required for the production of pro-inflammatory cytokines [Hou et al., 2010]. *E. dispar* genome lacks EhCP-A5 [Bruchhaus et al., 1996]. Inhibition of CP activity prevented trophozoites from destroying the epithelium surface, the collagen network and invading the lamina propria. When the human colon was challenged with CP-A5-deficient *E. histolytica* strain, the epithelial layer was destroyed but the collagen structures encountered in the tissue remained intact, thus abolishing tissue invasion [Thibeaux et al., 2012].

Furthermore, inflammatory responses triggered by pro-mature CP-A5 may have a major role in collagen network degradation. It has been suggested that fibroblasts, epithelial and immune cells in situ release MMPs, thus contributing to the extensive matrix lysis observed during intestinal invasion and facilitating tissue penetration by *E. histolytica.* These alternations of the immune response contribute to ineffective host defenses and thereby excessive inflammation, tissue damage and amoeba spreading in the host [Muńoz et al., 1982].

Trypanosoma

About thirty percent of people infected by *T. cruzi,* transmitted mainly by hematophagous triatomine, develop the major chronic clinical manifestations of Chagas' disease as cardiomiopathies and digestory system disorders [Engman and Leon, 2002]. It is estimated that 9 millions of people are infected by the *T. cruzi* and 20.000 deaths occur per year mostly in Latina America [Schofield et al., 2006]. An essential feature of *T. cruzi* in host cells is its ability to infect and replicate within many cellular types [Burleigh and Woolsey, 2002]. The success of the infection depends, at first, on parasite capacity to migrate through the ECM thus gaining access to the host cell surface. It is postulated that the secreted *T. cruzi* prolyl oligopeptidase (POP Tc80) may take part in parasite dissemination since it hydrolyzes types I and IV collagens [Santana et al., 1997] and fibronectin [Grellier et al., 2001]. POP Tc80 collagenolytic activity was demonstrated *in situ* on rat mesentery, rich in type I collagen, and comparable to that mediated by collagenases from *C. histolyticum* [Santana et al., 1997]. Prolyl oligopetidase integrates the S9 family of serine proteases and has the ability to hydrolyze the substrates after proline residues especially in oligopeptides of up to 30 residues.

Its abnormal activity seems to be involved in the pathogenesis of several hormone and neurologic disorders as blood pressure regulation, homeostasis, glycemia, neurotransmission, and memory formation [Dresdner et al., 1982].

The role of POP Tc80 in the process of active infection by the parasite was demonstrated through the use of specific and selective inhibitors, which inhibit the entry of trypomastigotes into different nonphagocytic cell types [Grellier et al., 2001]. Since collagen binds to the host cell membrane via integrins, its hydrolysis by POP Tc80 could trigger the signals that rearrange the cytoskeleton [Tardieux et al., 1992] in favor of parasite entry (Figure 3). As the main function of POPs is the cleavage of biologically active peptides, POP Tc80 could also contribute to the maturation/activation of parasite factors required for invasion.

Beside POP Tc80, collagenolytic activities have been attributed to other *T. cruzi* proteases as cathepsin B and MMP-9-like. Cathepsin B, a lysosomal cysteine protease expressed in all parasite developmental forms, degrades type I collagen and its role in parasite nutrition and virulence has been proposed [Garcia et al., 1998]. Nogueira de Melo and collegues [2010] suggested that the secreted MMP-9-like, detected in *T. cruzi* culture supernatant may play a role in myocarditis induction [Nogueira de Melo et al., 2010].

As well as Chagas disease, sleep sickness is a neglected tropical disease endemic in Sub-Saharan Africa countries, caused by *T. brucei* via tsetse infected flies' bite. One of the most dramatic abilities of *T. brucei* is that it may cross the blood-brain barrier and invade the central nervous system. It has been showed that *T. brucei* cysteine proteases drive parasite transmigration through the blood-brain barrier by calcium dependent signaling events [Grab et al., 2009; Nikolskaia et al., 2006]. Evidence from both animal models and human studies supports a role for MMPs in the blood–brain barrier disruption in neuroinflammatory diseases [Yong et al., 2001].

A collagenolytic prolyl oligopeptidase has also been described in *T. brucei* (POP Tb) [Bastos et al., 2010] and this activity could help the parasite to penetrate the capillary endothelium [Goodwin, 1971] contributing to its propagation within the host. *In vivo* infection in mice revealed that POP Tb is released in host plasma, a natural environment of the parasite, where it keeps its full activity for hours. Similar to several POPs, POP Tb readily hydrolyses hormone peptides such as some deregulated in sleep sickness [Ndung'u et al., 1992]. Among them, abnormal levels of thyrotropin-releasing hormone (TRH) and gonadotropin-releasing hormone (GnRH) seem to correlate with hypothyroidism and hypogonadism, frequent symptoms seen in sleeping sickness [Hublart et al., 1988]. POP Tb could contribute to the blood-brain barrier disruption by cleaving entire collagen and/or its fragment over the course of a trypanosome infection.

Fasciola hepatica

Outbreaks of fasciolosis have become widespread in mammalians (either humans or cattles and sheeps), estimating that over 2.4 million people are infected with *F. hepatica* [Keiser and Utzinger, 2005], the aetiological agent of the disease. Despite its historical association with domestic areas, fasciolosis is known as an emerging foodborne zoonotic disease occurring mainly in South America [Robinson and Dalton, 2009]. This fact turned fasciolosis into a disease economically important in temperate zones, where *F. hepatica* distribution is predominant [Mitchell, 2002].

The establishment of *F. hepatica* infection occurs due to the overcoming of intrinsic obstacles, such as immune system and invasion of several tissues in human body. The infective form ingested by the vertebrate host is the metacercariae, which excysts in the small intestine and the juvenile worm penetrates through the gut wall into the peritoneal cavity in order to reach the liver parenchyma and, finally, the bile ducts to mature itself [Andrews, 1999].

As the path of *F. hepatica* within the body involves the penetration in several tissues, attempting to establish effectively the infection, this liver fluke developed powerful proteolytic machinery that plays an important role in the parasite virulence [Irving et al., 2003; Robinson et al., 2008b]. In 1965, Thorsell e Bjorkman reported for the first time that the adult *F. hepatica* was able to secrete proteases identified as papain-like cysteine proteases. Currently it is known that cathepsin L and cathepsin B represent the major proteases secreted by *F. hepatica* parasites [Robinson et al., 2008a] and they are responsible for the success of the major mechanisms of invasion, such as the parasite migration through host tissues, the degradation of host macromolecules in order to provide amino acids [Dalton et al., 2003], and the suppression of host-immune responses [Berasain et al., 2000; Smith et al., 1993].

Although the involvement of both cathepsin L and cathepsin B in the penetration of infective juveniles in gut wall [McGonigle et al., 2008] was demonstrated, they are restricted to different life stages of the worm. Cathepsin B is present only in infective juveniles and immature liver stages [Meemon et al., 2004; Wilson et al., 1998] and along with cathepsin-L, these proteases add sufficient proteolytic capacity for the parasite to penetrate both the intestinal wall and the bulk of the liver, and to protect itself from the immune attack [Morphew et al., 2007; Robinson et al., 2008b]. In contrast, proteolytic activity in adults is due only to cathepsin L, which degrades hemoglobin to provide necessary nutrients for worm survival [Dalton et al., 2003; Stack et al., 2008]. The family of cathepsins L was formed from successive genes duplications in *F. hepatica* which resulted in a large family of monophyletic origin consisting of 5 clades [Irving et al., 2003]. These data together make the cathepsin L cysteine proteases family an important virulence factor correlated with *F. hepatica* migration and entry in order to establish fasciolosis.

Conclusion

Successful infection depends on the capacity of a pathogen to migrate through host tissues. For this, infective agents must cross many tissue barriers such as skin, bones, vessels and extracellular matrix that possess a variety of collagens. Since these challenging molecules have a particular three-dimensional structure, it is not surprising that only specialized enzymes can recognize their forms and degrade them. The evolution have selected a number of microorganisms and worms that are able to counteract the presence of collagens and thus to infect thousands of different hosts, resulting in the establishment of many still incurable diseases that affect millions of people around the world. The scientific knowledge in this field reveals that collagenases are important virulence factors and their specific or selective inhibition can result in new chemotherapeutical agents to treat those diseases. However, exactly where, when and how those charming enzymes work must be fully understood to search for powerful inhibitors that could be experimentally assayed *in vivo*. For this, interdisciplinary research involving cell biology, molecular biology, biochemistry, bioinformatics and structural biology must to be carried out in a coordinated way. Cutting collagens is a hard task, but understanding how it takes place is even harder.

References

Abad, A., Fernández-Molina, J. V., Bikandi, J., Ramírez, A., Margareto, J., Sendino, J., Hernando, F. L., Pontón, J., Garaizar, J., and Rementeria, A. (2010). What makes *Aspergillus fumigatus* a successful pathogen? Genes and molecules involved in invasive aspergillosis. *Rev. Iberoam. Micol.* 27, 155-182.

Abrahamson, D. R. (1986). Recent studies on the structure and pathology of basement membranes. *J. Pathol.* 149, 257-278.

Ahsan, M. M., Kimura, T., Karita, S., Sakka, K., and Ohmiya, K. (1996). Cloning, D. N. A. sequencing, and expression of the gene encoding *Clostridium* thermocellum cellulase CelJ, the largest catalytic component of the cellulosome. *J. Bacteriol.* 178, 5732-5740.

Andrews, S. J. (1999). The life cicle of *Fasciola hepatica*. Oxford, U. K.: C. A. B. I. edn.

Ankri, S., Stolarsky, T., Bracha, R., Padilla-Vaca, F., and Mirelman, D. (1999). Antisense inhibition of expression of cysteine proteinases affects *Entamoeba histolytica*-induced formation of liver abscess in hamsters. *Infect. Immun.* 67, 421-422.

Arhets, P., Olivo, J. C., Gounon, P., Sansonetti, P., and Guillén, N. (1998). Virulence and functions of myosin II are inhibited by overexpression of light meromyosin in Entamoeba histolytica. *Mol. Biol. Cell* 9, 1537-1547.

Armstrong, D. G., and Jude, E. B. (2002). The role of matrix metalloproteinases in wound healing. *J. Am. Podiatr. Med. Assoc.* 92, 12-18.

Arnold, L. H., Butt, L. E., Prior, S. H., Read, C. M., Fields, G. B., and Pickford, A. R. (2011). The interface between catalytic and hemopexin domains in matrix metalloproteinase-1 conceals a collagen binding exosite. *J. Biol. Chem.* 286, 45073-45082.

Atley, L. M., Mort, J. S., Lalumiere, M., and Eyre, D. R. (2000). Proteolysis of human bone collagen by cathepsin K: characterization of the cleavage sites generating by cross-linked N-telopeptide neoepitope. *Bone* 26, 241-247.

Balloy, V., and Chignard, M. (2009). The innate immune response to Aspergillus fumigatus. *Microbes Infect.* 11, 919-927.

Baronas-Lowell, D., Lauer-Fields, J. L., and Fields, G. B. (2004). Induction of endothelial cell activation by a triple helical alpha2beta integrin ligand, derived from type I collagen alpha1(I)496-507. *J. Biol. Chem.* 279, 952-962.

Bastos, I. M., Grellier, P., Martins, N. F., Cadavid-Restrepo, G., de Souza-Ault, M. R., Augustyns, K., Teixeira, A. R., Schrével, J., Maigret, B., da Silveira, J. F., et al. (2005). Molecular, functional and structural properties of the prolyl oligopeptidase of Trypanosoma cruzi (POP Tc80), which is required for parasite entry into mammalian cells. *Biochem. J. 388*, 29-38.

Bastos, I. M., Motta, F. N., Charneau, S., Santana, J. M., Dubost, L., Augustyns, K., and Grellier, P. (2010). Prolyl oligopeptidase of Trypanosoma brucei hydrolyzes native collagen, peptide hormones and is active in the plasma of infected mice. *Microbes Infect.* 12, 457-466.

Bauvois, B., Sancéau, J., and Wietzerbin, J. (1992). Human U937 cell surface peptidase activities: characterization and degradative effect on tumor necrosis factor-alpha. *Eur. J. Immunol.* 22, 923-930.

Beauvais, A., Monod, M., Debeaupuis, J. P., Diaquin, M., Kobayashi, H., and Latgé, J. P. (1997a). Biochemical and antigenic characterization of a new dipeptidyl-peptidase isolated from Aspergillus fumigatus. *J. Biol. Chem.* 272, 6238-6244.

Beauvais, A., Monod, M., Wyniger, J., Debeaupuis, J. P., Grouzmann, E., Brakch, N., Svab, J., Hovanessian, A. G., and Latgé, J. P. (1997b). Dipeptidyl-peptidase IV secreted by Aspergillus fumigatus, a fungus pathogenic to humans. Infect Immun. 65, 3042-3047.

Beck, D. L., Doğan, N., Maro, V., Sam, N. E., Shao, J., and Houpt, E. R. (2008). High prevalence of *Entamoeba moshkovskii* in a Tanzanian H. I. V. population. Acta Trop. 107, 48-49.

Beecher, D. J., Olsen, T. W., Somers, E. B., and Wong, A. C. (2000). Evidence for contribution of tripartite hemolysin B. L., phosphatidylcholine-preferring phospholipase C, and collagenase to virulence of Bacillus cereus endophthalmitis. *Infect Immun.* 68, 5269-5276.

Behnsen, J., Lessing, F., Schindler, S., Wartenberg, D., Jacobsen, I. D., Thoen, M., Zipfel, P. F., and Brakhage, A. A. (2010). Secreted Aspergillus fumigatus protease Alp1 degrades human complement proteins C3, C4, and C5. *Infect Immun.* 78, 3585-3594.

Bejarano, P. A., Langeveld, J. P., Hudson, B. G., and Noelken, M. E. (1989). Degradation of basement membranes by *Pseudomonas aeruginosa* elastase. *Infect Immun.* 57, 3783-3787.

Berasain, P., Carmona, C., Frangione, B., Dalton, J. P., and Goñi, F. (2000). Fasciola hepatica: parasite-secreted proteinases degrade all human IgG subclasses: determination of the specific cleavage sites and identification of the immunoglobulin fragments produced. *Exp. Parasitol.* 94, 99-110.

Berman, E. (1991). Biochemistry of the eye. New York, N. Y.: Plenum Press.

Bertini, I., Fragai, M., Luchinat, C., Melikian, M., Toccafondi, M., Lauer, J. L., and Fields, G. B. (2012). Structural basis for matrix metalloproteinase 1-catalyzed collagenolysis. *J. Am. Chem. Soc.* 134, 2100-2110.

Bidwell, E., and Van Heyningen, W. E. (1948). The biochemistry of the gas gangrene toxins; the kappa-toxin, collagenase, of Clostridium welchii. *Biochem. J.* 42, 140-151.

Birkedal-Hansen, H., Moore, W. G., Bodden, M. K., Windsor, L. J., Birkedal-Hansen, B., DeCarlo, A., and Engler, J. A. (1993). Matrix metalloproteinases: a review. *Crit. Rev. Oral. Biol. Med.* 4, 197-250.

Blackwood, L. L., Stone, R. M., Iglewski, B. H., and Pennington, J. E. (1983). Evaluation of Pseudomonas aeruginosa exotoxin A and elastase as virulence factors in acute lung infection. *Infect Immun.* 39, 198-201.

Bodey, G. P., Bolivar, R., Fainstein, V., and Jadeja, L. (1983). Infections caused by Pseudomonas aeruginosa. *Rev. Infect. Dis.* 5, 279-313.

Bond, M. D., and Van Wart, H. E. (1984). Purification and separation of individual collagenases of Clostridium histolyticum using red dye ligand chromatography. *Biochemistry* 23, 3077-3085.

Bottone, E. J. (2010). Bacillus cereus, a volatile human pathogen. *Clin. Microbiol. Rev.* 23, 382-398.

Brodsky, B., and Persikov, A. V. (2005). Molecular structure of the collagen triple helix. *Adv. Protein. Chem.* 70, 301-339.
Bruchhaus, I., Jacobs, T., Leippe, M., and Tannich, E. (1996). Entamoeba histolytica and Entamoeba dispar: differences in numbers and expression of cysteine proteinase genes. *Mol. Microbiol.* 22, 255-263.
Burleigh, B. A., and Woolsey, A. M. (2002). Cell signalling and Trypanosoma cruzi invasion. *Cell Microbiol.* 4, 701-711.
Bycroft, M., Bateman, A., Clarke, J., Hamill, S. J., Sandford, R., Thomas, R. L., and Chothia, C. (1999). The structure of a P. K. D. domain from polycystin-1: implications for polycystic kidney disease. *E. M. B. O. J.* 18, 297-305.
Callegan, M. C., Booth, M. C., Jett, B. D., and Gilmore, M. S. (1999). Pathogenesis of gram-positive bacterial endophthalmitis. *Infect Immun.* 67, 3348-3356.
Camargo, A. C., Caldo, H., and Reis, M. L. (1979). Susceptibility of a peptide derived from bradykinin to hydrolysis by brain endo-oligopeptidases and pancreatic proteinases. *J. Biol. Chem.* 254, 5304-5307.
Chapman, J. A., Tzaphlidou, M., Meek, K. M., and Kadler, K. E. (1990). The collagen fibril--a model system for studying the staining and fixation of a protein. *Electron Microsc. Rev.* 3, 143-182.
Chen, X. L., Zhang, Y. Z., Lu, J. T., Xie, B. B., Sun, C. Y., and Guo, B. (2007). Autolysis of a novel multidomain subtilase-cold-adapted deseasin MCP-01 is pH-dependent and the surface loops in its catalytic domain, the linker, and the P_proprotein domain are susceptible to proteolytic attack. *Biochem. Biophys. Res. Commun.* 358, 704-709.
Cheng, H. C., Abdel-Ghany, M., Elble, R. C., and Pauli, B. U. (1998). Lung endothelial dipeptidyl peptidase IV promotes adhesion and metastasis of rat breast cancer cells via tumor cell surface-associated fibronectin. *J. Biol. Chem.* 273, 24207-24215.
Chung, L., Dinakarpandian, D., Yoshida, N., Lauer-Fields, J. L., Fields, G. B., Visse, R., and Nagase, H. (2004). Collagenase unwinds triple-helical collagen prior to peptide bond hydrolysis. *E. M. B. O. J.* 23, 3020-3030.
Clark, C. G., Alsmark, U. C., Tazreiter, M., Saito-Nakano, Y., Ali, V., Marion, S., Weber, C., Mukherjee, C., Bruchhaus, I., Tannich, E., et al. (2007). Structure and content of the Entamoeba histolytica genome. *Adv. Parasitol.* 65, 51-190.
Clark, I. M., and Cawston, T. E. (1989). Fragments of human fibroblast collagenase. Purification and characterization. *Biochem. J.* 263, 201-206.
Coudrier, E., Amblard, F., Zimmer, C., Roux, P., Olivo-Marin, J. C., Rigothier, M. C., and Guillén, N. (2005). Myosin II and the Gal-GalNAc lectin play a crucial role in tissue invasion by Entamoeba histolytica. *Cell Microbiol.* 7, 19-27.
Dalton, J. P., Neill, S. O., Stack, C., Collins, P., Walshe, A., Sekiya, M., Doyle, S., Mulcahy, G., Hoyle, D., Khaznadji, E., et al. (2003). Fasciola hepatica cathepsin L-like proteases: biology, function, and potential in the development of first generation liver fluke vaccines. *Int. J. Parasitol.* 33, 1173-1181.
Das, S., Mandal, M., Chakraborti, T., Mandal, A., and Chakraborti, S. (2003). Structure and evolutionary aspects of matrix metalloproteinases: a brief overview. *Mol. Cell Biochem.* 253, 31-40.
Davey, R. T., and Tauber, W. B. (1987). Posttraumatic endophthalmitis: the emerging role of Bacillus cereus infection. *Rev. Infect Dis.* 9, 110-123.

Di Lullo, G. A., Sweeney, S. M., Korkko, J., Ala-Kokko, L., and San Antonio, J. D. (2002). Mapping the ligand-binding sites and disease-associated mutations on the most abundant protein in the human, type I collagen. *J. Biol. Chem.* 277, 4223-4231.

Diacovich, L., and Gorvel, J. P. (2010). Bacterial manipulation of innate immunity to promote infection. *Nat. Rev. Microbiol.* 8, 117-128.

Docherty, A. J., and Murphy, G. (1990). The tissue metalloproteinase family and the inhibitor T. I. M. P.: a study using cDNAs and recombinant proteins. *Ann. Rheum. Dis.* 49 Suppl. 1, 469-479.

Dresdner, K., Barker, L. A., Orlowski, M., and Wilk, S. (1982). Subcellular distribution of prolyl endopeptidase and cation-sensitive neutral endopeptidase in rabbit brain. *J. Neurochem.* 38, 1151-1154.

Ducka, P., Eckhard, U., Schönauer, E., Kofler, S., Gottschalk, G., Brandstetter, H., and Nüss, D. (2009). A universal strategy for high-yield production of soluble and functional clostridial collagenases in E. coli. *Appl. Microbiol. Biotechnol.* 83, 1055-1065.

Döring, G., Maier, M., Müller, E., Bibi, Z., Tümmler, B., and Kharazmi, A. (1987). Virulence factors of Pseudomonas aeruginosa. *Antibiot. Chemother.* 39, 136-148.

Eckhard, U., Schönauer, E., Ducka, P., Briza, P., Nüss, D., and Brandstetter, H. (2009). Biochemical characterization of the catalytic domains of three different Clostridial collagenases. *Biol. Chem.* 390, 11-18.

Eckhard, U., Schönauer, E., Nüss, D., and Brandstetter, H. (2011). Structure of collagenase G. reveals a chew-and-digest mechanism of bacterial collagenolysis. *Nat. Struct. Mol. Biol.* 18, 1109-1114.

Engman, D. M., and Leon, J. S. (2002). Pathogenesis of Chagas heart disease: role of autoimmunity. *Acta Trop.* 81, 123-132.

Fotedar, R., Stark, D., Marriott, D., Ellis, J., and Harkness, J. (2008). Entamoeba moshkovskii infections in Sydney, Australia. *Eur. J. Clin. Microbiol. Infect. Dis.* 27, 133-137.

French, M. F., Bhown, A., and Van Wart, H. E. (1992). Identification of Clostridium histolyticum collagenase hyperreactive sites in type I, II, and III collagens: lack of correlation with local triple helical stability. *J. Protein. Chem.* 11, 83-97.

French, M. F., Mookhtiar, K. A., and Van Wart, H. E. (1987). Limited proteolysis of type I collagen at hyperreactive sites by class I and II Clostridium histolyticum collagenases: complementary digestion patterns. *Biochemistry* 26, 681-687.

Fülöp, V., Böcskei, Z., and Polgár, L. (1998). Prolyl oligopeptidase: an unusual beta-propeller domain regulates proteolysis. *Cell* 94, 161-170.

Garcia, M. P., Nóbrega, O. T., Teixeira, A. R., Sousa, M. V., and Santana, J. M. (1998). Characterisation of a Trypanosoma cruzi acidic 30 kDa cysteine protease. *Mol. Biochem. Parasitol.* 91, 263-272.

Gelbard, M. K., James, K., Riach, P., and Dorey, F. (1993). Collagenase versus placebo in the treatment of Peyronie's disease: a double-blind study. *J. Urol.* 149, 56-58.

Geurts, N., Opdenakker, G., and Van den Steen, P. E. (2012). Matrix metalloproteinases as therapeutic targets in protozoan parasitic infections. *Pharmacol. Ther.* 133, 257-279.

Goodwin, L. G. (1971). Pathological effects of Trypanosoma brucei on small blood vessels in rabbit ear-chambers. *Trans. R. Soc. Trop. Med. Hyg.* 65, 82-88.

Grab, D. J., Garcia-Garcia, J. C., Nikolskaia, O. V., Kim, Y. V., Brown, A., Pardo, C. A., Zhang, Y., Becker, K. G., Wilson, B. A., de A Lima, A. P., et al. (2009). Protease activated receptor signaling is required for African trypanosome traversal of human brain microvascular endothelial cells. *PLoS Negl. Trop. Dis.* 3, e479.

Granum, P. E. (1994). Bacillus cereus and its toxins. *Soc. Appl. Bacteriol. Symp. Ser.* 23, 61S-66S.

Granum, P. E., and Lund, T. (1997). Bacillus cereus and its food poisoning toxins. *F. E. M. S. Microbiol. Lett.* 157, 223-228.

Grellier, P., Vendeville, S., Joyeau, R., Bastos, I. M., Drobecq, H., Frappier, F., Teixeira, A. R., Schrével, J., Davioud-Charvet, E., Sergheraert, C., et al. (2001). Trypanosoma cruzi prolyl oligopeptidase Tc80 is involved in nonphagocytic mammalian cell invasion by trypomastigotes. *J. Biol. Chem.* 276, 47078-47086.

Haque, R., Huston, C. D., Hughes, M., Houpt, E., and Petri, W. A. (2003). Amebiasis. *N. Engl. J. Med.* 348, 1565-1573.

Heck, L. W., Morihara, K., McRae, W. B., and Miller, E. J. (1986). Specific cleavage of human type III and IV collagens by Pseudomonas aeruginosa elastase. *Infect Immun.* 51, 115-118.

Hergenrother, P. J., and Martin, S. F. (1997). Determination of the kinetic parameters for phospholipase C. (Bacillus cereus) on different phospholipid substrates using a chromogenic assay based on the quantitation of inorganic phosphate. *Anal. Biochem.* 251, 45-49.

Hesse, F., Burtscher, H., Popp, F., and Ambrosius, D. (1995). Recombinant enzymes for islet isolation: purification of a collagenase from Clostridium histolyticum and cloning/expression of the gene. *Transplant. Proc.* 27, 3287-3289.

Hou, Y., Mortimer, L., and Chadee, K. (2010). Entamoeba histolytica cysteine proteinase 5 binds integrin on colonic cells and stimulates NFkappaB-mediated pro-inflammatory responses. *J. Biol. Chem.* 285, 35497-35504.

Hublart, M., Lagouche, L., Racadot, A., Boersma, A., Degand, P., Noireau, F., Lemesre, J. L., and Toudic, A. (1988). Endocrine function and African trypanosomiasis. Evaluation of 79 cases. *Bull. Soc. Pathol. Exot. Filiales.* 81, 468-476.

Hurst, D. R., Schwartz, M. A., Ghaffari, M. A., Jin, Y., Tschesche, H., Fields, G. B., and Sang, Q. X. (2004). Catalytic- and ecto-domains of membrane type 1-matrix metalloproteinase have similar inhibition profiles but distinct endopeptidase activities. *Biochem. J.* 377, 775-779.

Irving, J. A., Spithill, T. W., Pike, R. N., Whisstock, J. C., and Smooker, P. M. (2003). The evolution of enzyme specificity in Fasciola spp. *J. Mol. Evol.* 57, 1-15.

Jensen, G. B., Hansen, B. M., Eilenberg, J., and Mahillon, J. (2003). The hidden lifestyles of Bacillus cereus and relatives. *Environ. Microbiol.* 5, 631-640.

Kadler, K. E., Holmes, D. F., Trotter, J. A., and Chapman, J. A. (1996). Collagen fibril formation. *Biochem. J.* 316 (Pt 1), 1-11.

Kafienah, W., Brömme, D., Buttle, D. J., Croucher, L. J., and Hollander, A. P. (1998). Human cathepsin K cleaves native type I and II collagens at the N-terminal end of the triple helix. *Biochem. J.* 331 (Pt 3), 727-732.

Katayama, S., Dupuy, B., Daube, G., China, B., and Cole, S. T. (1996). Genome mapping of Clostridium perfringens strains with I-CeuI shows many virulence genes to be plasmid-borne. *Mol. Gen. Genet.* 251, 720-726.

Keene, W. E., Petitt, M. G., Allen, S., and McKerrow, J. H. (1986). The major neutral proteinase of Entamoeba histolytica. *J. Exp. Med.* 163, 536-549.

Keiser, J., and Utzinger, J. (2005). Emerging foodborne trematodiasis. *Emerg. Infect. Dis.* 11, 1507-1514.

Khairnar, K., Parija, S. C., and Palaniappan, R. (2007). Diagnosis of intestinal amoebiasis by using nested polymerase chain reaction-restriction fragment length polymorphism assay. *J Gastroenterol* 42, 631-640.

Knäuper, V., Osthues, A., DeClerck, Y. A., Langley, K. E., Bläser, J., and Tschesche, H. (1993). Fragmentation of human polymorphonuclear-leucocyte collagenase. *Biochem. J.* 291 (Pt 3), 847-854.

Kolattukudy, P. E., Lee, J. D., Rogers, L. M., Zimmerman, P., Ceselski, S., Fox, B., Stein, B., and Copelan, E. A. (1993). Evidence for possible involvement of an elastolytic serine protease in aspergillosis. *Infect Immun.* 61, 2357-2368.

Kurup, V. P., and Grunig, G. (2002). Animal models of allergic bronchopulmonary aspergillosis. *Mycopathologia* 153, 165-177.

Labruyère, E., Zimmer, C., Galy, V., Olivo-Marin, J. C., and Guillén, N. (2003). EhPAK, a member of the p21-activated kinase family, is involved in the control of Entamoeba histolytica migration and phagocytosis. *J. Cell Sci.* 116, 61-71.

Landis, B. N., Grouzmann, E., Monod, M., Busso, N., Petak, F., Spiliopoulos, A., Robert, J. H., Szalay-Quinodoz, I., Morel, D. R., and Lacroix, J. S. (2008). Implication of dipeptidylpeptidase IV activity in human bronchial inflammation and in bronchoconstriction evaluated in anesthetized rabbits. *Respiration* 75, 89-97.

Lauer-Fields, J. L., Chalmers, M. J., Busby, S. A., Minond, D., Griffin, P. R., and Fields, G. B. (2009). Identification of specific hemopexin-like domain residues that facilitate matrix metalloproteinase collagenolytic activity. *J. Biol. Chem.* 284, 24017-24024.

Leikina, E., Mertts, M. V., Kuznetsova, N., and Leikin, S. (2002). Type I collagen is thermally unstable at body temperature. *Proc. Natl. Acad. Sci.* US 99, 1314-1318.

Lemichez, E., Lecuit, M., Nassif, X., and Bourdoulous, S. (2010). Breaking the wall: targeting of the endothelium by pathogenic bacteria. *Nat. Rev. Microbiol.* 8, 93-104.

Lund, T., De Buyser, M. L., and Granum, P. E. (2000). A new cytotoxin from Bacillus cereus that may cause necrotic enteritis. *Mol. Microbiol.* 38, 254-261.

Lund, T., and Granum, P. E. (1999). The 105-kDa protein component of *Bacillus cereus* non-haemolytic enterotoxin (Nhe) is a metalloprotease with gelatinolytic and collagenolytic activity. *F. E. M. S. Microbiol. Lett.* 178, 355-361.

Löster, K., Zeilinger, K., Schuppan, D., and Reutter, W. (1995). The cysteine-rich region of dipeptidyl peptidase IV (CD 26) is the collagen-binding site. *Biochem. Biophys. Res. Commun.* 217, 341-348.

MacLennan, J. D. (1962). The histotoxic clostridial infections of man. *Bacteriol. Rev.* 26, 177-276.

MacLennan, J. D., Mandl, I., and Howes, E. L. (1953). Bacterial digestion of collagen. *J. Clin. Invest.* 32, 1317-1322.

Martinez, M. F., Haines, T., Waller, M., Tingey, D., and Gomez, W. (2007). Probable occupational endophthalmitis from Bacillus cereus. *Arch. Environ. Occup. Health* 62, 157-160.

Maschmeyer, G., Haas, A., and Cornely, O. A. (2007). Invasive aspergillosis: epidemiology, diagnosis and management in immunocompromised patients. *Drugs* 67, 1567-1601.

Matsushita, O., Yoshihara, K., Katayama, S., Minami, J., and Okabe, A. (1994). Purification and characterization of Clostridium perfringens 120-kilodalton collagenase and nucleotide sequence of the corresponding gene. *J. Bacteriol.* 176, 149-156.

McGonigle, L., Mousley, A., Marks, N. J., Brennan, G. P., Dalton, J. P., Spithill, T. W., Day, T. A., and Maule, A. G. (2008). The silencing of cysteine proteases in Fasciola hepatica newly excysted juveniles using R. N. A. interference reduces gut penetration. *Int. J. Parasitol.* 38, 149-155.

Meemon, K., Grams, R., Vichasri-Grams, S., Hofmann, A., Korge, G., Viyanant, V., Upatham, E. S., Habe, S., and Sobhon, P. (2004). Molecular cloning and analysis of stage and tissue-specific expression of cathepsin B encoding genes from Fasciola gigantica. *Mol. Biochem. Parasitol.* 136, 1-10.

Mentlein, R., Dahms, P., Grandt, D., and Krüger, R. (1993). Proteolytic processing of neuropeptide Y and peptide YY by dipeptidyl peptidase IV. *Regul. Pept.* 49, 133-144.

Miller, E. J., and Gay, S. (1982). Collagen: an overview. *Methods Enzymol.* 82 Pt A, 3-32.

Minor, R. R. (1980). Collagen metabolism: a comparison of diseases of collagen and diseases affecting collagen. *Am. J. Pathol.* 98, 225-280.

Mitchell, G. (2002). Update on Fasciolosis in Cattle and Sheep. *In Practice* 24(7), 378.

Miyamoto, K., Nukui, E., Itoh, H., Sato, T., Kobayashi, T., Imada, C., Watanabe, E., Inamori, Y., and Tsujibo, H. (2002). Molecular analysis of the gene encoding a novel chitin-binding protease from Alteromonas sp. strain O-7 and its role in the chitinolytic system. *J. Bacteriol.* 184, 1865-1872.

Moncada, D., Keller, K., and Chadee, K. (2003). Entamoeba histolytica cysteine proteinases disrupt the polymeric structure of colonic mucin and alter its protective function. *Infect Immun.* 71, 838-844.

Morjhara, K., and Homma, J. (1985). *Pseudomonas* proteases. In: Holder I, ed. Bacterial enzymes and virulence. Boca Raton, Fl: C. R. C. Press.

Morphew, R. M., Wright, H. A., LaCourse, E. J., Woods, D. J., and Brophy, P. M. (2007). Comparative proteomics of excretory-secretory proteins released by the liver fluke Fasciola hepatica in sheep host bile and during in vitro culture ex host. *Mol. Cell Proteomics* 6, 963-972.

Murphy, G., Allan, J. A., Willenbrock, F., Cockett, M. I., O'Connell, J. P., and Docherty, A. J. (1992). The role of the C-terminal domain in collagenase and stromelysin specificity. *J. Biol. Chem. 267*, 9612-9618.

Muńoz, M. L., Calderón, J., and Rojkind, M. (1982). The collagenase of Entamoeba histolytica. *J. Exp. Med.* 155, 42-51.

Nagase, H., Visse, R., and Murphy, G. (2006). Structure and function of matrix metalloproteinases and TIMPs. *Cardiovasc. Res.* 69, 562-573.

Ndung'u, J. M., Wright, N. G., Jennings, F. W., and Murray, M. (1992). Changes in atrial natriuretic factor and plasma renin activity in dogs infected with Trypanosoma brucei. *Parasitol. Res.* 78, 553-556.

Netzel-Arnett, S., Salari, A., Goli, U. B., and Van Wart, H. E. (1994). Evidence for a triple helix recognition site in the hemopexin-like domains of human fibroblast and neutrophil interstitial collagenases. *Ann. N. Y. Acad. Sci.* 732, 22-30.

Nikolskaia, O. V., de A. Lima, A. P., Kim, Y. V., Lonsdale-Eccles, J. D., Fukuma, T., Scharfstein, J., and Grab, D. J. (2006). Blood-brain barrier traversal by African trypanosomes requires calcium signaling induced by parasite cysteine protease. *J. Clin. Invest.* 116, 2739-2747.

Nogueira de Melo, A. C., de Souza, E. P., Elias, C. G., dos Santos, A. L., Branquinha, M. H., d'Avila-Levy, C. M., dos Reis, F., Costa, T. F., Lima, A. P., de Souza Pereira, M. C., et al. (2010). Detection of matrix metallopeptidase-9-like proteins in Trypanosoma cruzi. *Exp. Parasitol.* 125, 256-263.

Oakley, C. L., Warrack, G. H., and Van Heyningen, W. E. (1946). The collagenase (kappa toxin) of Cl. welchii type A. *J. Pathol. Bacteriol.* 58, 229-235.

Oda, K., Ito, M., Uchida, K., Shibano, Y., Fukuhara, K., and Takahashi, S. (1996). Cloning and expression of an isovaleryl pepstatin-insensitive carboxyl proteinase gene from Xanthomonas sp. T-22. *J. Biochem.* 120, 564-572.

Ohuchi, E., Imai, K., Fujii, Y., Sato, H., Seiki, M., and Okada, Y. (1997). Membrane type 1 matrix metalloproteinase digests interstitial collagens and other extracellular matrix macromolecules. *J. Biol. Chem.* 272, 2446-2451.

Orikoshi, H., Nakayama, S., Hanato, C., Miyamoto, K., and Tsujibo, H. (2005). Role of the N-terminal polycystic kidney disease domain in chitin degradation by chitinase A from a marine bacterium, Alteromonas sp. strain O-7. *J. Appl. Microbiol.* 99, 551-557.

Overall, C. M. (2002). Molecular determinants of metalloproteinase substrate specificity: matrix metalloproteinase substrate binding domains, modules, and exosites. *Mol. Biotechnol.* 22, 51-86.

Palmer, G. E., Askew, D. S., and Williamson, P. R. (2008). The diverse roles of autophagy in medically important fungi. *Autophagy* 4, 982-988.

Park, S. J., and Mehrad, B. (2009). Innate immunity to Aspergillus species. *Clin. Microbiol. Rev.* 22, 535-551.

Perrakis, A., Tews, I., Dauter, Z., Oppenheim, A. B., Chet, I., Wilson, K. S., and Vorgias, C. E. (1994). Crystal structure of a bacterial chitinase at 2.3 A resolution. *Structure* 2, 1169-1180.

Peterkofsky, B. (1982). Bacterial collagenase. *Methods Enzymol.* 82, 453–471.

Pflugfelder, S. C., and Flynn, H. W. (1992). Infectious endophthalmitis. *Infect Dis. Clin. North Am.* 6, 859-873.

Pollack, M. (1984). The virulence of Pseudomonas aeruginosa. *Rev. Infect Dis.* 6 Suppl. 3, S617-626.

Pollack, M. (1985). *Pseudomonas aeruginosa.* In: Mandell G., Douglas R., and Bennett J., eds. Principles and practice of infectious diseases. New York: John Wiley and Sons.

Prockop, D. J., Kivirikko, K. I., Tuderman, L., and Guzman, N. A. (1979). The biosynthesis of collagen and its disorders (first of two parts). *N. Engl. J. Med.* 301, 13-23.

Rawlings, N. D., Barrett, A. J., and Bateman, A. (2012). M. E. R. O. P. S.: the database of proteolytic enzymes, their substrates and inhibitors. *Nucleic. Acids. Res.* 40, D343-350.

Reed, S. L., Keene, W. E., McKerrow, J. H., and Gigli, I. (1989). Cleavage of C3 by a neutral cysteine proteinase of Entamoeba histolytica. *J. Immunol.* 143, 189-195.

Reichard, U., Büttner, S., Eiffert, H., Staib, F., and Rüchel, R. (1990). Purification and characterisation of an extracellular serine proteinase from Aspergillus fumigatus and its detection in tissue. *J. Med. Microbiol.* 33, 243-251.

Reyes, C. D., and García, A. J. (2004). Alpha2beta1 integrin-specific collagen-mimetic surfaces supporting osteoblastic differentiation. *J. Biomed. Mater. Res.* A 69, 591-600.

Robinson, M. W., Corvo, I., Jones, P. M., George, A. M., Padula, M. P., To, J., Cancela, M., Rinaldi, G., Tort, J. F., Roche, L., et al. (2011). Collagenolytic activities of the major secreted cathepsin L peptidases involved in the virulence of the helminth pathogen, Fasciola hepatica. *PLoS Negl. Trop. Dis.* 5, e1012.

Robinson, M. W., and Dalton, J. P. (2009). Zoonotic helminth infections with particular emphasis on fasciolosis and other trematodiases. *Philos. Trans. R. Soc. Lond. B. Biol. Sci.* 364, 2763-2776.

Robinson, M. W., Dalton, J. P., and Donnelly, S. (2008a). Helminth pathogen cathepsin proteases: it's a family affair. *Trends. Biochem. Sci.* 33, 601-608.

Robinson, M. W., Tort, J. F., Lowther, J., Donnelly, S. M., Wong, E., Xu, W., Stack, C. M., Padula, M., Herbert, B., and Dalton, J. P. (2008b). Proteomics and phylogenetic analysis of the cathepsin L protease family of the helminth pathogen Fasciola hepatica: expansion of a repertoire of virulence-associated factors. *Mol. Cell Proteomics.* 7, 1111-1123.

Rojkind, M. (1979). Chemistry and biosynthesis of collagen. *Bull. Rheum. Dis.* 30, 1006-1010.

Rood, J., McClane, B., Songer, J., and Titball, R. (1997). *The Clostridia: Molecular Biology and Pathogenesis.* London: Academic, 533.

Sanchez-Lopez, R., Alexander, C. M., Behrendtsen, O., Breathnach, R., and Werb, Z. (1993). Role of zinc-binding- and hemopexin domain-encoded sequences in the substrate specificity of collagenase and stromelysin-2 as revealed by chimeric proteins. *J. Biol. Chem.* 268, 7238-7247.

Santana, J. M., Grellier, P., Schrével, J., and Teixeira, A. R. (1997). A Trypanosoma cruzi-secreted 80 kDa proteinase with specificity for human collagen types I and IV. *Biochem. J.* 325 (Pt 1), 129-137.

Schofield, C. J., Jannin, J., and Salvatella, R. (2006). The future of Chagas disease control. *Trends Parasitol.* 22, 583-588.

Shen, H. D., Tam, M. F., Chou, H., and Han, S. H. (1999). The importance of serine proteinases as aeroallergens associated with asthma. *Int. Arch. Allergy Immunol.* 119, 259-264.

Shi, L., Ermis, R., Garcia, A., Telgenhoff, D., and Aust, D. (2010). Degradation of human collagen isoforms by Clostridium collagenase and the effects of degradation products on cell migration. *Int. Wound J.* 7, 87-95.

Singh, B., Fleury, C., Jalalvand, F., and Riesbeck, K. (2012). Human pathogens utilize host extracellular matrix proteins laminin and collagen for adhesion and invasion of the host. *F. E. M. S. Microbiol. Rev.*

Smith, A. M., Dowd, A. ., Heffernan, M., Robertson, C. D., and Dalton, J. P. (1993). Fasciola hepatica: a secreted cathepsin L-like proteinase cleaves host immunoglobulin. *Int. J. Parasitol.* 23, 977-983.

Smith, L. D. (1979). Virulence factors of Clostridium perfringens. *Rev. Infect Dis.* 1, 254-262.

Springman, E. B., Angleton, E. L., Birkedal-Hansen, H., and Van Wart, H. E. (1990). Multiple modes of activation of latent human fibroblast collagenase: evidence for the role of a Cys73 active-site zinc complex in latency and a "cysteine switch" mechanism for activation. *Proc. Natl. Acad. Sci.* US 87, 364-368.

Stack, C. M., Caffrey, C. R., Donnelly, S. M., Seshaadri, A., Lowther, J., Tort, J. F., Collins, P. R., Robinson, M. W., Xu, W., McKerrow, J. H., et al. (2008). Structural and functional relationships in the virulence-associated cathepsin L proteases of the parasitic liver fluke, Fasciola hepatica. *J. Biol. Chem.* -9908.

Stanley, S. L., and Reed, S. L. (2001). Microbes and microbial toxins: paradigms for microbial-mucosal interactions. VI. Entamoeba histolytica: parasite-host interactions. *Am. J. Physiol. Gastrointest Liver Physiol.* 280, G1049-1054.

Starkweather, K. D., Lattuga, S., Hurst, L. C., Badalamente, M. A., Guilak, F., Sampson, S. P., Dowd, A., and Wisch, D. (1996). Collagenase in the treatment of Dupuytren's disease: an in vitro study. *J. Hand Surg. Am.* 21, 490-495.

Stenfors Arnesen, L. P., Fagerlund, A., and Granum, P. E. (2008). From soil to gut: Bacillus cereus and its food poisoning toxins. *F. E. M. S. Microbiol. Rev.* 32, 579-606.

Sternlicht, M. D., and Werb, Z. (2001). How matrix metalloproteinases regulate cell behavior. *Annu. Rev. Cell Dev. Biol.* 17, 463-516.

Sweeney, S. M., DiLullo, G., Slater, S. J., Martinez, J., Iozzo, R. V., Lauer-Fields, J. L., Fields, G. ., and San Antonio, J. D. (2003). Angiogenesis in collagen I requires alpha2beta1 ligation of a GFP*GER sequence and possibly p. 38 M. A. P. K. activation and focal adhesion disassembly. *J. Biol. Chem.* 278, 30516-30524.

Sweeney, S. M., Orgel, J. P., Fertala, A., McAuliffe, J. D., Turner, K. R., Di Lullo, G. A., Chen, S., Antipova, O., Perumal, S., Ala-Kokko, L., et al. (2008). Candidate cell and matrix interaction domains on the collagen fibril, the predominant protein of vertebrates. *J. Biol. Chem.* 283, 21187-21197.

Tallant, C., Marrero, A., and Gomis-Rüth, F. X. (2010). Matrix metalloproteinases: fold and function of their catalytic domains. *Biochim. Biophys. Acta.* 1803, 20-28.

Tardieux, I., Webster, P., Ravesloot, J., Boron, W., Lunn, J. A., Heuser, J. E., and Andrews, N. W. (1992). Lysosome recruitment and fusion are early events required for trypanosome invasion of mammalian cells. *Cell* 71, 1117-1130.

Thibeaux, R., Dufour, A., Roux, P., Bernier, M., Baglin, A. C., Frileux, P., Olivo-Marin, J. C., Guillén, N., and Labruyère, E. (2012). Newly visualized fibrillar collagen scaffolds dictate Entamoeba histolytica invasion route in the human colon. *Cell Microbiol.* 14, 609-621.

Thorsell, W., Björkman, N., and Wittander, G. (1965). Studies on the action of some enzymes on the cyst wall of isolated metacerkariae from the liver fluke, Fasciola hepatica L. *Experientia* 2, 587-589.

Tillack, M., Biller, L., Irmer, H., Freitas, M., Gomes, M. A., Tannich, E., and Bruchhaus, I. (2007). The Entamoeba histolytica genome: primary structure and expression of proteolytic enzymes. *B. M. C. Genomics* 8, 170.

Vahey, J. B., and Flynn, H. W. (1991). Results in the management of Bacillus endophthalmitis. *Ophthalmic Surg.* 22, 681-686.

Van Wart, H. E., and Birkedal-Hansen, H. (1990). The cysteine switch: a principle of regulation of metalloproteinase activity with potential applicability to the entire matrix metalloproteinase gene family. *Proc. Natl. Acad. Sci.* US 87, 5578-5582.

Vermout, S., Baldo, A., Tabart, J., Losson, B., and Mignon, B. (2008). Secreted dipeptidyl peptidases as potential virulence factors for Microsporum canis. *F. E. M. S. Immunol. Med. Microbiol.* 54, 299-308.

Wang, Y. K., Zhao, G. Y., Li, Y., Chen, X. L., Xie, B. B., Su, H. N., Lv, Y. H., He, H. L., Liu, H., Hu, J., et al. (2010). Mechanistic insight into the function of the C-terminal P. K. D. domain of the collagenolytic serine protease deseasin MCP-01 from deep sea

Pseudoalteromonas sp. SM9913: binding of the P. K. D. domain to collagen results in collagen swelling but does not unwind the collagen triple helix. *J. Biol. Chem.* 285, 14285-14291.

Wilson, J. J., Matsushita, O., Okabe, A., and Sakon, J. (2003). A bacterial collagen-binding domain with novel calcium-binding motif controls domain orientation. *E. M. B. O. J.* 22, 1743-1752.

Wilson, L. R., Good, R. T., Panaccio, M., Wijffels, G. L., Sandeman, R. M., and Spithill, T. W. (1998). Fasciola hepatica: characterization and cloning of the major cathepsin B protease secreted by newly excysted juvenile liver fluke. *Exp. Parasitol.* 88, 85-94.

Wolf, K., Mazo, I., Leung, H., Engelke, K., von Andrian, U. H., Deryugina, E. I., Strongin, A. Y., Bröcker, E. B., and Friedl, P. (2003). Compensation mechanism in tumor cell migration: mesenchymal-amoeboid transition after blocking of pericellular proteolysis. *J. Cell Biol.* 160, 267-277.

Woods, D. E., Cryz, S. J., Friedman, R. L., and Iglewski, B. H. (1982). Contribution of toxin A and elastase to virulence of Pseudomonas aeruginosa in chronic lung infections of rats. *Infect Immun.* 36, 1223-1228.

Woods, D. E., and Iglewski, B. H. (1983). Toxins of Pseudomonas aeruginosa: new perspectives. *Rev. Infect. Dis.* 5 Suppl. 4, S715-722.

Wretlind, B., and Pavlovskis, O. R. (1983). Pseudomonas aeruginosa elastase and its role in pseudomonas infections. *Rev. Infect Dis.* 5 Suppl. 5, S998-1004.

Yong, V. W., Power, C., Forsyth, P., and Edwards, D. R. (2001). Metalloproteinases in biology and pathology of the nervous system. *Nat. Rev. Neurosci.* 2, 502-511.

Yoshihara, K., Matsushita, O., Minami, J., and Okabe, A. (1994). Cloning and nucleotide sequence analysis of the colH gene from Clostridium histolyticum encoding a collagenase and a gelatinase. *J. Bacteriol.* 176, 6489-6496.

Zhao, B., Janson, C. A., Amegadzie, B. Y., D'Alessio, K., Griffin, C., Hanning, C. R., Jones, C., Kurdyla, J., McQueney, M., Qiu, X., et al. (1997). Crystal structure of human osteoclast cathepsin K complex with E-64. *Nat. Struct. Biol.* 4, 109-111.

Zhao, G. Y., Chen, X. L., Zhao, H. L., Xie, B. B., Zhou, B. C., and Zhang, Y. Z. (2008). Hydrolysis of insoluble collagen by deseasin MCP-01 from deep-sea Pseudoalteromonas sp. SM9913: collagenolytic characters, collagen-binding ability of C-terminal polycystic kidney disease domain, and implication for its novel role in deep-sea sedimentary particulate organic nitrogen degradation. *J. Biol. Chem.* 283, 36100-36107.

In: Type I Collagen
Editors: Maria Eduarda Henriques and Marcio Pinto
ISBN: 978-1-62257-625-8

Chapter III

TYPE I COLLAGEN AND ITS UTILITY AS SPECIFIC BONE MARKER

***S. M. Friedman*[1] *and S. N. Zeni*[2]**

[1]Head of Department of Oral Biochemistry, School of Dentistry, Buenos Aires University, Buenos Aires, Argentina

[2]Department of Oral Biochemistry, School of Dentistry and Osteopathy Medical Section. Clinical Hospital "Jose de San Martin," Buenos Aires University; Laboratory of Bone Metabolic Diseases. Institute of Inmmunology, Genetic and Metabolism (INIGEM), CONICET, Argentina

ABSTRACT

Collagens are proteins centrally involved in the formation of fibrillar and microfibrillar networks of the extracellular matrix. The biosynthesis of collagens starting with gene transcription within the nucleus, to the aggregation of collagen heterotrimers into large fibrils is a complex multistep process. It is characterized by the presence of a large number of co- and post-translational modifications, many of them being unique to collagens or collagen-like proteins. The fibril-forming collagens are synthesized as procollagens which is released to the extracellular space where undergo several modifications: removal of large procollagen N- and C-terminal peptides, ordered aggregation, crosslink formation. Biochemically, collagen is composed of a triple helix which consists of three α-chains. The amino acid composition of collagen is atypical for proteins, particularly with respect to its high hydroxyproline (Hyp) content. However, their size, function and tissue distribution vary considerably among collagens. To date, more than twenty genetically distinct collagen types have been described; being type I collagen the most abundant and best studied collagen of the body. It forms more than 90% of the organic mass of bone and is the major collagen of tendons, skin, ligaments, cornea, and many interstitial connective tissues with the exception of very few tissues such as hyaline cartilage, brain, and vitreous body. The collagen type I triple helix is usually formed as a heterodimer by two identical α1(I)-chains and one α2(I)-chain. In most organs and notably in tendons and fascia, type I collagen gives tensile stiffness and in bone, it defines substantial biomechanical properties regarding load bearing, tensile strength, and torsional stiffness in particular after calcification. The post-translational modifications of the collagenous matrix are important for both its structural and mechanical properties, and disruption of the cross-linking can result in severe dysfunction of the tissue. Both, biosynthesis and breakdown products are used in medicine as specific and sensitive bone markers to evaluate bone remodelling. In this regard N-terminal procollagen type I (PICP) is used as a bone formation marker while the crosslinks and the N and C-telopeptides (NTX and CT, respectively) are used as bone resorption markes.

BACKGROUND

Collagens can be defined as "structural proteins of the ECM which contain one or more domains harboring the conformation of a collagen triple helix (van der Rest M, Garrone R, 1991). It is probably the most abound protein in the human body and the major constituent in the extracellular matrix (ECM) of most connective tissues. To date, more than twenty genetically distinct collagen types have been described. Biochemically, all collagens shear an unusual amino acid composition containing in three polypeptide chains which constitutes the basic unit named tropocollagen. Each collagen polypeptide, designated as α chain, exists as a left-handed helical polypeptide about 1000 residues long in which every third residue is glycine (Gly) resulting in a (Gly-X-Y) n sequence (Kielty CM, Shuttlewort CA, 1993). The three α-chains are intertwined in a right-handed helix to form the triple helix in which the Gly residues occupy the center of the structure; the other amino acids are in the outer positions (van der Rest M, Garrone R. 1991). About one-third of the X positions are occupied by proline and a similar number of Y positions are hydroxyproline (Hyp) (a posttranslationally modified form of proline). These amino acids have their side chains pointing outward of the helix, at the surface of the protein offering an exceptional potential for lateral interactions, particularly with other triple helices which is a unique characteristic of collagen molecules (Ramachandra GN, Reddi AH, 1976). The triple helix wound around each other in a unique type of helical structure to form a thin rigid rod with a molecular mass of around 300,000 Da which provides specific properties and functions to each type of collagen in the body.

Collagens can be classified into subfamilies based on their quaternary structure. These subfamilies include fibrillar, fibril associated with interrupted triple-helices (FACIT), short chain, basement membrane, multiplexins, and membrane associated with interrupted triple-helices (MACIT) (Cole W, 1994). The fibrous types represent the first members of the collagen superfamily to be discovered and the major products synthesized by connective tissue cells (fibroblasts, osteoblasts and chondrocytes). In all the fibrillar collagen the monomeric molecules polymerise to form striated fibers that are stabilized by intermolecular cross-links, thereby preventing the long rod-like collagen molecules from sliding past each other under stress (Bailey AJ. et al., 1980). As a consequence, they form virtually inextensible fibers, providing exceptional tensile strength and resistance to external mechanical forces. The major supporting fibrillar collagen are types I, II, III which represent more than the 80 – 90 percent of this protein in the body, and the minor fibrillar collagens are V and XI. The fibrillar collagens are all composed of a large continuous triple helix (COL1) bordered by non-triple-helical (NC) globular domains that form N- and C-terminal extensions called N- and C-propeptides respectively (Hohenester E, Domain J, 2002). The C-propeptide is referred to as the NC1 domain; the N-propeptide is divided into sub-domains: a short sequence (NC2) that links the major triple helix to the minor one (COL2), and a globular N-terminal end (NC3). Whereas the NC1 domains are well conserved among the fibrillar collagen members, the NC3 domains show significant variations. The NC3 domains of α1(I), α1(IIA) and α1(III) chains all harbor a cystein-rich repeat domain characterized by the presence of 10 cysteine residues in their sequence, which form disulfide bonds (Bornstein P, 2002). Fibrillar collagens are associates with the FACIT collagens (Type IX, XII and XIV) which could mediate interactions between fibrillar collagens and other components, or the ECM, or between fibrillar collagens and cells. The type I collagen is associated with XII and XIV collagens molecules.

TYPE I COLLAGEN

Type I collagen is the most abundant and best studied collagen of the body. It comprises 90% of the organic matrix of bone and, together with the mineral, governs the biomechanical properties and functional integrity of this tissue. It is also found in tendon, skin and vascular system. The fundamental structural unit of type I collagen is a long (300-nm), thin (1.5-nm-diameter) heterodimer molecule. Its triple helical structure consists of two identical α1(I)- and one α2(I)-domains that, together with the primary sequence, are identical to type I collagen found elsewhere in the body, although it has distinctive features of posttranslational chemistry, notably in its profile of cross-linking amino acids (Eyre et al., 1988). The polypeptide chains are synthesized individually with identical length triple helix $(Gly\text{-}X\text{-}Y)^{338}$ structural domains, but the α1- and α2-chains have distinctive amino (N-) and carboxyl (C-) terminal extension both, telo- and pro-peptides. Type I collagen is particularly synthesized by fibroblasts and osteoblasts as a soluble molecule called procollagen. The biosynthesis of such molecule is a complex process as a number of posttranslational modification reactions are needed to render the protein with the characteristics necessary for its correct conformation and cross-link formation. The biosynthetic pathway includes two steps: one intracellular and other extracellular. In humans, the gene coding for the α1 chain of type I collagen (COL1A1) is located on the long arm of chromosome 17 (17q21.3-q22), and the gene coding for the α2 chain (COL1A2) is located on the long arm of chromosome 7 (7q21.3-q22). After transcription of both, α1 and α2 chains, the mature mRNAs are translated into membrane bound ribosomes. The nascent polypeptide chains undergo extensive enzymatic posttranslational modifications (Prockop DJ, Kivirikko K, 1984). In the cisternae of the rough endoplasmic reticulum (ER) both, the pro-α1 and pro-α2 chains undergo first the hydroxylation of proline and lysine (Lys) to hydroxyproline (Hyp) and hydroxylisine (Hyl) by two different hydroxylase enzymes. These modifications are essential for assembly the type I collagen chains in a triple helix and then released into the ECM. The major triple helix of the molecule forms spontaneously; it starts from the C-terminal propeptide domains of the chains which is strengthened by intra and inter chains-disulfide bridges; the N-terminal propeptide, is the last to assume its native conformation and it only content intra disulfide bridges. The formation of the helix stops the posttranslational modification reactions in the ER. The hydroxyl groups in the Hyp residues give stability to the triple helix collagen by forming hydrogen bridges between different chains. In the absence of Hyp, the collagen chains cannot form a proper helical structure, and the resultant molecule is weak and quickly destroyed (Bienkowski RS et al., 1978). The Hyl is essential to support glycosylation which imparts unique chemical and structural characteristics to the newly formed collagen molecule and may influence fibril size (Kivirikko KI, Myllyla R, 1979). The highest activities of glycosylation enzymes are found in the very young people and decrease with aging (Anttinen H et al., 1977). Unlike the Hyp which is found only in helical regions of the molecule, the Hyl is present both in the helical region and in the small non-helical regions terminals; in this late region it has an important role in the formation of intermolecular cross-links. The content of Hyp residues per α-chain do not differ greatly among the type I collagen of different tissues (Clik EM, Bornstein P, 1970). Conversely Hlp content can vary from 4-15 residues per□□-chain (Barnes et al., 1973, Eyre and Muir 1975). It is low in dermis and bone and high in fibrocartilage. The Lys hydroxylation pattern within bone type I collagen presents different characteristic as compared to the skin and other non-mineralized tissues and is evidenced from the chemistry of the cross-links formed. The resulting peptide possesses N- and C-terminal extensions to the collagen helix called propeptides PINP and PICP, respectively (Figure 1). Both ends confer solubility to the procollagen to be transported easily within the cell to the site where this large precursor form is secreted into the ECM (Dehm P et al., 1972). As the procollagen is secreting out specific proteolytic enzymes called procollagen proteinases rapidly remove both propeptides (Lapiere CM et al., 1971). The removal of the bulky, globular PICP is a necessary prerequisite for the assembly of the collagen to fibrils, whereas the PINP, more rod-like propeptide can for some time remain attached to part of the collagen molecules, which are on the surface of the fibrils. As the fibril grows in thickness, the removal of the PINP also reaches completion.

The propeptides are two different proteins, yet produced in equimolar amounts with each other and with the collagen deposited in the tissue (Melkko J et al., 1996). Propeptide cleavage dramatically decreases the solubility of the resulting protein often called tropocollagen or simply collagen (Fessler LI et al., 1975). Excision of both propeptides allows the collagen molecules to polymerize into normal fibrils in the ECM. As the triple helical collagen molecules line up and begin to form fibrils and then fibers, another post-translational modification takes place. Indeed, during fibrillogenesis some Lys and Hyl residues are deaminated by other specialized enzymes called lysine and hydroxylisine oxidase to form the aldehyde derivatives, respectively which spontaneously associate with ε-NH_2 groups from lysyl or hydroxylysyl residue of adjacent molecules forming intra and inter chains cross-links. This step is called crosslink formation and is the critical step that increases the tensile strength of the fibrils (Bailey AJ et al., 1974). The three α-chains in the tropocollagen molecule are helical polypeptides however a non-helical of 15 to 20 amino acids named telopeptides are surrounding the N and C-terminal regions (figure 1).

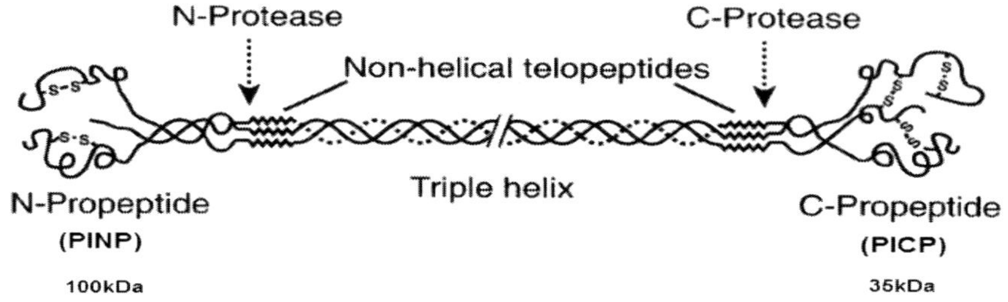

Figure 1. Type I procollagen molecule. Specific proteases cleave the N-terminal propeptide (PINP) and C-terminal propeptide (PICP) releasing these into the circulation (Modified fromf: Hale LV et al., 2007).

These regions are susceptible to proteolysis, while the triple helix is resistant to the attack of the majority of proteolytic enzymes. These telopeptides are involved in the covalent cross-linking of the collagen molecules as well as linking to other structures of the matrix. Although cross-linking occurs extracellularly, the nature of the cross-link also depends on the previous intracellular post-translational modifications to the collagen molecule, in particular, hydroxylation of Lys residues. The extent of their hydroxylation, both within the triple helical sequences and the terminal N- and C-telopeptides, varies greatly between collagen types and tissues. Hydroxylation of specific Lys governs the nature of the cross-link formed, and as a consequence, the biomechanical properties of the tissue_(Ebeling PR et al., 1992). For example, bone has a clear deficiency in the extent of cross-linking by the mature pyridinoline cross-links (only one cross-link per five collagen molecules). In addition, bone possesses highly hydroxylated cross-links, the ketoimines and the pyridinolines which are largely restricted to mineralizing tissues. The tropocollagen is characterized by the ability to assemble into highly orientated supramolecular aggregates with a characteristic supraestructure, the typical quarter-staggered fibril-array forming microfibrils. The resistance of these structures is due to covalent bond between different triple tropocollagen helix. Unlike the majority of proteins that are cross-linked by disulfide, collagen molecules, without cysteine residues, condense Lys and Hyl residues in adjacent chains to form cross-links.

Clinical Use of C- and N-Propeptides

Both, PINP and PICP are cleaved by specific proteinases before the collagen molecules are assembled into fibers. Both peptides can be found in the circulation where their concentrations reflect the rate of synthesis of type I collagen. PICP has a molecular weight (MW) of 115 kDa; it is composed of three equal peptide chains which are stabilized by disulphide bridges. It is globular in shape and due to post-translational glycosilation content high-mannose type oligosaccharides. It has a short serum half-life of 6–8 minutes because it is cleared shortly after synthesis by liver endothelial cells via the mannose receptor (Olsen BR et al., 1977; Smedsrod B et al., 1990). PINP has a MW of only 70 kDa. It is a partly helical, partly globular protein with two equal size alpha 1(I) chains and one shorter part of alpha 2(I) chain. The molecule is rich in proline and Hyp and is phosphorylated. The type I collagen is being synthesized in osteoblasts and deposited as osteoid in the resorption cavity, the release of the PINP may be somewhat delayed and takes place at the latest during the matrix maturation phase of osteoblast development. For that, it has a half-life longer than PICP and it is cleared from the circulation by liver endothelial cells scavenger receptor (Melkko J et al., 1994). Most of the 400 and 1200 g of collagen produced in the adult human body per year is type I collagen.

This indicates that between 150 and 500 g of propeptide material is set free in the same time, about one third of this being PINP and the rest PICP. Since both PICP and PINP are generated from newly synthesized collagen in a stoichiometric fashion, they are considered quantitative measures of newly formed type I collagen. Although type I collagen propeptides may also arise from other sources, most of the non-skeletal tissues exhibit a slower turnover than bone, and contribute very little to the circulating propeptide pool. Both propeptides are currently measured by specific immunoassays (Taubman MB et al., 1974; Melkko J et a., 1990). Different studies have shown good correlations between serum PICP levels and the rate of bone formation (Eriksen EF et at, 1993; Hassager C et al., 1991); however, the clinical relevance of PICP in metabolic bone diseases evaluation is still viewed with skepticism (Ebeling PR et a., 1992; Charles P. et al., 1994); conversely, the serum PINP appears to be of greater diagnostic validity. Serum PINP levels could be low in children suffering osteogenesis imperfecta, a bone genetic disorder caused by mutations in COL1 or COL2 gene (Lund AM et al., 1998). Recently, the joint Working Group on Bone Marker Standards (WG-BMS) of the International Federation of Clinical Chemistry and Laboratory Medicine (IFCC) and the International Osteoporosis Foundation (IOF) recommends the use of serum PINP as bone synthesis reference marker in the prediction of fracture risk and for monitoring treatment of osteoporosis. (Vasikaran S. et al., 2011). In addition, serum PINP is also a useful indicator of other bone diseases such as the activity of Paget disease or bone metastases of osteoblastic nature. In this regard, PINP levels have been shown to be helpful in the management of bone spread from various malignant disorders (particularly breast cancer, prostate carcinoma and multiple myeloma) at both early and advanced disease stages (Koizumi M et al., 2001; Klepzig M et al., 2009). Serum levels of PINP are also correlated to the bone loss after menopause in breast cancer patients without evidence of relapse (Saarto T. et al., 2007). The synthesis of type I collagen is avoid for glucocorticoids administration which can be evidenced by a decrease in concentration levels of PINP (Oikarinen A, et al., 1992; Autio A. et al.,1994). In this regard, the PINP levels could also be a useful marker for monitoring the response to alendronate or teriparatide in glucocorticoid-induced osteoporosis patients (Burshell AL, et al., 2010).

Ageing Molecular Changes in the Structural Components Type I Collagen

Aging affects intra and extra cellular proteins, which are subjected to a variety of spontaneous chemical degradation reactions under physiological conditions. Tropocollagen is susceptible to age-related changes which although have been known for several decades (Verzar F, 1964; Viidik A, 1982), the molecular mechanisms are only now being unraveled.

a) β-Aspartyl Isomerization and Racemization

The isomerization and racemization of aspartyll residues is an unusual modification of collagen occurring with age in long lived proteins (Clarke, 1987). ach of the two C-terminal telopeptide α1-chain of type I collagen consists of a 26-amino acid sequence (Kadler K, 1994) which contains an Asp-Gly (DG) sequence that is a potential site for β-isomerization (Figure 2). The biological role of β-isomerization is not known yet; however several studies had demonstrated that it is often accompanied by a decreased physiological protein/peptide activity (Hayakawa Y, 1994). By the process of □-isomerization, the peptide backbone is transferred from the aspartyl α-carboxyl group to the side chain β-carboxyl group, resulting in a perturbation of the peptide backbone (Fledelius C,et al., 1997). The peptide backbone nitrogen attack on the side chain carbonyl group of an adjacent Asp residue results in the formation of a five-member succinimide ring.

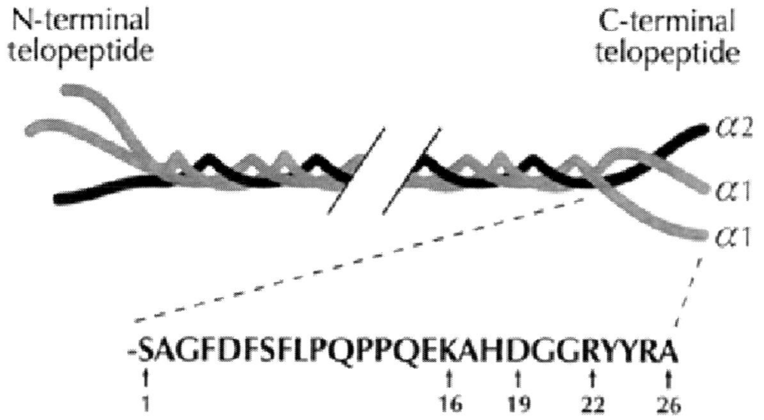

Figure 2. Amino acid composition of C-terminal telopeptide. Fledelius C et al., 1997).

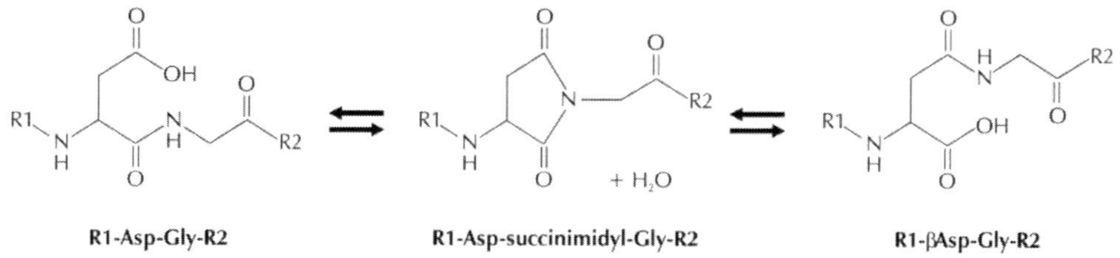

Figure 3. Asp–Gly Beta-isomerization in the collagen type I telopeptide with increasing age (Fledelius C et al., 1997).

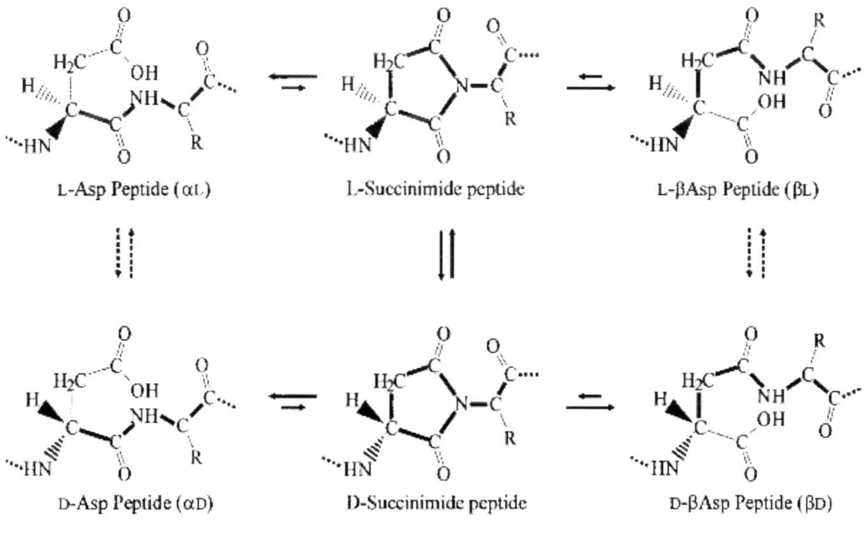

Figure 4. Schematic racemization and isomerization of the R1 As (Cloos PAC, Fledelius C, 2000).

A metastable succinimide forms after a spontaneous nucleophilic attack of the peptide bond α-amino group of the side-chain β-carboxyl group. This intermediate hydrolyzes to a mixture of Asp (α CTX) and isoaspartyl (β CTX) residues, as well as other minor biproducts (Figure 3). It has been shown that the specific $A^{1209}HDGGR^{1214}$ sequence of the C-telopeptide of the α1 chain of type I collagen can also undergo racemization (Fledelius, C et al., 1997; Cloos PAC, Fledelius C, 2000). When type I collagen molecules are synthesized, the Asp residue is in the native L-enantiomeric form. By the process of racemization there is a conversion of naturally occurring L-amino acids to the biologically rare D-isomers. The initial step appears to be the nucleophilic attack of the Asp side-chain carbonyl group by the peptide-bond nitrogen, to form an unstable five-membered L-succinimide ring which is prone to hydrolysis and racemization. This reaction yields peptides and β-Asp peptides in both the D and L configurations leading to the formation of four end-products (Figure 4). The spontaneous non-enzymatic chemical reaction of isomerization and racemization, occur in several proteins in vivo and their end-products could represent a potential biochronological tool for investigating bone turnover in vivo (Figure 4). In addition, most experimental evidence currently suggests that the processes of Asp racemization and isomerization (RI) are interdependent reactions, and that the accumulation of D-Asp in polypeptides is determined primarily by the rate of succinimide formation (Geiger T, Clarke S, 1987; Brennan TV, Clarke S, 1995; Radkiewicz J L et al., 1996). The N-telopeptides suffer these modifications too (Brady J. et al., 1999). However, the Asp-Gly sequence in the α2(I) N-telopeptide is located directly adjacent to the cross-linking Lys which would confer some additional resistance to proteolysis.

b) Intermolecular Cross-Linking

Perhaps the most important changes in bone type I collagen with age involve the formation of intermolecular cross-links. These cross-links are initially formed to provide an optimum function but can subsequently over-stiffen the fibres when present in excess. The two major cross-link processes are:

1) *Enzymatic Cross-Links*: this process occurring at N- and C- terminal telopeptides induces an initial fibres stabilization to provide positive effects on the bone mechanical properties (Figure 5).
2) *Glycation - or Oxidation-Induced Non-Enzymatic Cross-Links:* [advanced glycation end products (AGEs)]: this process is based on the reaction with glucose or its metabolites that occurs with age and lead to microdamage and bone fragility.

1. Lysyl Oxidase-Derived Cross-Links

The cross-linking mechanism occurs at specific Lys and Hyl residues and is based upon aldehyde formation by the enzyme lysyl-oxidase which activity decreases with age (Figure 6). Although type I collagen is genetically identical in all tissues, its heterogeneity is attributed mainly to the quantitative differences in the conversion of Lys and Hyl residues that, in turn, depends on the lysyl-oxidase activity. This EC enzyme acts only upon telopeptide residues when bound to a highly conserved amino acid sequence (Hyl-Gly-His-Arg-Gly). This sequence is a conserved feature of the fibrous collagens and in bone type I collagen is located in two intermolecular sites: one linking two C-terminal telopeptides to residue 87 of the triple helix α1 or α2 chain, and the other linking two N-terminal telopeptides to residue 930 of the triple helix α1 chain (Kühn K, 1982). After this initial enzymatic step, the telopeptide Lys-aldehydes condense with either Lys or Hyl residues at the two intermolecular sites of the triple helix to form reducible Schiff bases. The amino acid Lys (K), located at position 9N and at the position 16C in the telopeptides, reacts and condensate with Lys or Hyl residues in the two triple helical region of an adjacent collagen molecule to give characteristic divalent immature cross-links called dehydro-hydroxylysino-norleucine (deH-HLNL) and dehydro-lysine-norleucine (DeH-LNL) (Eyre DR. et al.,1984).

They spontaneously undergo Amadori rearrangement to form hydroxylysino-5-k-ketonorleucine (HLKNL) and lysino-ketonorleucine (LKNL), respectively. As bone is less hydroxylated than tendon, skin or cartilage, the immature cross-links are primarily derived from the telopeptide hydroxylysyl-aldehydes, the major cross-link being the keto-imine HLKNL. In soft connective tissues such as skin, cornea and sclera, which lack significant telopeptide lysyl hydroxylase activity, the divalent aldimine-type cross-links predominate (Robins SP, Brady JD, 2002). A portion of divalent immature cross-links is considered to undergo a spontaneous reaction with another telopeptide Lys or Hyl aldehyde to form trivalent mature pyridinium or pyrrole cross-links (figure 3). However, while the pyrrole crosslinks probably form between three adjacent collagen molecules, the pyridinium crosslinks connect two collagen molecules together (Robins SP, Duncan A, 1983).

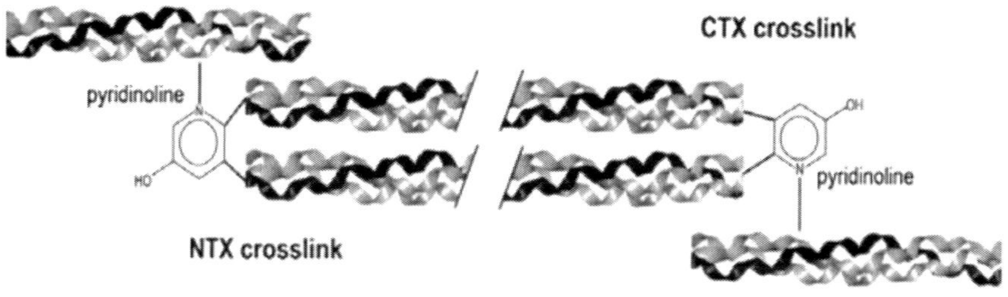

Figure 5. N - and C - terminal pyridinoline crooslinks (Modified from Cloos PAC, Fledelius C, 2000).

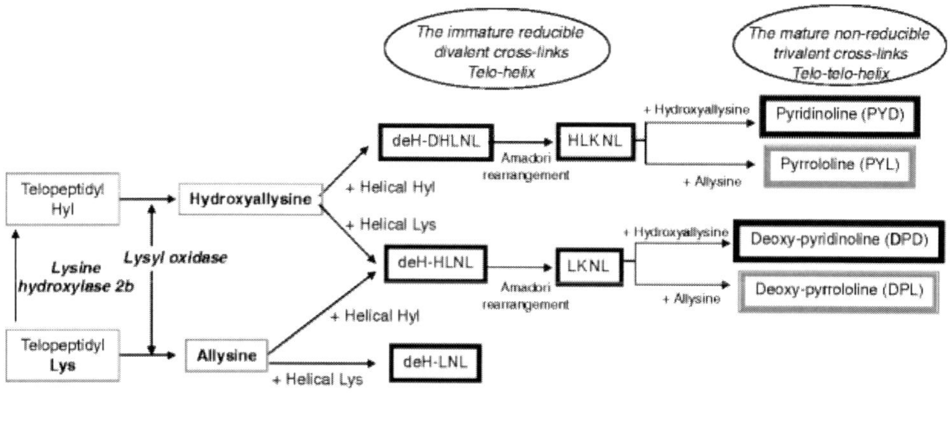

Figure 6. Enzymatic pathway of cross-link formation in bone collagen (Modified from Saito M, Marumo K, 2010).

The trivalent mature pyridinoline cross-links are hydroxylysyl-pyridinoline also known as pyridinoline (PYD) and lysyl-pyridinoline also known as deoxypyridinoline (DPD) (Eyre DR, Oguchi H, 1980). The proposed mechanism of pyridinium cross-link formation is thought to be derived from an immature divalent cross-link by reaction with another immature divalent cross-link or with a free hydroxyallysine in another collagen telopeptide. However, this reaction has not been demonstrated directly (Saito M, Marumo K, 2010). When the lysyl hydroxylase activity is lower the telopeptide Lys are not completely hydroxylated, leading to the reaction of a lysyl aldehyde with HLKNL resulting in a pyrrole derivative (Figures 6-7). Unfortunately, the concentration of pyrrole is difficult to determine because of its instability. Human bone appears to contain similar amounts of pyrrole and pyridinoline crosslinks (Ristelli J et al., 1994). The proportion of divalent keto-imine cross-links has been reported to be approximately 1 mol/mol of collagen in young bones and to decrease with age to 0.4 mol/mol of collagen (Eyre DR, 1987). With time, they can mature to trivalent forms, which include the hydroxylysyl-(HP) and lysyl-(LP) pyridinolines, hydroxylysyl- and lysyl pyrroles and most likely other, as yet, uncharacterised cross-links (Brady JD, Robins SP, 2001; Eyre DR, 1987; Hansen DA, Eyre DR, 1996; Yamauchi M, Mechanic GL, 1988). The total amount of pyridinium cross-links (HP + LP) in bone collagen, assessed by chemical cross-link analyses, has been found to be as low as 0.2–0.3 mol/mol of collagen (Eyre DR, 1987; Hansen DA, Eyre DR, 1996). From this, it has been estimated that majority of the cross-links in bone collagen are immature in their nature (Oxlund H, et al. 1996). Pyridinium crosslinks are located at both N- and C-terminal ends of collagen, DPD predominate at the N-terminal region (Hanson DA, Eyre DR, 1996), and is found primarily in calcified tissues (Eyre DR, 1981). Pyrrole, as DPD, also seems to be preferentially located at the N-terminal ends of the molecule (Hansen DA, Eyre DR, 1996).

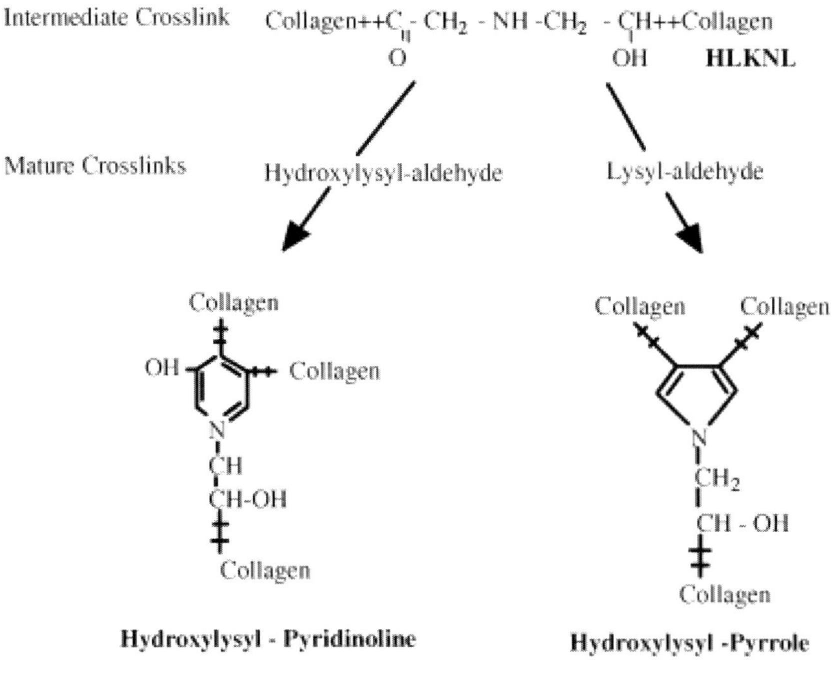

Figure 7. Maturation of lysyl-oxidase induced cross-links (Avery NC, Bailey AJ, 2005).

The difference in location of the pyridinoline crosslinks and pyrrole suggests different functions for each of these molecules. Knott L and Bailey AJ and colleagues speculated that pyrrole forms interfibrillar crosslinks, whereas the pyridinoline would preferentially form intrafibrillar crosslinks (Knott L, Bailey AJ, 1998; Bailey AJ, et al., 1998). Collagen crosslinking is important to the biomechanical properties, to the strength, and to the mineralization of bone (Wassen MHM et al., 2000; Saito M, Marumo K, 2010). In fact, the DPD/PYR ratio correlated with the cancellous bone strength and stiffness determined by compression test, the higher the ratio the stronger and stiffer the bone (Banse X et al., 2002). Although with increasing age there is a significant loss of bone that lead to a decrease in the mechanical strength, the composition of bone collagen and cross-links nature remains constant (Bailey AJ et al., 1999). In adults, the PYD/DPD ratio remains constant at about 3.5 although their concentrations are lower in trabecular bone than in cortical bone (Eyre DR et al., 1988). In contrast, there was no difference in the content of pyrrole cross-links between cortical and cancellous bone (Knott L, Bailey AJ, 1999).

2. Non-Enzymic Glycosylation-Derived Cross-Links (Glycation)

The glycation is likely to be more important in proteins possessing a long biological half-life, such as mature collagen, and plays a central role in the pathogenesis of ageing (Cerami A. et al., 1987; Paul RG, Bailey AJ, 1996). The non-enzymatic glycation of the side-chains of Lys and Arg results in advanced glycation end-products (AGEs) cross-links. The initial reaction is a Schiff base formation followed by a spontaneous Amadori rearrangement (figure 8); these reactions occurs in a time-dependent manner, are regulated by tissue turnover rate (Saito M. et al., 2008; Saito M et al., 2010), oxidative stress (Saito M. et al. 2006), or glycation level (Vashishth D, 2007; Garnero P, et al. 2006). Modifications of Lys or Arg side-chains, without involvement of telopeptides, by reaction with glucose clearly alter the charge profile of the molecules. The glycation reactions are enhanced in diabetic subjects due to hyperglycemia; they occur during ageing and affect several properties of collagen such as its optimal biochemical functioning, interaction with cells, remodeling or even it action as an oxidizing agent. Both, the Schiff base and the Amadori product subsequently undergo oxidation, particularly in the presence of metal ions and reactive oxygen species (ROS). The resulting products of glycoxidation may fragment to more reactive species such as 3-deoxyglucosome, glyoxal (GO) and methyl glyoxal (MGO), both of which react rapidly with Lis and Arg to form AGEs (Figure 9). The most damaging types of AGEs are probably those forming intermolecular cross-links; this effect decreases the critical flexibility and permeability of the tissues and renders it more resistant to enzymes reducing the turnover. The only well-characterized glycation cross-link shown to be present in tissues in vivo is pentosidine which derived from Lys, Arg and ribose; it is a well-established intermolecular cross-linking AGE used as a surrogate marker of whole AGEs (Saito M, Marumo K, 2010; Viguet-Carrin S et al., 2006; Garnero P, et al., 2006) (Figure 8). Glycated collagen has the ability to accelerate the oxidation of compounds such as lipids, and produce the potential cross-linking compound, malondialdehide (MDA) (Hicks M. et al., 1988). MDA can diffuse from their site of origin in membranes and react with intracellular or extracellular targets, such as protein and, it will not only have a direct affect upon collagen function but may also act as a link between glycation and further lipid peroxidation.

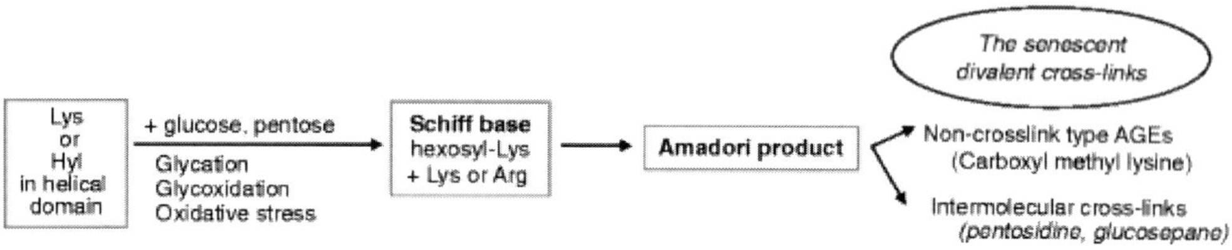

Figure 8. Non-enzymatic pathway of AGEs formation in bone collagen (Modified from: Saito M, Marumo K, 2010).

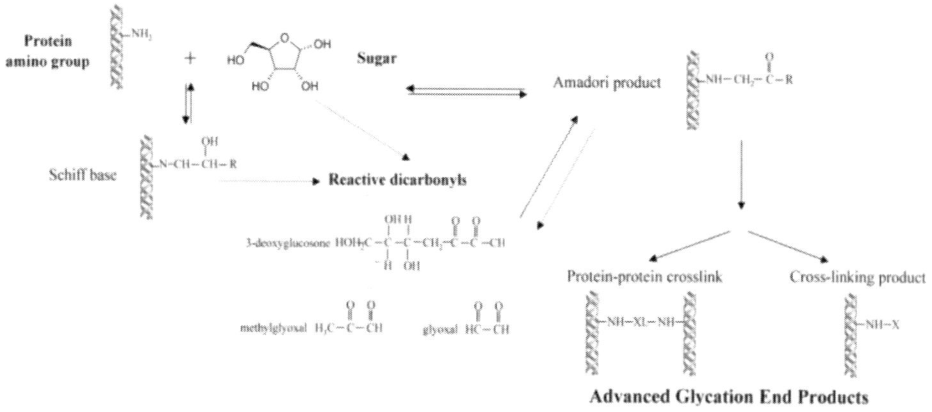

Figure 9. Pathways of advanced glycation end products (Viguet-Carrin S. et al. 2006).

In addition, MDA type cross linking will decrease the turnover of the collagen and consequently result in an increase in its susceptibility to further glycation propagating a vicious circle of protein and fatty acid damage. This possible important aspect of glycation reactions of collagen have recently expanded to include the action of the aldehydic products derived from lipid oxidation (Baynes JW, Thorpe SR, 2000) known as ALEs; although there is no evidence of an age-accumulation of ALEs yet. There have been described several AGEs specific receptors (RAGEs); the mechanism involves in the interaction AGE-RAGE has also been linked to the development of pathological conditions resulting from AGE formation. In this regard, several pharmaceutical interventions were evaluated to attempts or inhibit AGEs formation and hence alleviate the glycation effect during ageing. Some agents were assessed as drug to inhibit the detrimental effects of excessive protein cross-linking, although with different efective results. Among them, pyridoxamine has also been shown to be an effective inhibitor of both AGEs (Onorato JM et al., 2000) and ALEs (Metz TO et al., 2003) although the primary mechanism is as yet unknown.

Collagen Breakdown

In the collagen metabolism the complex process of degradation is as important as the step of formation. In this regard, type I collagen, like other proteins, undergoes continues turnover to ensure the replacement of old tissue with new one (Chan GK, Duque G, 2002). Under normal healthy conditions, type I collagen turnover occurs at a very slow and controlled rate. Indeed, when type I collagen is fully hydroxylated and in a triple helical structure, it is resistant to the most proteases attack, and only specialized enzymes, called collagenases, can degraded the collagen molecule (Gross J. et al., 1974). However, the extent of collagen degradation could be quite extensive during rapid growth and several disease states (i.e osteoporosis, Paget disease, arthritis and cancer among others). Bone type I collagen is degraded after the hydroxyapatite dissolution that occurs at the very low pH generated by the release of hydrochloric acid by the osteoclast. The molecule is cleaved into several fragments in the extracellular phagolysosomal-like resorption compartment of the osteoclast. There are two types of proteolytic enzymes that breakdown the organic matrix of type I collagen: lysosomal cathepsins and matrix metalloproteinases (MMPs) (Everts V et al., 1998). At acidic pH, cathepsin K (cat K), attacks at multiple sites of the type I collagen, including several sites at the helical region (Garnero P et al. 1998). Thus, the triple helix becomes susceptible to further action of proteolytic enzymes, including MMPs 2, 9, 13, 14 at neutral pH later in the resorption process (Everts V et al., 1998). Cat K is selectively expressed by osteoclasts and appears to be the critical cysteine proteinase, is rate limiting for bone resorption, and is extremely efficient in type I collagen degradation; however, several data suggest that other proteolytic enzymes, either belonging or not belonging to the class of cysteine proteinases, could be involved in matrix degradation by osteoclasts (Brage M et al., 2005).

All the fragments induced by proteolysis are taken up by the cell and further digested intracellularly and/or excreted at the baso-lateral membrane (Chambers TJ, 2000); they enter into the circulation and are excreted by the urine (Bonde M et al., 1994, and 1996). Several fragments derived from mature type I collagen do not further metabolize by the liver and/or the kidney; their posttranslational modifications (i.e. cross-linking, glycosylation, etc.) protect them against a complete degradation securing their survival into urine (Cloos PAC et al., 1996). The subsequent detection of these fragments in serum or urine provides an index of collagen degradation (Bonde, M et al., 1996; Cloos PAC, et al., 1996; Rosenqvist, C et al., 1998). There are several biochemical bone-related molecules with more or less specificity for evaluating bone resorption which have been applied in the diagnosis and management of bone metabolic diseases (Delmas, P. D, 1993). It is important to take into account that urinary degradation products might also be derived from non-skeletal sources, as type I collagen is widely distributed in most connective tissues throughout the body; however, fragments derived from non-skeletal sources may often lack the post-traslational modifications and may consequently be unprotected against proteolysis, resulting in complete metabolism of such fragments (Cloos PAC et al., 1996).

Hyp is the major component of type I collagen in bone as well as in other tissues. It is released during bone resorption, and although not reutilized, 80–90% of the free form is metabolized in the liver. Only 1% of urinary Hyp is present as free amino acid while 90% is in the form of small peptides, the rest in larger peptides that are thought to be formed during bone formation rather than degradation. The urine Hyp levels were the first available bone resorption marker from type I collagen breakdown, however it can be originated by several sources. Indeed, only 50% of the Hyp in urine is from bone degradation, the other sources are collagen of other tissues, including skin, and other proteins like C1q fraction of complement. Moreover, the urinary levels of Hyp are affected by a diet containing meat, gelatin, etc (Robins SP, 1982). When bone turnover increase urinary Hyp increase although, the lack of tissue specificity, and the obstructive sensitivity to diet and other factors make it an unspecific bone resorption marker. Hyl is glycosylated and two glycosides are formed, galactosyl–hydroxylysine (Gal–Hyl) and glucosyl–galactosyl–hydroxylysine (Glc–Gal–Hyl), which also appear in the urine (Segrest JP, 1982). While Hyl and its glycosides are less abundant than Hyp in bone collagen, certain properties make Hyl theoretically a better marker of bone turnover than urinary Hyp. Gal–Hyl is not metabolized and not influenced by dietary factors (Prockop DJ, Kivirikko K, 1995). In normal urine, 80% of the total Hyl is in the form of Hyl, 10% is free and unglycosylated, and the remainder is peptide-bound, which suggests that free Hyl is largely metabolized and not excreted (Eyre DR, 1997). However, in addition to all structural collagens, both Hyp and Hyl are also found in certain serum proteins, such as the C1q component of complement. This disadvantage and others make Hyl a less specific indice of bone resorption and therefore it has been largely replaced by newer markers. Type I collagen fibers are stabilized by covalent pyridinium cross-links between molecules which render the corresponding parts of the polypeptide chains relatively resistant to the action of degrading enzymes. These cross-links are formed during the collagen maturation and the end products of DPD and PYD are released into circulation during breakdown of bone and cartilage. They are no further metabolized (Eyre DR, 1992) and are cleared by the urine. Forty percent of them are found in the free form while the rest are peptide-bound; they are normally excreted into urine in a PYD/DPD ratio of 3.8-6.0, which is almost comparable to that found in bone.

This indicates that the majority of these urinary pyridinium cross-links are mainly derived from bone (Delmas PD, 1993; Eyre DR, 1993). Unlike Hyp excretion, pyridinium cross-links excretion is not influenced by the diet, a fact that may partly explain its improved performance compared to Hyp when measured in 24- hour collections. In early 90's, a commercially enzyme immunoassay (ELISA) for measuring pyridinolines as bone resorption marker became available (Robins SP, 1982). This assay measured both, DPD and PYD, either free or peptide-bound with a MW less than 1000 Daltons (Seyedin SM et al., 1993). However, DPD is almost exclusively found in bone and dentin whereas PYD is also found in cartilage, ligaments and vessels. For that reason, assays for measuring only free DPD were further developed (Robins SP et al., 1994; Rosano TG et al., 1998). The main molecular sites involved in collagen cross-linking are the short non-helical peptides at both ends of the collagen molecule, termed amino- (N) and carboxy- (C) terminal telopeptides. In normal collagen, these telopeptides are each linked via pyridinium or pyrrole compounds to the helical portion of neighbouring collagen molecules (Herrmann M, Seibel M, 2008). During collagen breakdown, N- and C-terminal telopeptide fragments of various sizes, still attached to the helical portions of a nearby molecule by a pyridinium or pyrrole cross-link, are released into the circulation and cleared by the kidney. The N-terminal cross-linking telopeptide of type I collagen called NTX is a breakdown product of Cat K action. The NTX urine assay is based on a monoclonal antibody that specifically recognizes an epitope embedded in the α2(I)-chain of the N-telopeptide fragment. The peptide has the sequence QYDGKGVG where K is involved in a trivalent PYD or DPD cross-linking site (Hanson DA et al., 1992). The crosslink at the N-terminal telopeptide region forms predominantly between α1(I) and α2(I) or α2(I) and *a*2(I) chains of collagen, a feature that is found only in type I collagen in bone. The urinary NTX assay (Osteomark ®) (Hanson DA, et al., 1992) uses an antibody that recognizes a crosslink containing sequence from the α2(I) N-telopeptide. The crosslink itself is not involved in the epitope (Robins SP, 1995). The antibody does not react with the linear peptide sequence, but needs to have the conformation of the crosslink peptide; the binding is not dependent on the nature of the cross-link because the antibody does not recognize PYD or DPD per se (Figure 10). Although an assay for measuring NTX in serum had been developed which has not become as widely used as urinary NTX. Related to the crosslink at the C-terminal telopeptide region, two degradation fragments have been characterized: the C-terminal cross-linking telopeptide of type I collagen (CTX) and the pyridinoline cross-linked C-telopeptide domains of type I collagen (ICTP), now termed CTX-MMP (Delmas PD, 2001) (Figure 11).CTX and ICTP or CTXMMP respond differently according to the clinical situations and treatments. In this regard, urinary CTX levels are markedly increased in postmenopausal women compared with premenopausal controls, and their values decrease markedly and shortly after initiation of antiresorptive therapy to postmenopausal women with osteoporosis; conversely, only slight and non-significant changes of serum CTX-MMP in the same conditions were observed (Delmas PD et al., 2000). The reason for such differences is that both fragments are released through different collagenolytic pathways.

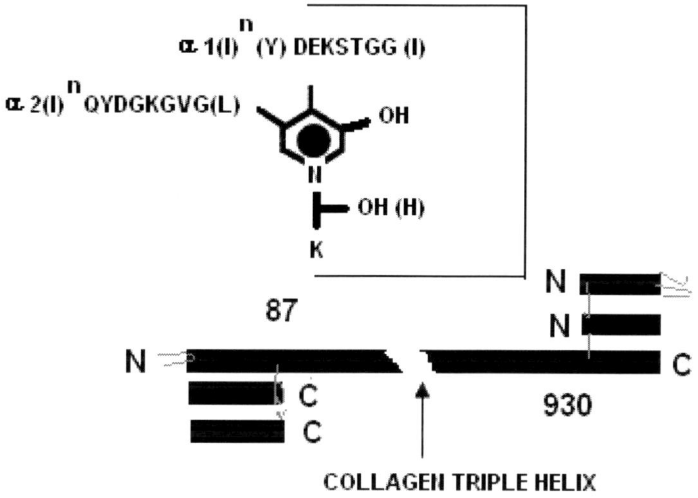

Figure 10. The structure of NTX antigen (Hanson DA et al., 1992).

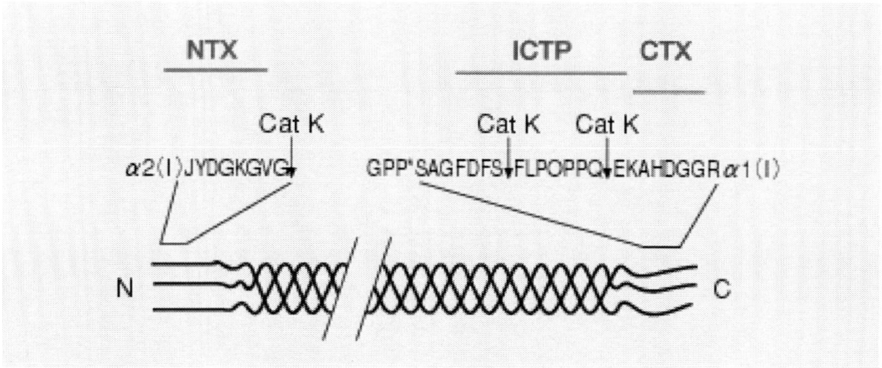

Figure 11. Different amino- (N) and carboxy- (C) terminal telopeptides; cat K sites of action (Soisumi M et al., 1999).

While CTX is generated by the Cat K–related pathway and functions in physiological bone turnover (Garnero P et al., 1998); CTXMMP antigen is generated by the MMPs pathway, which is typically involved in pathologic bone degradation (Garnero P, et al., 2003). Cat K destroys the ICTP epitope (Sassi ML et al., 2000). The serum assay for ICTP was the first of the telopeptides markers to be developed, but since the helical part of the α-chains is strongly conserved among different types of collagen, the specificity of this assay in reflecting bone resorption is not the best and it had been found to be less sensitive than other assays in clinical use (Risteli L et al., 1993; Garnero P. et al. 1994). For example, serum ICTP decreased in patients on estrogen replacement therapy (ERT) but did not return to baseline after ERT as did other markers of bone resorption, suggesting that it is not as sensitive as the other assays (Garnero P et al., 1994). MMP enzymes are expressed mainly in increased bone remodeling associated with neoplasic conditions.

In this regard, serum ICTP has however shown to be a valuable index of bone turnover in other pathological situations, including patients with bone metastases of breast, prostate and lung cancer cells and multiple myeloma (Koizumi M et al., 1999; Garnero P et al., 2003). CTX, like NTX are small enough to be readily clear by the kidney and then can be measured in serum or urine. The urinary CTX assay was first developed as an enzyme immunoassay (ELISA) using a synthetic antibody against an 8-aminoacid sequence from the C-telopeptide of α1 chains of human type I collagen which only requires one α1 chain to react (Bonde M et al., 1994) (Figure 12). This octapeptide contains the epitope with the Asp-Gly (DG) motif that is synthesized as αCTX (Alexandersen P et al., 2005) and can be isomerizated to βCTX in an age-dependent process (Chan GK et al., 1997; Fledelius C et al., 1997). The α and β form of CTX can be separately measured in urine (Bonde M et al. 1994; Fledelius C et al. 1997; Takahashi M et al., 1999) and each isoform per se provides a dynamic index of the rate at which bone is resorbed. Indeed, in urine from children only the 50% of the CTX is β-isomerized, whereas in urine from adults and in collagenase digests from old trabecular and cortical bone this β-isomerization reaches 70-80%. This seems to indicate that equilibrium with respect to β-isomerization is reached in old bone; it was suggest that in mineralized tissues such as bone almost reached equilibrium within a period of 3 years (Fledelius C. et al., 1997).

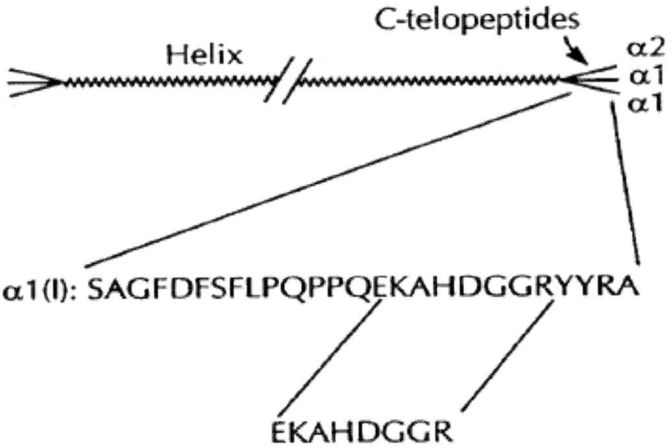

Figure 12. CTX telopeptide and antibody sequence (Pedersen BJ et al., 1998).

As αCTX and βCTX reflect degradation of young and old bone, respectively, quantification of the relative amounts of the newly synthesized α CTX form compared with the age-modified β CTX form (α/β ratio) can give an estimate of the average age of the resorbed bone collagen. The α/β ratio seems to be markedly increased in diseases characterized by significant localized increases in bone turnover at local skeletal sites. In this regard, Paget's disease is characterized by very high bone turnover in restricted areas of the skeleton, resulting in a disorganized mosaic of woven and lamellar bone at the affected sites (Siris ES, 1993). It is characterized by a highly increased rate of bone turnover, resulting in degradation of relatively newly formed (young) bone. The urinary ratio found in patients with Paget's disease is markedly elevated compared with that of age-matched healthy controls because the contribution of αCTX from the diseased areas is very high compared with βCTX (Fledelius C et al., 1997). In contrast, some conditions of highly increased systemic bone turnover (e.g., hyperparathyroidism) do not seem to involve significant changes in α/β ratios, although total CTX-levels (i.e., α and β CTX) are increased to approximately the same extent as in Paget's disease (Cloos PAC et al., 2003). The α/β ratio is also altered in clinical situations characterized by a marked increase in new bone formation such as skeletal fractures (Hoshino H et al., 1999), growing skeleton (Fledelius C et al., 1997; Cloos PAC, Fledelius C, 2000), bone metastases (Cloos PAC et al., 2003a; Cloos PAC, Christgau S, 2002; Cloos PAC et al., 2004; Garnero P et al., 1997).

The native form of CTX is ααCTX, composed of two crosslinked αCTX peptides (one from each of the two α(I)- chains of a collagen molecule), originates from newly synthesized collagen type I, whereas ββCTX is released from aged collagen type I. Thus, the ratio between αα and ββ CTX gives an indication of the bone matrix age, maturation, and possibly quality (Fledelius C et al., 1997). The urinary ratio between αα and ββ CTX represents the sum of all sites where bone is being remodeled. It has been shown that the mean age of bone assessed by αα/ββ CTX is lower in bone that is highly remodeled (trabecular bone) versus higher in less remodeled bone (cortical bone) (Cloos PA, Fledelius C, 2000) (Figure 13). It is known that the bone matrix age decreases as bone turnover is decreased during antiresorptive treatments. In this way, bisphosphonates, which markedly reduce bone resorption and bone turnover, induce a decrease in the αα/ββ CTX ratio, indicating an increase in bone tissue age (Leeming DJ et al., 2009). CTX fragments derived from newly synthesised collagen are of the native peptide form (L-aspartyl peptide (αL) where the Asp residue (D^{1211}) is on the L-enantiomeric form and is linked to the Gly residue (G^{1212}) through a peptide bond. With age CTX fragments will rearrange to three age-modified forms: the isomerized form (L-isoaspartyl peptide (βL), where the bond between the Asp and Gly residue goes through the β-carboxyl group of the aspartyl residue; the racemised form (D-aspartyl peptide [αD]), where the Asp (D1211) is on a D-enantiomeric form; and the isomerized and racemised form (D-isoaspartyl peptide [βD]) (Cloos PAC, Fledelius C, 2000) (Figure 4). The relative accumulation of the three age-modified forms is dependent on the balance between anabolic and catabolic processes in bone, and pathologic situations affecting these processes may thus also affect the relative amounts of the four CTX forms. Healthy adults had αL/βL CTx ratios <5 in a narrow, well defined range; osteoporotic patients an increase significant in this ratio while all patients with Paget's disease displayed αL/βL CTX ratios more than three standard deviation (SD) above the normal mean (Cloos PAC, Fledelius C, 2000).

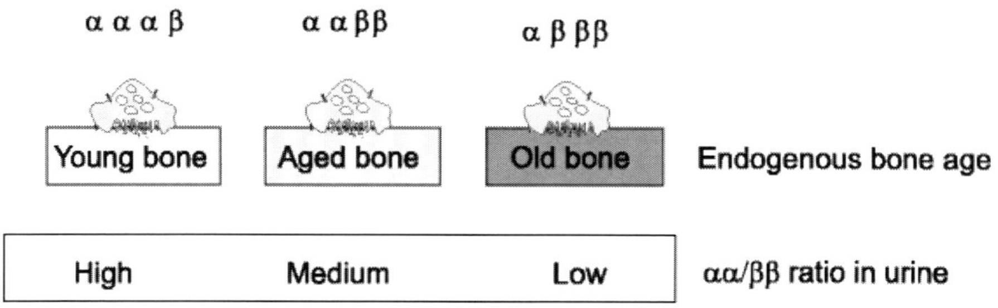

Figure 13. Schematic overview of the bone collagen age profile measured as the ratio between ααCTX and ββCTX (Modified from Leeming DJ et al., 2009).

The e urinary excretion of native αLCTX was more predictive of fracture risk than the age-related isoforms (βL, αD, and βD) of type I collagen. The accumulation of the age-related CTX isoforms in bone matrix depends on both the inversion rate of the different isoforms and the rate of bone turnover. This indicates that for a given inversion rate, a higher bone turnover rate will be associated with lower levels of age-related CTX isoforms and higher levels of native αLCTX, a concept that is in agreement with the positive correlation we found between the urinary ratios of native αLCTX on age-related isoforms and serum bone ALP. Thus, the measurement of native αLCTX may be more sensitive to detect small increases of bone turnover, which have been shown to be associated with increased risk of fracture (Garnero P et al., 2002).

CONCLUSION

Collagens constitute a family of proteins present in the ECM of connective tissues. Collagen triple-helices are well known to interact and form higher order structures, such as fibrils. Type I collagen {[α1(I)]2α2(I)} is the most abundant type of collagen and is widely distributed in almost all connective tissues with the exception of hyaline cartilage. In all connective tissues, collagen has mechanical functions, providing elasticity and structure for the component tissues. Type I collagen comprises approximately 95% of the entire collagen content of bone and about 80% of the total proteins present in bone. Changes in posttranslational modifications of collagen (occurring during maturation and aging of bone collagen) are associated with mechanical properties of bone.

It seems that an increase in enzymatic collagen crosslinks (PYD, DPD, and pyrrole) may be associated with increased ultimate stress and stiffness, whereas the content of AGEs due to the age-related nature of this modification is associated with post-yield energy absorption. Together, these findings support the notion that the extent and nature of collagen crosslinking are important contributors to bone quality. Bone turnover can be evaluated by noninvasive biochemical markers of bone resorption. However, with the used of new bone markers it can be assessed not only the rate of bone turnover but the collagen ''quality'' (such as crosslinking and isomerization pattern). Finally, bone turnover evaluation may be also important in determining bone strength because it influences the pattern of mature/immature crosslinking in bone.

REFERENCES

Alexandersen P, Peris P, Guañabens N, Byrjalsen I, Alvarez L, Solberg H, Cloos PA. Non-isomerized C-telopeptide fragments are highly sensitive markers for monitoring disease activity and treatment efficacy in Paget´s disease of bone. *J. Bone Miner Res.* 2005; 20:588-95.

Anttinen H, Oikarinen A, Kivirikko KI. Age-related changes in human skin collagen galactosyltransferase and collagen glucosyltransferase activities. *Clin. Chim. Acta.* 1977; 76:95-101.

Autio P, Oikarinen A, Melkko J, Risteli J, Risteli L. Systemic glucocorticoids decrease the synthesis of type I and type III collagen in human skin in vivo, whereas isotretinoin treatment has little effect. *Br. J. Dermatol.* 1994;131,660–663.

Avery NC, Bailey AJ. Enzymic and non-enzymic cross-linking mechanisms in relation to turnover of collagen: relevance to aging and exercise. *Scand. J. Med. Sci. Sports* 2005; 15(4):231-40.

Bailey AJ, Light ND, Atkins ED. Chemical cross-linking restrictions on models for the molecular organization of the collagen fibre. *Nature* 1980; 288 (5789):408-10.

Bailey AJ, Paul RG, Knott L. Mechanisms of maturation and ageing of collagen. *Mech. Ageing Dev.* 1998; 106:1–56.

Bailey AJ, Robins SP, Balian G. Biological significance of the intermolecular crosslinks of collagen. *Nature* 1974; 251:105-9.

Bailey AJ, Sims TJ, Ebbesen EN, Mansell JP, Thomsen JS, Moskilde Li. Age-related changes in the biochemical properties of human cancellous bone collagen*:* relationships to bone strength. *Calcif. Tissue Int.* 1999*;* 65*:* 203–210.

Banse X, Devogelaer JP, Lafosse JPA, Sims TJ, Grynpas M, Bailey AJ. The cross-link profile of bone collagen correlates with the structural organization of the trabeculae. *Bone* 2002; 31*:* 70–76.

Barnes MJ, Constable BJ, Morton LF, Kodicek E., Bone collagen metabolism in vitamin D deficiency. *Biochem. J.* 1973; 132(1):113-5.

Baynes JW, Thorpe SR. Glycoxidation and lipoxidation in atherogenesis. *Free Radic. Biol. Med.* 2000; 28(12): 1708-16.

Bienkowski RS, Baum BJ, Crystal RG. Fibroblasts degrade newly synthesized collagen within the cell before secretion. *Nature* 1978; 276:413-6.

Bonde M, Fledelius C, Qvist P, Christiansen C. Coated-tube radioimmunoassay for C-telopeptides of type I collagen to assess bone resorption. *Clin. Chem.* 1996; ***42***:1639–44.

Bonde M, Qvist P, Fledelius C, Riis BJ, Christiansen C. Immunoassay for quantifying type I collagen degradation products in urine evaluated. *Clin. Chem.* 1994; ***40***:2022–5.

Bornstein P. The NH(2)-terminal propeptides of fibrillar collagens: highly conserved domains with poorly understood functions. *Matrix Biol.* 2002; 21, 217–226.

Brady J, Ju J, Robins SP. Isoaspartyl bonds in the N-terminal sequence of collagen type I. Implications for their use as markers of collagen degradation. *Clin. S Furthmayr H.,* ed), pp. 1–30, CRC Press, Inc., Boca Raton, FL.1982ci 1999*:* 96*:* 209–215.

Brady JD, Robins SP. Structural characterization of pyrrolic cross-links in collagen using a biotinylated Ehrlich's reagent. *J. Biol. Chem.* 2001; 276: 18812–18818.

Brage M, Abrahamson M, Lindstrom V, Grubb A, Lerner UH. Different cysteine proteinases involved in bone resorption and osteoclast formation. *Calcif. Tissue Int. 2005;* 76*:* 439–447.

Brennan TV, Clarke S. Effect of adjacent histidine and cysteine residues on the spontaneous degradation of asparaginyl- and aspartyl-containing peptides. *Int. J. Pept. Protein Res.* 1995 45(6):547-53.

Burshell AL, Möricke R, Correa-Rotter R, Chen P, Warner MR, Dalsky GP, Taylor KA, Krege JH. Correlations between biochemical markers of bone turnover and bone density responses in patients with glucocorticoid-induced osteoporosis treated with teriparatide or alendronate. *Bone* 2010; 46:935-99.

Cerami A, Vlassara H, Brownlee M. Glucose and aging. *Sci. Am.* 1987; 256, 82–88.

Chan GK, Duque G. Age-related bone loss: old bone, new facts. *Gerontology* 2002; 48:62–71.

Chan GK, Fledelius C, Johnsen AH, Cloos PA, Bonde M, Qvist P. Characterization of urinary degradation products derived from type I collagen. Identification of a beta-isomerized Asp-Gly sequence within the C-terminal telopeptide (alpha1) region. J Biol Chem 1997; ***272***:9755–63.

Chambers TJ. Regulation of the differentiation and function of osteoclasts. *J. Pathol.* 2000; 192: 4–13.

Charles P, Mosekilde L, Risteli L, et al. Assessment of bone remodeling using biochemical indicators of type I collagen synthesis and degradation: relation to calcium kinetics. *Bone Miner* 1994; 24: 81–94.

Clarkes S. Propensity for spontaneous succinimide formation from aspartyl and asparaginyl residues in cellular proteins. *Int. J. Peptide Prot. Res.* 1987; 30, 808–821.

Click EM, Bornstein P. Isolation and characterization of the cyanogen bromide peptides from the alpha 1 and alpha 2 chains of human skin collagen. *Biochemistry* 1970;9(24):4699-706.

Cloos PAC, Bonde M, Fledelius C, Christgau S, Christiansen C. In: Osteoporosis (Papapoulos SE, Lips P, Pols HAP, Johnston CC, Delmas PD., eds.), *Elsevier Science*, Amsterdam Rosenqvist C., pp. 227-231, 1996.

Cloos PAC, Christgau S. Non-enzymatic covalent modifications of proteins: Mechanisms, physiological consequences and clinical applications. *Matrix Biol.* 2002; 21: 39–52.

Cloos PAC, Christgau S, Lyubimova N, Body JJ, Qvist P, Christiansen C. Breast cancer patients with bone metastases are characterised by increased levels of non-isomerized type I collagen fragments. *Breast Cancer Res.* 2003a; 5: R103–R1.

Cloos PAC, Fledelius C. Collagen fragments in urine derived from bone resorption are highly racemized and isomerized. A biological clock of protein ageing with clinical potential. *Biochem. J.* 2000; 345: 473–480.

Cloos PAC, Fledelius C, Christgau S, Christiansen C, Engsig M, Delmas P, Body JJ, Garnero P. Investigation of bone disease using osomerized and racemized fragments of type I collagen. *Calcif. Tissue Int.* 2003; 72*:* 8–17.

Cloos PAC, Lyubimova N, Solberg H, Qvist P, Christiansen C, Christgau S An immunoassay for measuring fragments of newly synthesized collagen type I produced during metastatic invasion of bone. *Clin. Lab.* 2004; 50*:* 279–289.

Cole WG. Collagen genes: mutations affecting collagen structure and expression. *Prog. Nucl. Acid Res. Mol. Biol.* 1994; 47: 29–80.

Dehm P, Jimenez SA, Olsen BR, Prockop DJ. A transport form of collagen from embryonic tendon: electron microscopic demonstration of an NH 2 -terminal extension and evidence suggesting the presence of cystine in the molecule (chick embryo-tropocollagen-gel filtration). *Proc. Natl. Acad. Sci. USA*. 1972; 69(1):60-4.

Delmas PD. Markers of bone formation and resorption. In Favus MJ, Ed. *Primer on Metabolic Bone Diseases and Disorders of Mineral Metabolism.* New York: Raven Press, pp 108–112, 1993.

Delmas PD. Committee of scientific advisors of the International Osteoporosis Foundation. Bone marker nomenclature. *Bone* 2001; 28:575-576.

Delmas PD, Eastell R, Garnero P, Seibel MJ, Stepan J The use of biochemical markers of bone turnover in osteoporosis. *Osteoporos Int.* 2000; 11(Suppl 6):S2–S17.

Ebeling PR, Peterson JM, Riggs BL. Utility of type I procollagen propeptide assays for assessing abnormalities in metabolic bone diseases. *J. Bone Miner Res.* 1992; 7:1243–50.

Eriksen EF, Charles P, Meisen F, et al. Serum markers of type 1 collagen formation and degradation in metabolic bone disease: correlation with bone histomorphometry. *J. Bone Miner Res.* 1993; 8:127–32.

Everts V, Delaissé JM, Korper W, Beertsen W. Cysteine proteinases and matrix metalloproteinases play distinct roles in the subosteoclastic resorption zone. *J. Bone Miner Res.* 1998; 13:1420-1430.

Eyre DR. Crosslink maturation in bone collagen. In: Veiss, A. (Ed.). The Chemistry and Biology of Mineralised Connective Tissues. *Elsevier North Holland,* New York, pp. 51–55, 1981.

Eyre DR. Collagen cross-linking amino acids. *Methods Enzymol.* 1987; 144:115–139.

Eyre D. New biomarkers of bone resorption. *J. Clin. Endocrinol. Metab.* 1992; 74:470A–470C.

Eyre DR. The specificity of collagen cross-links as markers of bone and connective tissue degradation. *Acta. Orthop. Scand. Suppl.* 1995;266:166-70.

Eyre DR. Bone biomarkers as tools in osteoporosis management. *Spine* 1997; 22 (Suppl.24):17S–24S.

Eyre DR, Dickson IR, Van Ness K. Collagen cross-linking in human bone and articular cartilage. Age-related changes in the content of mature hydroxypyridinium residues. *Biochem. J.* 1988; 252(2):495-500.

Eyre DR, Muir H. The distribution of different molecular species of collagen in fibrous, elastic and hyaline cartilages of the pig. *Biochem. J.* 1975; 151(3):595-602.

Eyre DR, Paz A, Gallop PM. Cross-linking in collagen and elastin. *Ann. Rev. Biochem.* 1984; 53:717–74.

Eyre DR, Oguchi H. The hydroxypyridinium crosslinks of skeletal collagens: their measurement, properties and a proposed pathway of formation. *Biochem. Biophys. Res. Commun.* 1980; 92:403–41.

Fessler LI, Morris NP, Fessler JH. Procollagen: biological scission of amino and carboxy extension peptides. *Proc. Nat. Acad. Sci. USA* 1975; 72: 4905–9.

Fledelius C, Johnsen AH, Cloos PAC, Bonde M, Qvist P. Characterization of urinary products derived from type I collagen. Identification of the β-isomerised asp-gly sequence within the C-terminal telopeptide α1 region. *J. Biol. Chem.* 1997*:* 272*:* 9755–9763.

Garnero P, Borel O, Byrjalsen I, Ferraras M, Drake FH, McQueney MS et al. The collagenolytic activity of cathepsin K is unique among mammalian proteinases. *J. Biol. Chem.* 1998; ***273***: 32347–52.

Garnero P, Borel O, Byrjalsen I, Ferreras M, Drake FH, McQueney MS, Foged NT, Delmas PD, Delaissé JM. The collagenolytic activity of cathepsin K is unique among mammalian proteinases. *J. Biol. Chem. 1998; 273:32347-32352.*

Garnero P, Borel O, Gineyts E Duboeuf F, Solberg H, Bouxsein ML, Christiansen C, Delmas PD. Extracellular posttranslational modifications of collagen are major determinants of biomechanical properties of fetal bovine cortical bone. *Bone* 2006; 38:300–309.

Garnero P, Cloos PA.C, Sornay-Rendu E, Qvist P, Delmas PD. Type I Collagen Racemization and Isomerization and the Risk of Fracture in Postmenopausal Women: The OFELY Prospective Study. *J. bone Miner Res.* 2002; 17: 826-833.

Garnero P, Fledelius C, Gineyts E, Serre CM, Vignot E, Delmas PD Decreased beta-isomerization of the C-terminal telopeptide of type I collagen alpha 1 chain in Paget's disease of bone. *J. Bone Miner Res.* 1997; 12: 1407–1415.

Garnero P, Ferraras M, Karsdal MA, NicAmhlaoibh R, Risteli J, Borel O, et al. The type I collagen fragments ICTP and CTX reveal distinct enzymatic pathways of bone collagen degradation. *J. Bone Miner Res.* 2003; 18:859-867.

Garnero P, Shih WJ, Gineyts E, Karpf D, Delmas PD Comparison of new biochemical markers of bone turnover in late postmenopausal osteoporotic women in response to alendronate. *J. Clin. Endocrinol. Metab.* 1994; 79:1693–1700.

Geiger T, Clarke S. Deamidation, isomerization, and racemization at asparaginyl and aspartyl residues in peptides. Succinimide-linked reactions that contribute to protein degradation. *J. Biol. Chem. 1987* 15; *262*(2): *785*-94.

Gross J, Harper E, Harris ED, McCroskery PA, Highberger JH, Corbett C, Kang AH. Animal collagenases: Specificity of action, and structures of the substrate cleavage site. *Biochem. Biophys. Res. Commun.* 1974; 61: 605-12.

Hansen DA, Eyre DR. Molecular site specificity of pyridinoline and pyrrole crosslinks in type I collagen of humanbone. *J. Biol. Chem.* 1996; 271:26508–26516.

Hanson DA, Weiss MAE, Bollen A-M, Maslan SL, Singer FR, Eyre DR. A specific immunoassay for monitoring human bone resorption: quantitation of type I collagen cross-linked N-telopeptides in urine. *J. Bone Miner Res.* 1992; 7:1251-8.

Hassager C, Jensen LT, Johansen JS, et al. The carboxy-terminal propeptide of type 1 procollagen in serum as a marker of bone formation: the effect of nandrolone decanoate and female sex hormones. *Metabolism* 1991; 40:205–8.

Hayakawa Y. Inclusion of a beta-aspartyl peptide bond causes the loss of inherent physiological activities. *J. Biochem.* 1994; 115(1):15-7.

Herrmann M, Seibel M. The amino- and carboxyterminal cross-linked telopeptides of collagen type I, NTX-I and CTX-I: A comparative review. *Clin. Chim. Acta.* 2008; 393: 57–75.

Hicks M, Delbridge L, Yue DK, Reeve TS. Catalysis of lipid peroxidation by glucose and glycosylated collagen. *Biochem. Biophys. Res. Commun.* 1988; 151, 649–655.

Hoshino H, Takahashi M, Kushida K, Ohishi T, Inoue T. The relationship between the degree of β-isomerization of type I collagen degradation products in the urine and ageing, menopause and osteoporosis with fractures. *Osteoporos. Int.* 1999; 9:405–409.

Kadler K Protein Profiles: *Extracellular Matrix* 1: Fibril-forming Collagens (Sheterline P., ed), Ac. Press, London, pp. 512–63, 1994.

Kivirikko KI, Myllyla R. Collagen glycosyltransferases. Int Rev Connect Tissue Res 1979;8:23-72.

Kielty CM, Shuttleworth CA Synthesis and assembly of fibrillin by fibroblasts and smooth muscle cells. *J. Cell Sci.* 1993;106 (Pt 1):167-73.

Klepzig M, Jonas D, Oremek GM. Procollagen type 1 amino-terminal propeptide: a marker for bone metastases in prostate carcinoma. *Anticancer Res.* 2009; 29, 671-3.

Knott L, Bailey AJ. Collagen cross-links in mineralizing tissues: a review of their chemistry, function, and clinical relevance. Bone 1998; 22: 181–187.

Knott L, Bailey AJ. Collagen biochemistry of avian bone: comparison of bone type and skeletal site. *Br. Poult. Sci.* 1999; 40:371–379.

Koizumi M, Matsumoto S, Takahashi S, Yamashita T, Ogata E. Bone metabolic markers in the evaluation of bone scan flare phenomenon in bone metastases of breast cancer. *Clin. Nucl. Med.* 1999; 24:15-20.

Koizumi M, Yonese J, Fukui I and Ogata E. The serum level of the amino-terminal propeptide of type I procollagen is a sensitive marker for prostate cancer metastasis to bone. *B. J. U. Int.* 7(4), 348-351.

Kühn KImmunochemistry of the Extracellular Matrix Furthmayr H., ed), CRC Press, Inc., Boca Raton, FL. pp. 1–30, 1982.

Hohenester E, Engel.Domain J. Structure and organisation in extracellular matrix proteins. *Matrix Biol.* 2002; 21, 115–128.

Lapiere CM, Lenaers A, Kohn LD. Procollagen peptidase: An enzyme excising the coordination peptides of procollagen. *Proc. Natl. Acad. Sci. USA* 1971; 68:3054-8.

Leeming DJ, Henriksen K, Byrjalsen I, Qvist P, Madsen SH, Garnero P, Karsdal MA. Is bone quality associated with collagen age? *Osteoporos. Int.* 2009; 20(9):1461-70.

Lund AM, Hansen M, Kollerup G, Juul A, Teisner B, Skovby F. Collagen-derived markers of bone metabolism in osteogenesis imperfecta. *Acta. Pediatr.* 1998; 87: 1131–11379.

Melkko J, Kauppila S, Niemi L, Risteli K, Haukipuro A. Jukkola et al. Immunoassay for intact amino-terminal propeptide of human type I procollagen. *Clin. Chem.* 1996; 42, 947–954.

Melkko J, Hellevik T, Risteli L, Risteli J, Smedsrod B. Clearance of the amino-terminal propeptides of types I and III procollagen is a physiological function of the scavenger receptor in liver endothelial cells. *J. Exp. Med.* 1994; 179:405-12.

Melkko J, Niemi S, Risteli L, Risteli J. Radioimmunoassay of the carboxyterminal propeptide of human type I procollagen. *Clin. Chem* 1990; 36: 1328–32.

Metz TO, Alderson NL, Thorpe SR,Thorpe JW. Pyridoxamine, aninhibitor of advanced glycation andlipoxidation reactions: a novel therapyfor treatment of diabeticcomplications. *Arch. Biochem. Biophys.* 2003; 419: 41–49.

Oikarinen A, Autio P, Vuori J, Väänänen K, Risteli L, Kiistala U, et al. Systemic glucocorticoid treatment decreases serum concentrations of carboxyterminal propeptide of type I procollagen (PICP) and aminoterminal propeptide of type III procollagen (PIIINP) in dermatological patients. *Brit. J. Dermatol.* 1992; 126,172–178.

Olsen BR, Guzman NA, Engel J, Condit C, Aase S. Purification and characterization of a peptide from the carboxy-terminal region of chick tendon procollagen type I. *Biochemistry* 1977;16:3030–6.

Onorato JM, Jenkins AJ, Thorpe SR,Baynes JW. Pyridoxamine, an inhibitorof advanced glycation reactions, also inhibits advanced lipoxidationreactions; mechanism of action ofpyridoxamine. *J. Biol. Chem.* 2000; 275:1177–21184.

Oxlund H., Mosekilde Li, Ørtoft G. Reduced concentration of collagen reducible cross links in human trabecular bone with respect to age and osteoporosis. *Bone* 1996; 19: 479–484.

Paul RG, Bailey AJ. Glycation of collagen: the basis of its central role in the late complications of ageing and diabetes. *Int. J. Biochem. Cell Biol.* 1996; 28, 1297–1310.

Pedersen BJ, Ravn P, Bonde M. Type I collagen C-telopeptide degradation products as bone resorption markers. *J. Clin. Ligand. Assay.* 1998; 21:118-27.

Prockop DJ. Kivirikko K. Heritable diseases of collagen. *N. Engl. J. Med.* 1984; 311(6):376-86.

Prockop DJ, Kivirikko K. Collagens: molecular biology, diseases, and potentials for therapy. *Annu. Rev. Biochem.* 1995; 64:403–434.

Radkiewicz JL, Zipse H, Clarke S, Houk KN. Neighboring side chain effects on asparaginyl and aspartyl degradation: an ab initio study of the relationship between peptide conformation and backbone NH acidity. *J. Am. Chem. Soc.* 2001 18;123(15):3499-506.

Ramachandran, G N, Reddi AH, eds *Biochemistry of collagen*. Plenum, New York, *pp. 45-84,* 1976.

Rosano TG, Peaston RT, Bone HG, Woitge HW, Francis RM, Seibel MJ. Urinary free deoxypyridinoline by chemiluminescence immunoassay: analytical and clinical evaluation. *Clin. Chem.* 1998; 44:2126-32.

Ristelli J, Eriksen H, Risteli L, Mansell JP, Bayley AJ . Pyrrolic crosslinks are as abundant in human bone type I collagen as pyridinolines. *J. Bone Miner Res.* 1994; 9(Suppl 1):S186.

Risteli L, Risteli J, Moniz C. Measuring collagen degredation. *Eur. J. Clin. Invest.* 1993; 23:339-340.

Robins SP. Turnover and cross-linking of collagen. In: Weiss JB, Jayson MV. Eds. *Collagen in Health and Disease*. Edinburgh: Churchill Livingstone, pp.160-178, 1982.

Robins SP. An enzyme-linked immunoassay for the collagen cross-link, pyridinoline. *Biochem. J.* 1982; 207:617-620.

Robins SP. Collagen cross-links in metabolic bone disease. *Acta. Ortbop. Scand.* 1995; 266:171-5.

Robins SP, Brady JD. Collagen cross-linking and metabolism, in: J.P. Bilezikian, L.G. Raisz, G.A. Rodan (Eds.), *Principles of Bone Biology*, vol. 1, second ed. Academic Press, San Diego, CA pp. 211–223, 2002.

Robins SP. Duncan A. Cross-linking of collagen. Location of pyridinoline in bovine articular cartilage at two sites of the molecule. *Biochem. J.* 1983; 215:175-82.

Robins SP, Woitge H, Hesley R, Ju J, Seyedin S, Seibel MJ. A direct enzyme-linked immunoassay for urinary deoxypyridinoline as a specificmarker for measuring bone resorption. *J. Bone Miner Res.* 1994; 9:1643-1649.

Rosenqvist C, Fledelius C, Christgau S, Pedersen BJ, Bonde M, Qvist P, Christiansen C . Serum CrossLaps one step ELISA. First application of monoclonal antibodies for measurement in serum of bone related degradation products from C-terminal telopeptides of type I collagen. *Clin. Chem.* 1998; 44*:* 2281–2289.

Saarto T, Blomqvist C, Risteli J, Risteli L, Sarna S and Elomaa I: Aminoterminal propeptide of type I procollagen (PINP) correlates to bone loss and predicts the efficacy of antiresorptive therapy in pre- and post-menopausal non-metastatic breast cancer patients. *Br. J. Cancer* (Anticancer Res) 2007; 78(2): 240 245.

Saito M, Fujii K, Marumo K. Degree of mineralization related collagen crosslinking in the femoral neck cancellous bone in cases of hip fracture and controls. *Calcif. Tissue Int.* 2006; 79:160–168.

Saito M, Marumo K. Collagen cross-links as a determinant of bone quality: a possible explanation for bone fragility in aging, osteoporosis, and diabetes mellitus. *Osteoporos. Int.* 2010; 21:195–214.

Saito M, Marumo K, Soshi S, Kida Y, Ushiku C, Shinohara A. Raloxifene ameliorates detrimental enzymatic and nonenzymatic collagen cross-links and bone strength in rabbits with hyperhomocysteinemia. *Osteoporos. Int.* 2010; 21:655–666.

Saito M, Mori S, Mashiba T, Komatsubara S, Marumo K. Collagen maturity, glycation induced-pentosidine, and mineralization are increased following 3-year treatment with incadronate in dogs. *Osteoporos. Int.* 2008; 19:1343–1354.

Sassi ML, Eriksen H, Risteli L, Niemi S, Mansell J, Gowen M, Risteli J. Immunochemical characterization of the assay for the carboxyterminal telopeptide of human type I collagen (ICTP): loss of antigenicity by treatment with cathepsin K. Bone 2000; 26:367-373.

Segrest JP.Urinary metabolites of collagen. *Meth. Enzymol.* 1982; 82:398–410.

Seyedin SM, Kung VT, Daniloff YI, Hesley RP, Gomez B, Nielsen LA, Rosen HN, Zuk RF. Immunoassay for urinary pyridinoline: The new marker of bone resorption. *J. Bone Miner Res.* 1993; 8:635-41.

Siris ES. In: *Primer on the Metabolic Bone Diseases and Disorders of the Mineral Metabolism* (Favus M. J., ed), Raven Press, Ltd., New York, pp. 375–384, 1993.

Smedsrod B, Melkko J, Risteli L, Risteli J. Circulating C-terminal propeptide of type I procollagen is cleared mainly via the mannose receptor in liver endothelial cells. *Biochem. J.* 1990; 271:345–50.

Takahashi M, Hoshino H, Kushida K. Measurements of urinary nonisomerized form of type I collagen degradation products (and[alpha]-CTx) in aging, menopause, and osteoporosis with fractures. ***Clin. Chim. Acta.*** 1999; 279:69-76.

Taubman MB, Goldberg B, Sherr C. Radioimmunoassay for human procollagen. *Science* 1974; 186:1115–7.

van der Rest M, Garrone R. Collagen family of proteins. *FASEB J.* 1991 5:2814-23.

Vashishth D. The role of the collagen matrix in skeletal fragility. *Curr. Osteoporos. Rep.* 2007; 5:62–66.

Vasikaran S, Cooper ., Eastell R, Griesmacher A, Morris HA, Trenti T. et al. International Osteoporosis Foundation and International Federation of Clinical Chemistry and Laboratory Medicine position on bone marker standards in osteoporosis. *Clin. Chem. Lab. Med.* 2011; 49, 1271–1274.

Verzar F. Ageing of the collagen fibre. *Int. Rev. Connect. Tiss. Res.* 1964; 2, 244–300.

Viguet-Carrin S, Garnero P, Delmas PD. The role of collagen in bone strength. *Osteoporos. Int.* 2006; 17:319–336.

Viidik A, Age-related changes in connective tissue. In: Viidik, A. (Ed.), Lectures in Gerontology. *Biology of Ageing Part 1.* Academic Press, London, pp. 173–21, 1982.

Wassen MHM, Lammens J, Tekoppele JM, Sakkers RJB, Liu Z, Verbout Aj, Bank RA. Collagen structure regulates fibril mineralization in osteogenesis as revealed by crosslink patterns in calcifying callus. *J. Bone Miner Res.* 2000; 15: 1776-85.
Yamauchi M, Mechanic GL. -linking of collagen. E. Nimni (Ed.), Collagen, CRC press, Boca Raton, FL, pp. 157–172, 1988.

In: Type I Collagen
Editors: Maria Eduarda Henriques and Marcio Pinto
ISBN: 978-1-62257-625-8

Chapter IV

Development of 3-D Collagen Gel Vascularized Tissue-Engineered Constructs for Bone Replacement and Regeneration Using Embryonic and Postnatal Progenitors

***Mani T. Valarmathi*[1,*] *and John W. Fuseler*[1]**

[1]Department of Cell Biology and Anatomy, School of Medicine,
University of South Carolina, Columbia, South Carolina, US

Abstract

Adult stem cell based tissue engineering for repair and regenerative purposes, has been an emerging area of intense investigation. The current major challenge to these approaches has been the inability to vascularize and perfuse in vitro engineered tissue constructs. Attempts to provide oxygen and nutrients to cells contained in biomaterial constructs have met with varying degrees of success. Engineering a tissue of clinically relevant magnitude requires the formation of extensive and stable microvascular networks within the tissue. Since most in vitro engineered tissue constructs do not contain the intricate microvascular structures of native tissue, the cells contained in scaffolds heavily rely on simple diffusion for oxygenation and nutritional delivery. The majority of cells need to be within 100-200 μm of a blood supply to receive adequate oxygen and nutrients for survival. Otherwise, due to limitations of diffusional transport, the cells in the interior regions of the artificial scaffold can experience hypoxia or anoxia and undergo cellular degeneration and necrosis. Hence, this necessitates the formation of appropriate in vitro three-dimensional (3-D) plexuses of new blood vessels within the pre-implanted biomaterial constructs through the process of in situ de novo vasculogenesis/angiogenesis for organ tissue engineering. To this end, here we demonstrate the application of 3-D matrix scaffolds composed of type I collagen to address these concerns.

---

* Corresponding author. Building 1 Room B-31, 6439 Garners Ferry Road, Laboratory of Stem Cell Biology and Tissue Engineering, Department of Cell Biology and Anatomy, School of Medicine, University of South Carolina, USA. Tel.: +1 803 216 3821; fax: +1 803 216 3846. E-mail addresses: valarmathi.thiruvanamalai @uscmed.sc.edu, valarmathi64@hotmail.com.

Keywords: Bone marrow stromal cells, Mesenchymal stem cells, Proepicardial cells, Osteogenesis, Vasculogenesis, Bone tissue engineering, Vascular tissue engineering, Type I collagen

1. Introduction

The extracellular matrix embodies as a natural scaffold for tissue development and reparative processes. Regenerative processes are profoundly dependent on interactions between the cells that participate in regeneration (cell-cell interactions) and the substrate on which they function (cell-matrix interactions). In tissue regenerative process, specific substrate requirements must often be met for regeneration to occur. This holds good for both natural regeneration and induced regeneration, the latter of which often involves virtually artificial or processed tissue substrates [Carlson, 2007]. In general, for any regenerative process the relationship between the regenerating or differentiating cells and their substrate is critical. It is this critical relationship that ultimately dictates the difference between true regeneration and a scarring response, degeneration [Carlson, 2007].

Angiogenesis and vascular invasion are a prerequisite to the process of organogenesis, both in development and during repair [Reddi, 1998; Carano and Filvaroff, 2003]. Developing vascularized tissue in vitro is important for clinical and surgical implications and is essential for the viability and functional integrity of any engineered tissue or organ [Lanza et al., 2000]. Most approaches to engineering new tissue have relied on the host for vascularization. Although this approach has been moderately successful, it has not proven effective in dense highly vascularized tissues such as bone or muscle [Leveber et al., 2005]. Therefore, strategies focused on the improvement of neovascularization of engineered tissues are of critical importance.

Organ tissue engineering offers a potential to develop in vitro functional equivalents of native tissue for tissue repair and to discover innovative approaches to treat and/or prevent various types of lesions. A major challenge for the transplantation of tissue-engineered constructs is insufficient oxygen and nutrient supply. Attempts to provide oxygen and nutrients to the cells contained in the biomaterial constructs have had varying degrees of success. Engineering a tissue of clinically relevant magnitude requires the formation of an extensive and stable microvascular networks within the tissue. Since most in vitro engineered tissue constructs do not contain the intricate microvascular structures of native tissue, the cells contained in scaffolds heavily rely on simple diffusion for oxygenation and nutritional delivery. Consequently, this necessitates the formation of appropriate in vitro three-dimensional (3-D) plexuses of new blood vessels within the pre-implanted biomaterial constructs through the process of in situ de novo vasculogenesis/angiogenesis for organ tissue engineering. And there exist a need for such a unique 3-D matrix scaffold that can provide a conducive microenvironment to sustain the developing microvascular structures.

The development of the vascular system is one of the earliest events in organogenesis. Given the complexity of the muscular and non-muscular organs such as heart and bone with respect to their structural organization and relationships between various different cell types, and its reliance on the vasculature, true differentiation cannot be readily achieved by any current in vitro protocols, including those that incorporate the cells within a 3-D structure.

However, some initial insight can be delineated from in vitro differentiation [Bianco et al., 2006]. One of the major challenges in engineering complex tissues such as bone and myocardium, which involves the reconstruction of 3-D shapes and internal architectures, is the need to vascularize the tissue in vitro for creating functionally competent vascular networks. Thus, a method to enhance graft vascularization requires the establishment of primitive vascular plexuses within the implant before transplantation by the use of cellular-based concepts [Finkenzeller et al., 2007].

In the case of bone, vascular cells have dramatic inductive osteogenic effects [Villanueva and Nimni, 1990]; reciprocally osteogenesis induces the expression of angiogenic factors [Carvalho et al., 2004]. Vascular arrangement of the overlying periosteum precedes and dictates the architecture of the new bone. It has been proposed that preconstruction of an appropriate vasculature and scaffold (collagen and non-collagen based) with pore size and surface architecture conducive to the growth of vessels is of paramount significance [Ripamonti et al., 2004; Ripamonti, 2004; Yoshikawa and Myoui, 2005]. Thus, appropriate vascularization of the scaffold in vitro could maintain cell viability during tissue growth, induce structural organization and promote further vascularization in the implant and adjacent host tissue following implantation.

In general, any successful tissue engineering approach to regeneration depends not only on the right choice of substrate and/or engineered scaffold but most importantly on the right source of initial cells, which will ultimately dictate and fill the defects and/or repair the lesions. For the aforementioned reasons, embryonic, fetal and postnatal stem cells as well as various types of progenitor cells, can be potential cellular sources for tissue engineering [Levenberg, 2005]. However, the source for the early-stage developmental cells is restricted. The utility of embryonic stem cells (ESCs) and induced pluripotent stem cells (iPSCs) in facilitating vascularized tissue/organ regeneration is still in its incipient stages. A number of issues, including a propensity for some implanted ESCs/iPSCs to form benign teratomas and/or malignant teratocarcinomas in the regenerating tissue/organ and their in vitro genomic instability during propagation, remain to be addressed [Pera, 2011].

It is well established that postnatal bone marrow acts as a central reservoir of adult stem/progenitor cells, such as hematopoietic stem cells (HSCs), bone marrow stromal cells/mesenchymal stem cells (BMSCs/MSCs), multipotent adult progenitor cells (MAPCs) and endothelial stem/progenitor cells (EPCs). BMSCs contain a phenotypically and functionally heterogeneous population of mesenchymal precursor cells that not only provide support for hematopoiesis but also contribute to the regeneration of bone, cartilage, adipose, muscle and other connective tissues both in vivo or in vitro [Bianco et al., 2001; Valarmathi et al., 2008a; 2008b; 2009; 2010; 2011; Fuseler and Valarmathi, 2012]. Bone marrow also contains cells that can differentiate into other cell types such as neuronal cells, hepatocytes, cardiomyocytes and epithelial cells of the lung, gastrointestinal tract, and skin [Moore, 1999; Lagasse et al., 2000; Orlic et al., 2001; Krause et al., 2001]. These results indicate that bone marrow-derived stem cells have a high degree of phenotypic plasticity. Importantly, it has been well established that in contrast to both ESCs/iPSCs, the adult stem cell, BMSCs exhibit multilineage differentiation potential in a well-controlled and predictable fashion.

Furthermore, unlike ESCs derivation, obtaining autologous or allogeneic BMSCs is feasible and can potentially be exploited to develop prevascularized tissue-engineered constructs for therapeutic purposes. Similarly, repeated isolation and rapid expansion of sufficient yield of autologous and/or allogeneic non-bone-marrow-derived resident stem cells/progenitors, especially from vital organs for routine therapeutic purposes are highly constrained. On the contrary, to certain extent autologous and/or allogeneic bone marrow-derived BMSCs are amenable for repeated isolation and reasonable in vitro expansion from the patients. In addition, the significant advantage of using these BMSCs is their low immunogenicity. These autologous or allogeneic BMSCs have been reported to be immunomodulatory and immunotolerogenic both in vitro as well as in vivo [Aggarwal and Pittenger, 2005]. Taken together, these data strongly indicate that BMSCs can represent the potential cell of choice for adult autologous and/or allogeneic stem cell based vascularized tissue regeneration.

In general, successful in vitro differentiation of cells depends on cell-cell as well as cell-matrix interactions. We therefore demonstrate that under appropriate in vitro physicochemical microenvironmental cues (combination of growth factors and extra cellular matrix, ECM) multipotent adult BMSCs alone or BMSCs in combination with embryonic-derived progenitors, on 3-D collagen gel based scaffolds engineered from aligned type I collagen strands and cultured in osteoinductive medium can generate numerous vascularized bone-like elements. These unique characteristics of bone marrow-derived cells make them an attractive source for tissue engineering that will be at the forefront for future technological developments [Bianco and Robey, 2001]. Consequently, this necessitates the development of appropriate in vitro models of 3-D functional vascularized tissues and prompts the development of 3-D vascularized tissue constructs for tissue engineering purposes, especially using the adult stem cell, BMSCs.

2. Significance and Role of ECM Materials During Tissue Regeneration and Development

It is well established that extracellular matrix (ECM) components play a critical role in morphogenesis. ECM molecules have potent effects on cell proliferation and differentiation, and direct the assembly of 3-D tissues in vitro. The physical nature of the substrate plays a significant role in regeneration. Different cell types have different reactions to the physical nature of their substrate. The substrate, however, is not simply a mechanical matrix. A variety of growth factors are bound to matrix molecules until they are released through the enzymatic activities of cells in the near vicinity [Taipale and Keski-Oja, 1997]. Other factors remain bound to the matrix and require local interactions with cells to exert their effects. Because of the potent effects of many of the growth factors, their localized binding to the substrate is a means of ensuring their availability in specific regions as requirements dictate, but at the same time serves to protect nearby cells from their indiscriminate activities. The substrate serves as a medium for the transmission of local chemical signals, whether bound growth factors or paracrine signals secreted from nearby cells. Under other circumstances the signaling molecules bound to the substrate serve as determinants of the pathway of the outgrowing or differentiating cells.

Collagenous proteins are a major constituent of all extracellular matrices. Traditionally, the role attributed to collagen has been mechano-architectural and structural. During the past several years, however, it has become obvious that collagen comprises a large heterogeneous class of molecules, some with structural properties classically attributed to "collagen," but numerous others with additional properties [Linsenmayer, 1991]. Until now, at least 28 types of collagen have been identified and described. These are found in unique tissue-specific patterns, arise during development in defined temporal and spatial patterns, and exhibit different functional properties. Also, collagens have been shown to be involved, either directly or indirectly, in cell attachment and differentiation, as chemotactic agents, as antigens in immunopathological processes, and as the defective component in certain pathological conditions [Linsenmayer, 1991]. Thus, in addition to their structural roles, collagens potentially have numerous developmental and physiological functions, many of which remain to be elucidated.

The most abundant type of collagen isolated from many adult connective tissues such as skin, bone, tendon, and cornea is type I collagen. Type I is the prototype fibrillar collagen. It is becoming increasingly evident that ECM can affect cell growth and differentiation not only by the direct attachment of its component molecules to receptors on the cell's surface, but also by binding and/or activating other molecules, in particular TGF-β and bFGF [Taub et al., 1990; Runyan et al., 1990; Vukicevic et al., 1992], that in turn also react with the cell. Cell proliferation, expansion and growth also demand flexibility in the growth matrix, such as that associated with tissue regeneration and during development. The matrix is also a reservoir of growth factors and possible morphogens, and serves to support rather specific cleavage reactions directed against carrier molecules like vitronectin and heparin sulfate that may have roles in determining the course of further cell growth and differentiation.

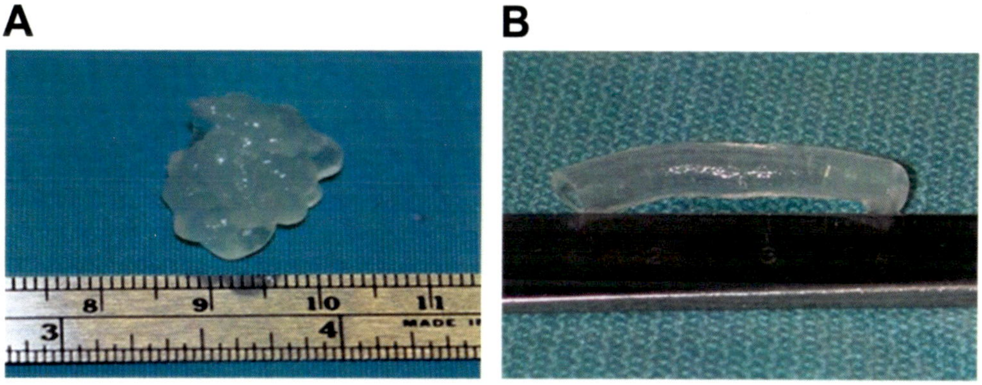

Figure 1. Fabrication of 3-D collagen gel based tubular scaffolds engineered from aligned type I collagen fibers. Type I collagen was extracted from bovine calf hides (A). Bovine collagen type I was extruded with a device that contained two counter-rotating cones to generate the 3-D collagen gel tubular scaffolds. The dimensions of tubes produced for this set of experiments had a length of 30 mm with a luminal diameter of 4 mm and an external diameter of 5 mm, leaving a wall thickness of 1 mm. The collagen tubes had a defined fiber angle of 18° relative to the central axis of the tube and had pores ranging from 1 to 10 μm (B). (A and B, courtesy of M.J. Yost).

3. Experimental Approach

The differentiation of rat BMSCs was carried out on a 3-D tubular scaffold made up of aligned type I collagen-gel fibers. Rat BMSCs were isolated from the tibial and femoral bone marrow of adult rats. The BMSCs isolated from the bone marrow were expanded, maintained and passaged to make sure that the attached marrow stromal cells were devoid of any non-adhering populations of cells. Phenotypic characterization of the BMSCs for cell surface markers was performed by confocal microscopy (qualitative evaluation) and single-color flow cytometry (quantitative analysis). This adherent population of cells were further purified and enriched by indirect magnetic cell sorting. The cells were subjected to CD90 positive selection. The resultant enriched $CD90^+/CD34^-/CD45^-$ fractions were expanded by subculturing and subjected to flow cytometric analysis to validate the proper phenotype. This population of purified BMSCs was used in all experiments. For osteogenic differentiation of BMSCs, the expanded and purified population of $CD90^+$ BMSCs was seeded into the collagen-gel tubular scaffold and cultured either in basal or osteogenic culture medium for up to 18 days. At regular intervals of 3, 6, 9, 12, 15 and 18 days the 3-D tube cultures as well as the 2-D standard Petri dish cultures were assayed by real-time reverse transcriptase quantitative polymerase chain reaction (RT-qPCR), immunohistochemical, cytochemical and biochemical analyses for various osteoblastic and vascular cell lineage specific differentiation markers as shown in table 1, 2 and 3. The time points at which these analyses were carried out cover the optimal range of both osteogenic and vasculogenic processes seen in vivo and/or in vitro and may mimic the progression of vascularized bone development.

4. Research Methods

4.1. Fabrication of Tubular Scaffold

The 3-D collagen type I tube served as a scaffold on which rat BMSCs differentiation cultures were carried out (Figure 1). The details of the production and properties of the collagen tubular scaffolds have previously been described [Yost et al., 2004]. Briefly, a 25 mg/ml solution of bovine collagen type I was extruded with a device that contained two counter-rotating cones. The liquid collagen was fed between the two cones and forced through a circular annulus in the presence of an NH_3-air (50-50 vol/vol) chamber. This process results in a hollow cylindrical tube of aligned collagen fibrils with an inner central lumen. The dimensions of tubes produced for this set of experiments had a length of 30 mm with a luminal diameter of 4 mm and an external diameter of 5 mm, leaving a wall thickness of 1 mm. The collagen tubes had a defined fiber angle of 18° relative to the central axis of the tube and had pores ranging from 1 to 10 μm. The rationale for the particular orientation of collagen fiber was based on our previous work on cardiovascular tissue engineering [Yost et al., 2004]. When proepicardial organ cells (PEs) were seeded onto this scaffold, they underwent maturation and differentiation and produced elongated vessel-like structures reminiscent of in vivo-like phenotype [Valarmathi et al., 2008b]. The tubes were sterilized using gamma radiation 1200 Gy followed by Stratalinker UV crosslinker 1800 (Stratagene) and then placed in Mosconas's solution (in mM: 136.8 NaCl, 28.6 KCl, 11.9 $NaHCO_3$, 9.4 glucose, 0.08 NaH_2PO_4, pH 7.4) (Sigma-Aldrich) containing 1 μl/ml gentamicin (Sigma-Aldrich) and incubated in 5% CO_2 at 37°C until cellular seeding [Valarmathi et al., 2010].

Table 1. Criteria to identify BMSCs/MSCs (Dominici et al., 2006)

Criteria to Identify BMSCs/MSCs			
1.	Adherence to plastic in standard culture conditions		
2.	Phenotype	Positive (≥95%+) CD73 CD90 CD105	Negative (≤2%+) CD11b or CD14 CD34 CD45 CD79α or CD19 HLA-DR
3.	In vitro differentiation: Osteoblasts, Chondroblasts and Adipocytes. (Demonstrated by staining of in vitro cell culture)		
International Society for Cellular Therapy (ISCT): Mesenchymal and Tissue Stem Cell Committee			

Table 2. Primary Antibodies Used in this Study (Valarmathi et al., 2008a; 2008b)

Primary Antibodies	Dilutions	Source	Cell Target
Characterization markers			
CD11b	1:250	BD Pharmingen	Leukocytes
CD31	1:10	Abcam	Endothelial
CD34	1:100	Santa Cruz Biotechnology	Endothelial
CD45	1:250	BD Pharmingen	Hematopoietic
CD73	1:50	BD Pharmingen	BMSCs
CD90	1:250	BD Pharmingen	BMSCs
OX43	1:50	Gene Tex, Inc	Endothelial
Osteogenic markers			
Osteonectin	1:100	DSHB	Osteoblasts
Osteopontin	1:100	DSHB	Osteoblasts
Osteocalcin	1:100	Santa Cruz Biotechnology	Osteoblasts
Alkaline phosphatase	1:100	R&D System	Osteoblasts
Vasculogenic markers			
Pecam-1	1:100	Santa Cruz Biotechnology	Endothelial
CD34	1:100	Santa Cruz Biotechnology	Endothelial
Flk-1	1:100	Santa Cruz Biotechnology	Endothelial
QCPN	1:100	DSHB	Quail Cells
QH1	1:100	DSHB	Quail Endothelial
Isolectin	1:100	Invitrogen	Endothelial
Tomato lectin	1:50	Vector Laboratories	Endothelial
α-SMA	1:100	Sigma-Aldrich	Smooth Muscle

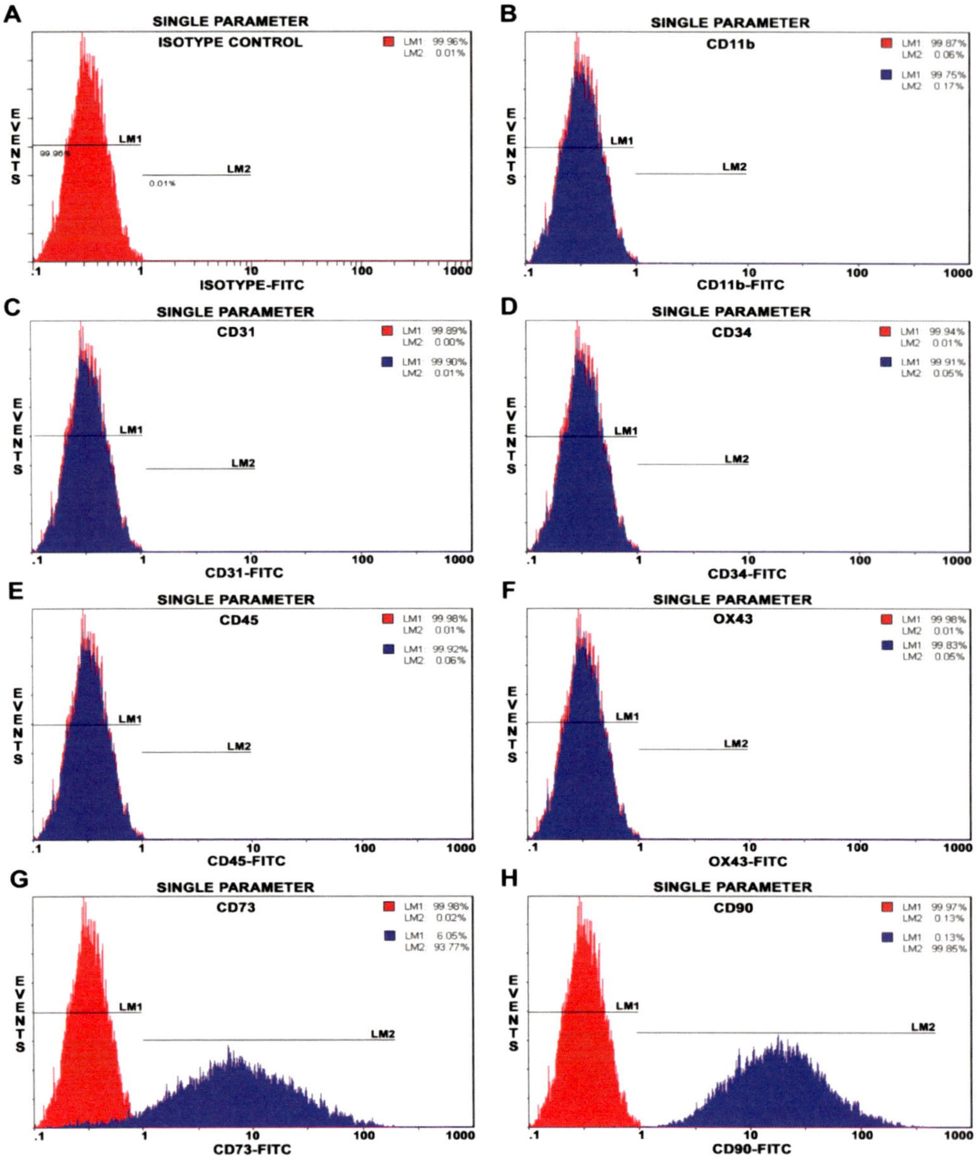

Figure 2. Immunophenotyping of undifferentiated rat BMSCs by flow cytometry. Single parameter histograms showing the relative fluorescence intensity of staining (abscissa) and the number of cells analyzed, events (ordinate). Isotype controls were included in each experiment to identify the level of background fluorescence (Panel A). The intensity and distribution of cells stained for hematopoietic and endothelial markers; CD11b, CD31, CD34, CD45 and OX43 (purple, shaded peaks) were not significantly different from those of isotype control (pink, shaded peaks) (Panels B-F), indicating that these cultures were devoid of any potential hematopoietic and/or endothelial cells of bone marrow origin. The fluorescent intensity was greater (shifted to right) when BMSCs were stained with either CD73 or CD90 (purple) compared to isotype control (pink) (Panels G, H). The predominant population of BMSCs consistently expressed CD73 and CD90 surface molecules, a property of rat bone marrow-derived mesenchymal/stromal stem cells. (Adapted from Valarmathi et al., 2011).

4.2. BMSCs isolation, Expansion and Maintenance (Nonclonal BMSC Culture)

Rat BMSCs were isolated from the bone marrow of adult 300g Sprague Dawley®™ SD®™ rats (Harlan Sprague Dawley, Inc.). Briefly, after euthanasia, the femoral and tibial bones were removed aseptically and cleaned extensively to remove associated soft connective tissues. The marrow cavities of these bones were flushed with Dulbecco's Modified Eagle Medium (DMEM; Invitrogen) and combined. The isolated marrow plugs were triturated, and passed through needles of decreasing gauge (from 18 gauge to 22 gauge) to break up clumps and cellular aggregates. The resulting single-cell suspensions were centrifuged at 200g for 5 minutes. Nucleated cells were counted using a Neubauer chamber. Cells were plated at a density of 5 X 10^6 – 2 X 10^7 cells per T75 cm^2 flasks in basal medium composed of DMEM supplemented with 10% fetal bovine serum (FBS, lot-selected; Atlanta Biologicals, Inc.), gentamicin (50 µg/ml) and amphotericin B (250 ng/ml) and incubated in a humidified atmosphere of 5% CO_2 at 37°C for 7 days. The medium was replaced, and changed three times per week until the cultures become ~70% confluent (between 12 and 14 days). The initial step is to isolate the mononuclear cells from the bone marrow by aspiration and centrifugation followed by plating and isolation of the cells based on differential adherence capacity to tissue culture dishes (passage 0 cells). Cells were trypsinized using 0.05% trypsin-0.1% EDTA and re-plated at a density of 1 x 10^6 cells per T75 cm^2 flasks. After three passages, attached marrow stromal cells were devoid of any non-adhering population of cells. These passaged BMSCs were cryopreserved and stored in liquid nitrogen until further use [Valarmathi et al., 2011].

4.3. Immunophenotyping of BMSCs by Flow Cytometry and Confocal Microscopy

BMSCs are a heterogeneous population of cells with varying degrees of cellular morphologies. Stringent characterization of BMSCs for the presence and/or absence of various specific cell surface markers/epitopes are required before these cells can be used in experimental procedures (Table 1). This meticulous characterization of BMSCs is to ensure that the employed population of cells contains solely stem/progenitor cells, and will obviate the possible contaminating marrow-derived endothelial cells and macrophages that are part of the adherent population of cultured cells. Therefore, characterization of BMSCs included qualitative evaluation for various specific cell surface markers and was performed on cells grown in the Lab-tek™ chamber slide system™ (Nunc) using a Zeiss LSM 510 Meta confocal scanning laser microscope (Carl Zeiss, Inc.), and quantitative analysis of the same set of markers was performed by single-color flow cytometry using a Coulter® EPICS® XL™ Flow Cytometer (Beckman Coulter, Inc.) as previously described [Valarmathi et al., 2009].

Immunophenotyping of undifferentiated BMSCs for various cell surface markers by flow cytometry revealed that the fluorescent intensity and distribution of the cells stained for CD11b (integrin α_m chain, Mac-1 α chain), CD31, CD34, CD45 (leukocyte common antigen) and OX43 (antigen expressed in all vascular endothelial cells of rat) were not significantly different from the intensity and distribution of cells stained with isotype controls (Figure 2A-F), signifying that these cultures were devoid of any possible hematopoietic stem and/or progenitor cells as well as differentiated bone-marrow-derived endothelial cells. In contrast, BMSCs exhibited high expression of CD73 and CD90 surface antigens (Figure 2G-H), which is a consistent characteristic of undifferentiated BMSCs. Phenotypic characterization using the same set of markers on BMSCs by confocal microscopy also revealed that these cells were negative for CD11b, CD31, CD34 and CD45 (Figure 3A-D) and, strongly positive for both CD73 and CD90 (Figure 3E-F). The expression profiles of these surface molecules were consistent with previous reports and meet the minimal criteria for defining multipotent mesenchymal stromal cells, set forth by the international society for cellular therapy (ISCT) position statement (Table 1 and 2) [Dominici et al., 2006; Valarmathi et al., 2009; Reyes et al., 2002].

4.4. Purification and Enrichment of $CD90^+$ BMSCs by Magnetic-activated Cell Sorting (MACS)

Purification and enrichment of input BMSCs (such as $CD45^-$, $CD34^-$, $CD90^+$, $CD105^+$) are mandatory either using MACS (magnetic activated cell sorter) or FACS (fluorescent activated cell sorter). Since the unpurified fraction may contain sizable number of contaminating adherent macrophages and bone marrow-derived endothelial progenitors and differentiated endothelial cells. The adherent populations of BMSCs were further purified by indirect magnetic cell labeling method using an autoMACS™ Pro Separator (Miltenyi Biotech). The cells were subjected to CD90 positive selection by incubating the cells with FITC- labeled anti-CD90 antibodies (BD Pharmingen), followed by incubation with anti-FITC magnetic microbeads (Miltenyi Biotech), and passed through the magnetic columns as per the manufacturer's instructions. The resultant enriched $CD90^+/CD34^-/CD45^-$ fractions were expanded by subcultivation and subjected to flow cytometric analysis as described previously [Valarmathi et al., 2010].

4.5. BMSCs Osteoblastic Differentiation

The isolated BMSCs were maintained and expanded for an additional two passages in basal media. Then, these cells were seeded into collagen-gel tubes at a density of $2x10^6$ cells/15mm tube and cultured either in basal medium or osteogenic medium consisting of DMEM supplemented with 10% FBS, 10 mM sodium β-glycerol phosphate (Sigma-Aldrich), 50 μg/ml L-ascorbic acid (Sigma-Aldrich), 10^{-8} M dexamethasone (Sigma-Aldrich) and 8 μg/ml gentamicin [Maniatopoulos et al., 1988] for 3, 6 and 9 days. In addition, BMSCs were seeded in 65 mm Petri dishes at a density of 3000 cells/cm^2 and cultured either in basal medium or osteogenic medium for 3, 6, 9, 12, 15 and 18 days.

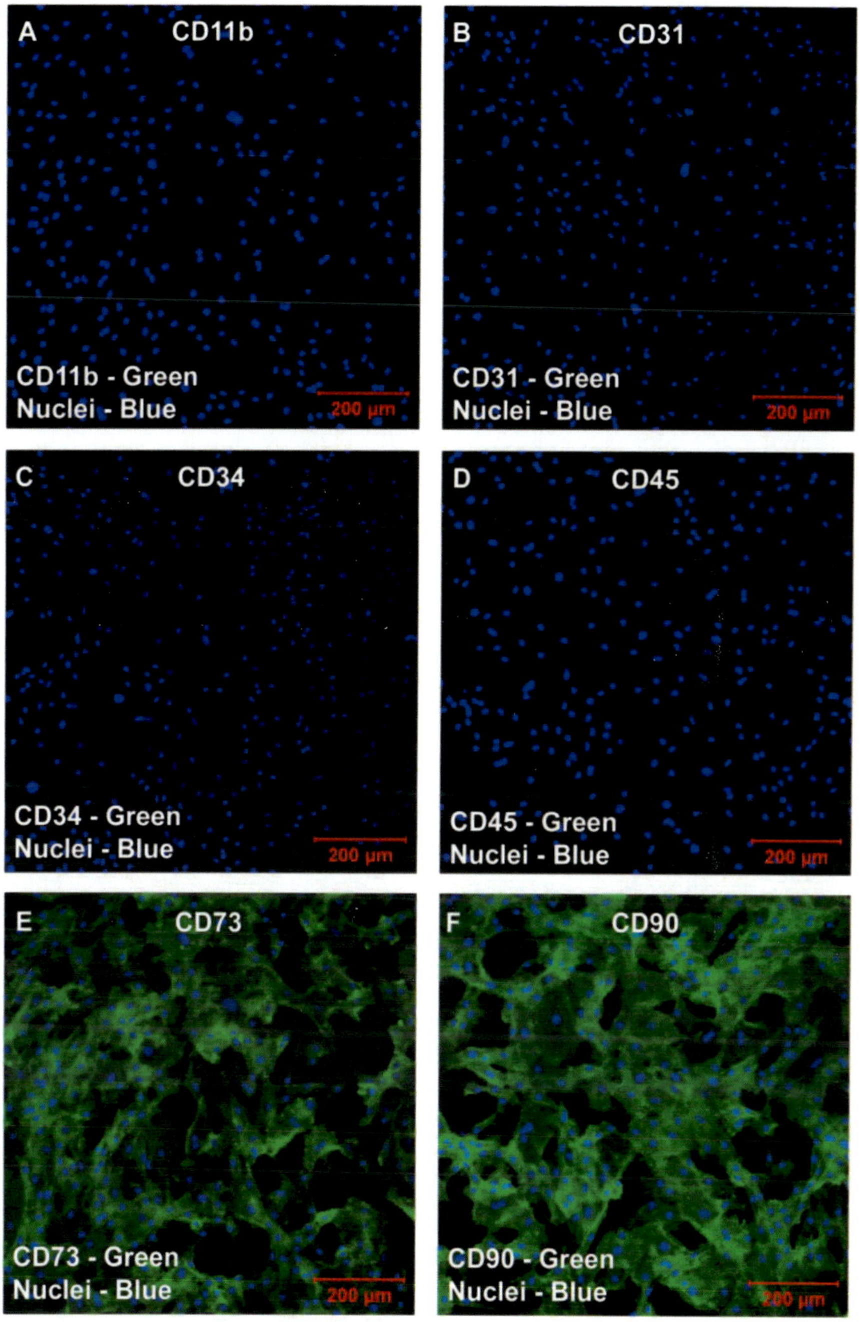

Figure 3. Immunophenotyping of undifferentiated rat BMSCs by confocal microscopy. Immunostaining and confocal microscopy revealed that BMSCs were negative for CD11b (A), CD 31 (B), CD 34 (C) and CD45 (D) and; were uniformly positive for CD73 (E) and CD90 (F) surface antigens, consistent with their undifferentiated state. Isotype and/or negative controls were included in each experiment to identify the level of background staining. Cells were also stained for nuclei (blue – DAPI, 4',6-diamidino-2-phenylindole). Merged images A-F (A-F, scale bar 200 μm).

4.6. Quail PE Isolation and BMSCs/PEs Co-culture

Pharaoh Quail eggs (Lake Cumberland, NC) were incubated at 38° for 65 h. Quail embryos staged according to Hamburger-Hamilton Staging (HH16-HH17) [Hamburger and Hamilton, 1951] were isolated and placed in Tyrode's buffer. The membranes around the embryo and heart were reflected back and the proepicardium was dissected using fine forceps. Passage 3 BMSCs were seeded into the tubular scaffold at a density of 2 x 10^6/15 mm tube by pipetting directly into the tubes and cultured in basal medium. On day 3 the majority of the media was removed from the BMSC tube culture and two proepicardial organs (PEs) were allowed to adhere to the tube surface for 12-16 h. After 12 – 16 h, fresh medium was again added to the culture. All explants and tube cultures were cultured either in basal medium or osteogenic medium for 3, 6 or 9 days as described above. In addition, BMSCs only were seeded in tubular scaffolds at a density of 2 x 10^6 cells/15 mm tube and cultured either in basal medium or in osteogenic medium for 3, 6 or 9 days.

All these BMSCs cultures and BMSCs/PEs co-cultures were terminated at these regular intervals and subsequently processed for RT-qPCR, immunohistochemical, cytochemical and biochemical analyses.

5. BMSCs and BMSCs/PEs Based Vascularied Bone Regeneration

In situ, bone is composed of a heterogeneous mixture of cell types (osteoid and endothelial lineages) embedded within a mineralized ECM, which serves to maintain its structural integrity [Heng et al., 2004]. Collagen type I is the most abundant protein in bone ECM. Numerous other collagen isoforms, non-collagenous proteins (i.e., osteocalcin, osteonectin, osteopontin, osteoadherin, fibronectin, bone sialoprotein, and thrombospondin), and proteoglycans are also found in bone ECM [Young et al., 1992; Robey, 1996]. Previous studies indicate that type I collagen promoted the osteogenic differentiation of undifferentiated mesenchymal stem cells in conventional two dimensional (2-D) monolayer cultures [Shi et al., 1996; Lan and Wang, 2003; Taira et al., 2003]. This indicates that the composition of the ECM substratum with which they are cultured influences the directed differentiation of these cells into the osteogenic lineage.

A reciprocal and functionally coupled relationship between cell growth and differentiation-related gene expression, three principle periods of the osteoblast developmental sequence are defined: proliferation, matrix development and maturation, and mineralization. During the proliferative phase of developing osteoblasts, several genes associated with formation of the ECM such as type I collagen, fibronectin, and transforming growth factor β (TGF-β) are actively expressed. These genes are then gradually down-regulated as the proliferative stage ends. However, collagen mRNA is continuously expressed at a low basal level here and during subsequent stages of osteoblastic differentiation. At the end of the proliferative period, genes that are associated with matrix development and maturation such as matricellular proteins (osteonectin, osteopontin and osteocalcin) are up-regulated. Progressive formation of the matrix down-regulates osteoblast proliferation, and subsequently matrix mineralization down-regulates the expression of genes that are associated with the ECM maturation period [Lian et al., 1992].

Proliferation of osteoblasts in a cell culture system depends on the density of the cultured cells and their inherent division potential as well as the type of substrates on which they are cultured. When primary diploid fetal calvarial-derived osteoblasts are cultured on type I collagen film or in collagen gel substrates, the cells receive support and/or inductive signals from the ECM which results in an accelerated progression and development of the osteoblastic phenotype, characterized by a decline in proliferative activity and the subsequent induction of genes associated with matrix maturation and mineralization of the developing osteoblasts [Stein et al., 1992].

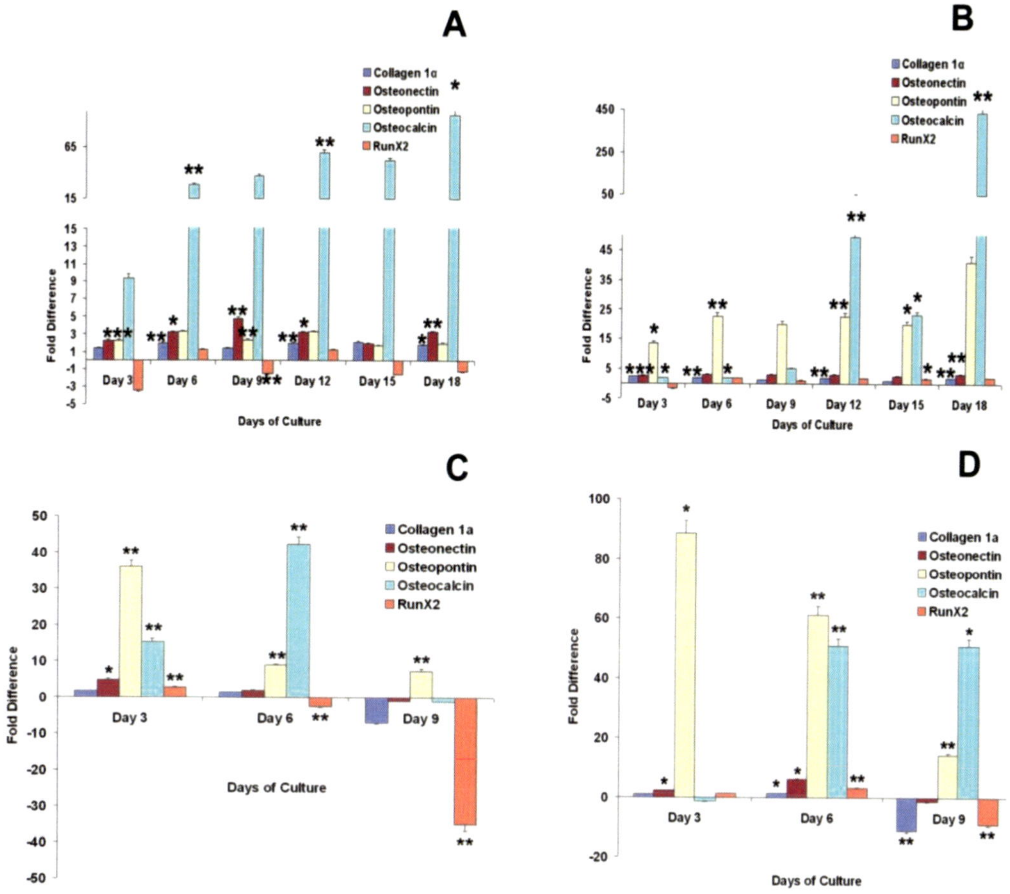

Figure 4. Quantitative real-time polymerase chain reaction (RT-qPCR) analysis of various key osteogenic markers, collagen 1α (Col1a1), osteonectin (Sparc), osteopontin (Spp1), osteocalcin (Bglap2) and runx2 (Runx2) as a function of time. BMSCs were cultured and maintained as described in Research Methods section and harvested at the time points indicated on the X-axis. BMSCs cultured in Petri dish in basal medium (A) and in osteo-inductive medium (B). BMSCs cultured in tubular scaffold in basal medium (C) and in osteo-inductive medium (D). The C_T (threshold cycle) values were calculated as the average of three replicate measurements for each sample analyzed. The expression ratio was calculated using the REST-XL version 2 software. The values are mean ± SE for three cultures (n=3), *$p < 0.05$; **$p < 0.001$ (Valarmathi et al., 2008a).

In any type of in vitro cellular differentiation, the cytodifferentiated cells need to be critically evaluated for their maturation and differentiation at transcriptional (mRNA level), translational (protein level) and functional levels. Consequently, in order to determine the osteogenic differentiation potential in this novel collagen-gel tubular scaffold, we have employed real-time quantitative RT-PCR assays for transcripts that code for osteoblast-related proteins including a major transcription factor for regulating osteogenesis, Runx2 (Table 3; Figure 4). Though gene expression studies have been done on osteogenic differentiation of BMSCs, these studies have been sparse and often contradictory. Byers et al. [1999] found that mRNA levels of osteopontin and osteocalcin increase with time in culture. We obtained similar results when BMSCs were differentiated under standard tissue culture conditions. Other groups have reported a decrease in the mRNA expression of either osteopontin [Malaval et al., 1994; Rickard et al., 1996] or osteocalcin [Cheng et al., 1994] during BMSCs differentiation. A similar decrease in expression pattern for osteopontin was observed in our tubular scaffold osteogenic cultures. These varied patterns of expression suggest that expression of these osteogenic markers may be substrate dependent.

The rapid induction of osteocalcin mRNA during the mineralization phase seen in our study is consistent with the maturation and differentiation of osteoblasts. Given that the scaffold is made of type I collagen and there was extensive mineralization, it suggests that there exists a down regulation of collagen type I mRNA by day 9. The Runx2 transcription factor appears to regulate the expression of numerous proteins specific to the osteogenic lineage [Zelzer et al., 2001]. There is also evidence that multiple signaling pathways converge on the Runx2 transcription factor to regulate osteoblast differentiation [Franceschi et al., 2003]. In our real-time PCR analysis, the level of Runx2 mRNA was progressively down regulated during the mineralization phase indicating that the terminal osteoblastic differentiation of BMSC was occurring in the osteogenic tube cultures.

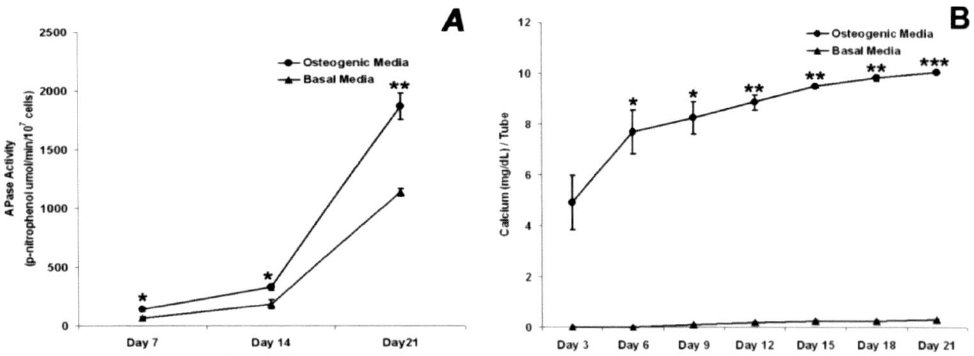

Figure 5. Osteogenic differentiation of BMSCs seeded in 3-D collagen-gel tubular scaffolds. Osteogenic differentiation of BMSCs over a period of three weeks was demonstrated by the increase in alkaline phosphatase and the deposition of minerals. (A) The quantification of alkaline phosphatase demonstrated an increase in activity over 21 days. * $p < 0.05$; ** $p < 0.01$ (compared to the basal medium values). The data represent the mean ± SEM of duplicate cultures (n=2). (B) The quantification of calcium indicated that the accumulation continued beyond 14 days. * $p < 0.05$; ** $p < 0.01$; *** $p < 0.001$ (compared to the basal medium values). The data represent the mean ± SEM of duplicate cultures (n=2). Adapted from Valarmathi et al., 2008a.

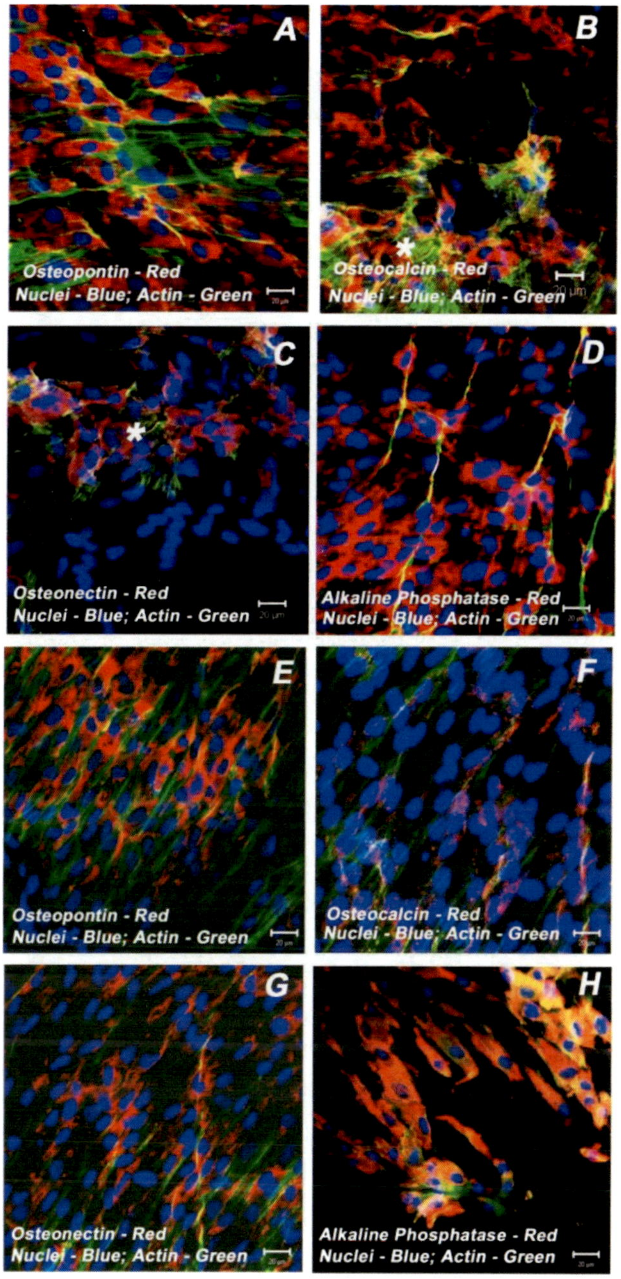

Figure 6. Expression pattern of various osteogenic markers in collagen tubes by immunostaining revealed highly differentiated sheets of mature osteoblasts represented by a distinctive phenotype (cuboidal to polygonal mononuclear cells) and biosynthetic activity (A-D). In addition, areas of multilayered cellular aggregates were seen (B-C, white asterisks). Localization of key osteoblastic phenotypic markers of day 9 osteoinductive tube culture sections demonstrated the expression of osteopontin (red, A), osteocalcin (red, B), osteonectin (red, C), and alkaline phosphatase (red, D). Similarly, localization of osteoblastic phenotypic markers of day 9 basal (E-H, controls) tube culture sections demonstrated the expression pattern of osteopontin (red, E), osteocalcin (red, F), osteonectin (red, G), and alkaline phosphatase (red, H). Cells were also stained for nuclei (blue, DAPI) and fibrillar actin (green, Alexa 488 phalloidin). Merged images A-H (A-H, Scale bar 20 μm). Adpated from Valarmathi et al., 2008a.

Table 3. RT-qPCR Primer Sequences Used in this Study (Valarmathi et al., 2008a; 2008b)

Genes	Forward Primer	Reverse Primer	Product Length (bp)	Annealing Temperature (°C)	GenBank Accession No
Col1a1	5'TCCTGCCGATGTC GCTATC3'	5'CAAGTTCCGGT GTGACTCGTG3'	234	58	XM_213440
Sparc	5'ACAAGCTCCACCT GGACTACA3'	5'TCTTCTTCACAC GCAGTTT3'	180	58	NM_012656
Spp1	5'GACGGCCGAGGTG ATAGCTT3'	5'CATGGCTGGTC TTCCCGTTGC3'	208	58	NM_012881
Bglap2	5'AAAGCCCAGCGAC TCT3'	5'CTAAACGGTGG TGCCATAGAT3'	232	58	NM_013414
Runx2	5'GCTTCTCCAACCC ACGAATG3'	5'GAACTGATAGG ACGCTGACGA3'	212	58	XM_346016
Arbp	5'CGACCTGGAAGTC CAACTAC3'	5'ATCTGCTGCAT CTGCTTG3'	109	58	Z29530

Under osteogenic conditions, the predominant population of cells in the tubular scaffold expressed osteopontin and osteonectin, whereas the number of osteocalcin and alkaline phosphatase expressing cells increased over time in osteogenic medium compared to basal tube cultures (Figure 5, 6). In addition, more cellular aggregates were seen at earlier time points in osteogenic medium. Some of these aggregates showed dense mineralization has previously been observed in other studies [Malaval et al., 1994; Rickard et al., 1996]. The observed upregulation of osteoblastic phenotypic markers and the earlier abundant mineralization seen in the BMSCs osteogenic tubular cultures more closely resembles the in vivo expression patterns, than the osteogenic differentiation of BMSCs under standard 2-D tissue culture conditions (Petri dishes).

It has been suggested that mineral formation which occurs in the presence of supersaturated β-glycerophosphate conditions (> 2mM) may be non-physiological. Chung and co-workers [1992] using a cell-free experimental system, pointed out that mineral particles formed spontaneously in the presence of alkaline phosphatase and β-glycerophosphate and were deposited into a collagen matrix. This phenomenon of mineral particle deposition was not observed when our cell-free collagen gel tubular scaffolds were incubated in osteogenic medium supplemented with 10mM β-glycerophosphate for 9 days. This indicates that the observed mineralization occurring in BMSCs collagen gel tubular constructs under osteogenic differentiation conditions is predominantly due to cell-mediated effect and substantiation of matricellular regulation of bone deposition (Figure 7).

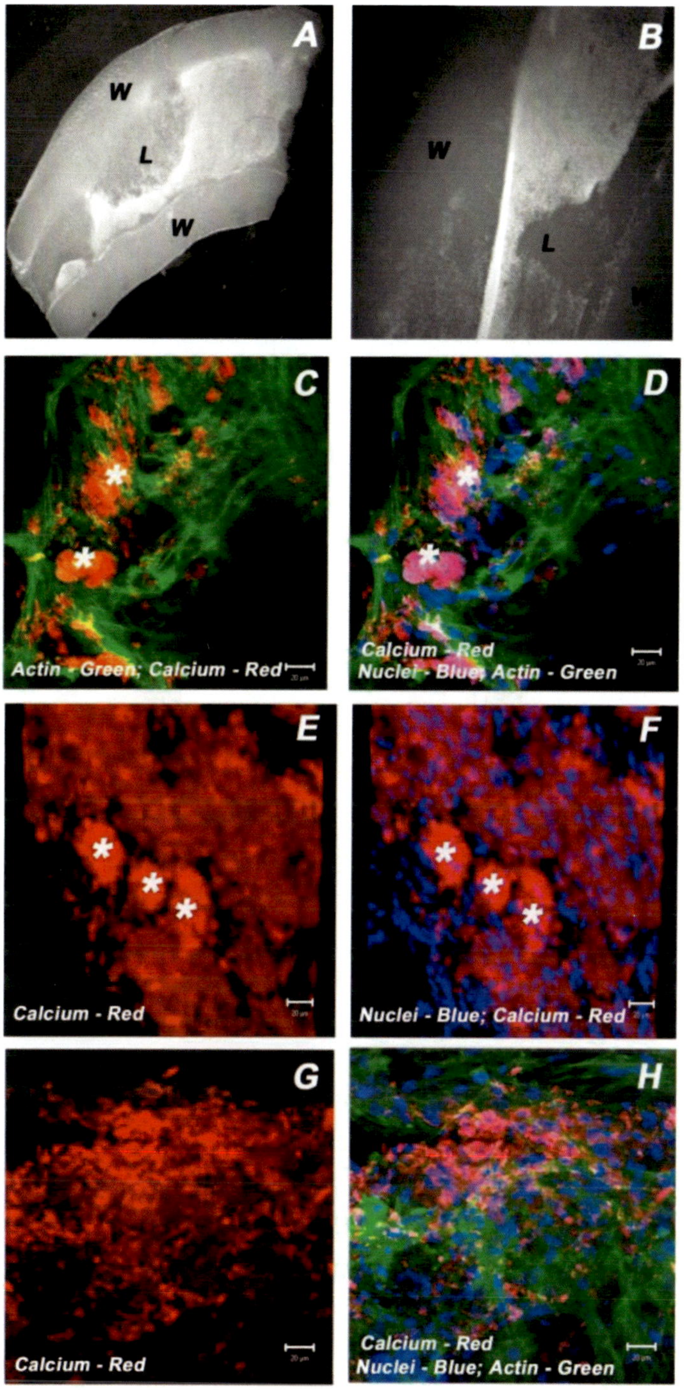

Figure 7. Pattern of mineralization and nodule formation. Longitudinal sections of the osteogenic tube cultures showing extensive areas of mineralization on the luminal surfaces (A-B) and streaks of calcification on the walls (A) (L, lumen; W, wall). Confocal scanning laser microscopic analysis of mineralized matrix by Alizarin red staining for calcium demonstrated extensive areas of diffuse and nodular (C-F, white asterisks) mineralization of the collagen-gel tubes. Sections of day 9 osteoinductive tube cultures were stained for calcium (red, Alizarin red) (C), (E), (G) revealing the mineralized extracellular matrix materials. Cells were also stained for nuclei (blue, DAPI) and fibrillar actin (green, Alexa 488 phalloidin). Figures E and F were projections representing 64 sections collected at 5.68 μm intervals. Figures G and H were projections representing 8 sections collected at 5 μm intervals. Merged images (C-D, F, H). (C-H, Scale bar 20 μm). Adapted from Valarmathi et al., 2008a.

Vasculogenesis is the de novo formation of blood vessels in which vascular precursor cells, angioblasts, differentiate from mesoderm to form endothelial cells, which then coalesce to form intact blood vessels. Angiogenesis is the process by which the vascular network is extended by the budding of preexisting vessels. In each of these processes, the blood vessels initially consist of a single layer of endothelial cells embedded in a scaffolding of extracellular matrix [Poole and Coffin, 1989]. Development of larger blood vessels, i.e., arteries, veins, arterioles and venules from these initial vessels involves recruitment of smooth muscle cell (SMC) precursor cells into the region surrounding the endothelial tubes with subsequent morphogenesis of the appropriate blood vessel. Apart from the two main vascular cell types (endothelial and smooth muscle cells), recent evidence indicates that bone marrow stem cells may also contribute to the process of angiogenesis, both in embryos and the adults. In addition, endothelial precursors have also been identified in the adult bone marrow. In vivo studies revealed that these endothelial precursors and other bone marrow-derived cells contribute to the angiogenesis as well as arteriogenesis in ischemic disease [Carmeliet and Luttun, 2001].

In our study [Valarmathi et al., 2008a], BMSCs cultured on the collagen type I tubular scaffold in osteogenic media showed a dramatic vascular morphogenesis (Figure 8). It appears that the specific structural organization of our collagen-gel 3-D tubular scaffolds and the supplements of osteogenic medium not only enhanced the osteoblastic differentiation but also supported the process of vasculogenesis as evidence by the formation of plexus of nascent capillary-structures. In addition, these elongated vessel-like structures were surrounded by SMCs. The α-SMA positive cells were not only recruited in juxtaposition to the aligned endothelial cells but they also wrapped around them in an orientation that mimics the formation of in vivo vessel-like structures. Furthermore, our osteogenic tube cultures produced both nascent endothelium lined capillary-like vessels and also microvessel-like structures containing smooth muscle cells. Both these types of microvascular structures could be originated from a common vascular progenitor of BMSCs. However, no definitive lumens were observed in our vessel-like tubes. Further work is ongoing to investigate whether our endothelial lined tubular structures seen in the walls of the tubular scaffold have a mature vascular phenotype.

Finally, since the phenotypic characterization and analysis of input BMSCs by flowcytometry and confocal microscopy demonstrated the lack of contaminating hematopoietic stem cells and other potential bone marrow-derived endothelial precursors as well as vascular-derived endothelial cells, the de novo vasculogenesis seen in this growth environment may be attributed to BMSCs. This behavior of BMSCs and their exhibition of vasculogenic potential can be attributed to the growth micro-environment provided by the aligned collagen-gel tubular scaffolds and the parameters set in these experimental conditions.

Similarly, a novel co-culture of two different types of plastic stem cells, BMSCs (postnatal) and PEs (embryonic), on a 3-D tubular scaffold engineered from aligned collagen type I strands and cultured in osteogenic medium can generate vascularized bone tissue. PE appears to have the potential to vascularize a variety of tissues that has not been adequately tested in vitro. Epicardial progenitors are an extremely plastic type of embryonic tissue that have been proposed and characterized to be a multipotent cellular lineage [Perez-Pomares et al., 2006].

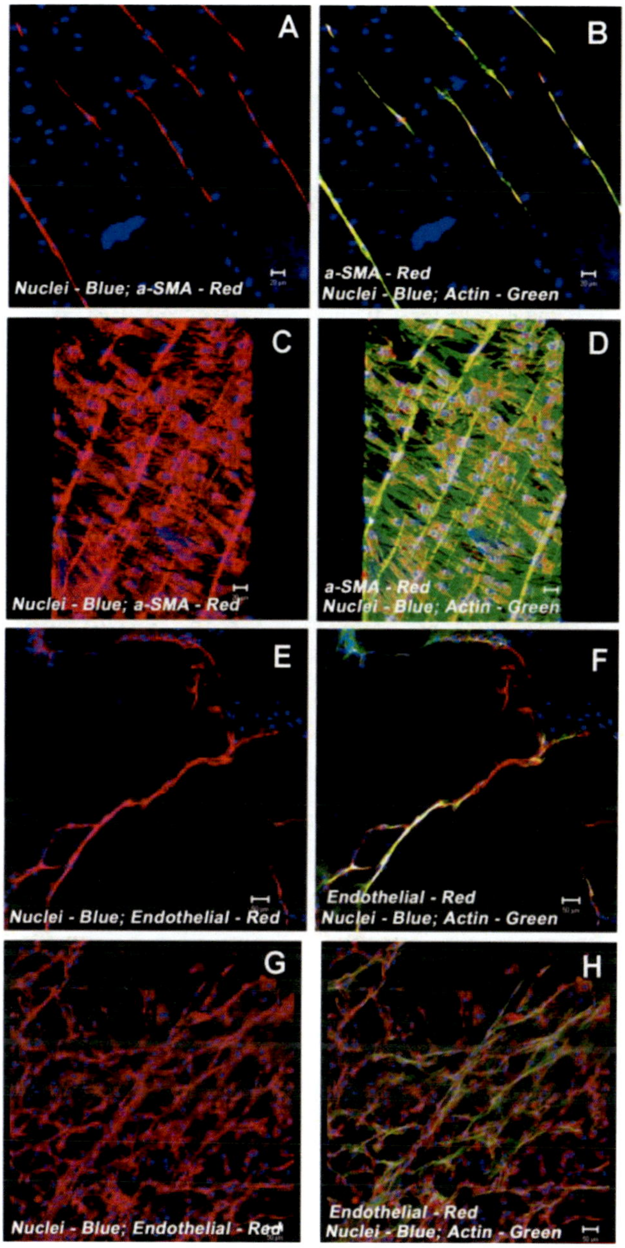

Figure 8. Expression pattern of vasculogenic markers α-SMA and tomato lectin (TL). Localization of BMSC-derived vascular progenitor cells on the collagen tube scaffold by confocal microscopy is seen in panels A, C, E, and G. The merged images showing the actin cytoskeleton are shown in panels B, D, F, H. Sections of a day 9 osteogenic tube culture demonstrated nascent capillary-like structures positive for α-SMA (red, A). These elongated cord-like structures showed strong colocalization of α-SMA and actin (merged, B). In the tubes nuclei appeared aligned (blue, DAPI). In adjacent fields, abundant sheets of parallel oriented α-SMA positive cells were abutting the nascent vessel-like structures (red, C). The merged image (D) shows actin and α-SMA in vessel-like structures that appear to be in different planes with almost a perpendicular alignment with the underlying α-SMA positive cells (D). Similar sections of osteogenic cultured tubes illustrate the sprouting and branching tubular structures positive for the rat endothelial marker tomato lectin (red, E-H). A plexus of arborizing endothelial cells was observed. These plexuses contained capillary-like vessels lined with endothelial cells (red, G). Similarly in the merged panel, the apparent multilayered nature of the vessels was observed. However in these fields, the plexuses of endothelial cells were not in a perpendicular arrangement but rather in a web-like orientation (merged, H). Figures C and D were projections representing 19 sections collected at 2 μm intervals. Figures G and H were projections representing 32 sections collected at 9 μm intervals. Merged images (A-H) (A-D, Scale bar 20 μm; E-H, Scale bar 50 μm). Adapted from Valarmathi et al., 2008a.

Several recent studies have demonstrated that progenitors of the epicardium and coronary vascular system are derived from extra cardiac tissue, the proepicardial organ (PEO). PEs (coronary progenitors) are easy to isolate and culture, and are shown to proliferate in different in vitro assays [Perez-Pomares, et al., 2002; Wessels and Perez-Pomares, 2004].

Fate mapping studies show that the proepicardium contains precursors for the endothelium, smooth muscle and adventitial cells (pericytes and fibroblasts) of the coronary vasculature [Tomanek, 2005]. Formation of coronary vessels occurs by an epithelial to mesenchymal transformation (EMT) of proepicardial cells at the surface of the heart, followed by vasculogenesis in the subepicardial layer, assembly and remodeling of a primitive coronary plexus, and investment by coronary smooth muscle cells [Majesky, 2004].

We hypothesized that embryonic PEs in the appropriate environment could be used to induce endothelial vessel networks in engineered bone tissue in vitro. Initial investigation used the avian PEs because it is readily amenable to isolation [Antin, 2004] and well developed antibodies are available for identifying specific vascular proteins. In addressing this hypothesis, first we developed a 3-D co-culture system in which rat BMSCs were co-seeded with quail PEs and cultured on a highly aligned, porous, biocompatible collagen-gel tubular scaffold for osteogenic and vasculogenic differentiation purposes. In these investigations, we compared the effects of two types of growth media, osteogenic and basal media on the osteogenic and vasculogenic fate of both BMSCs and PEs, in addition, we compared and specifically assessed the consequence of PEs presence on the expression of osteogenic markers in BMSCs. Osteogenic medium promoted the osteoblastic differentiation of the BMSCs and also supported the formation of endothelium lined tube-like structures within the constructs. In contrast, basal medium alone generated vessel-like structures within the constructs and did not support the differentiation of BMSCs into osteoblasts.

The expression pattern of key osteogenic gene transcripts in the 3-D tube constructs was determined by analysis of the expression of collagen type I, osteonectin, osteopontin, osteocalcin and Runx2 at mRNA level in the tube constructs (Figure 9). RT-qPCR results showed that osteoblastic differentiation of BMSCs in osteogenic conditions resulted in increased expression of non-collagenous proteins such as osteopontin (bone sialoprotein) and osteocalcin specific of osteoblasts. Moreover, co-cultures that included BMSCs/PEs had higher levels of osteopontin and osteocalcin mRNAs than BMSCs alone. The increased expression of the osteoblast-specific structural gene, osteocalcin, which is only expressed by fully differentiated osteoblasts by day 9, is consistent with the observed endothelial networks in the co-culture. This endothelialization could possibly be one of the necessary factors regulating the induction of mature osteoblasts and mineralization of the constructs and may not be sufficient on its own.

Identification and localization of various osteogenic markers by immunostaining and confocal microscopy of day 9 tube cultures showed that BMSCs were competent to adhere and undergo condensation in these tubular scaffolds. These BMSCs were also able to undergo complete maturation and differentiation into alkaline phosphatase and osteocalcin positive osteoblasts, and which formed highly cohesive cellular aggregates (Figure 10, 11, 12). Furthermore, these cellular aggregations culminated into mineralized bone-like nodules (Figure 13). When BMSCs and PEs were co-cultured on the scaffolds, the PEs organized into tube-like structures in association with the BMSC-derived developing osteoblasts throughout the construct, forming vessel-like networks within the engineered bone tissue in vitro. This illustrated the in vitro formation of vascularized bone-like element from undifferentiated progenitor cells (BMSCs/PEs).

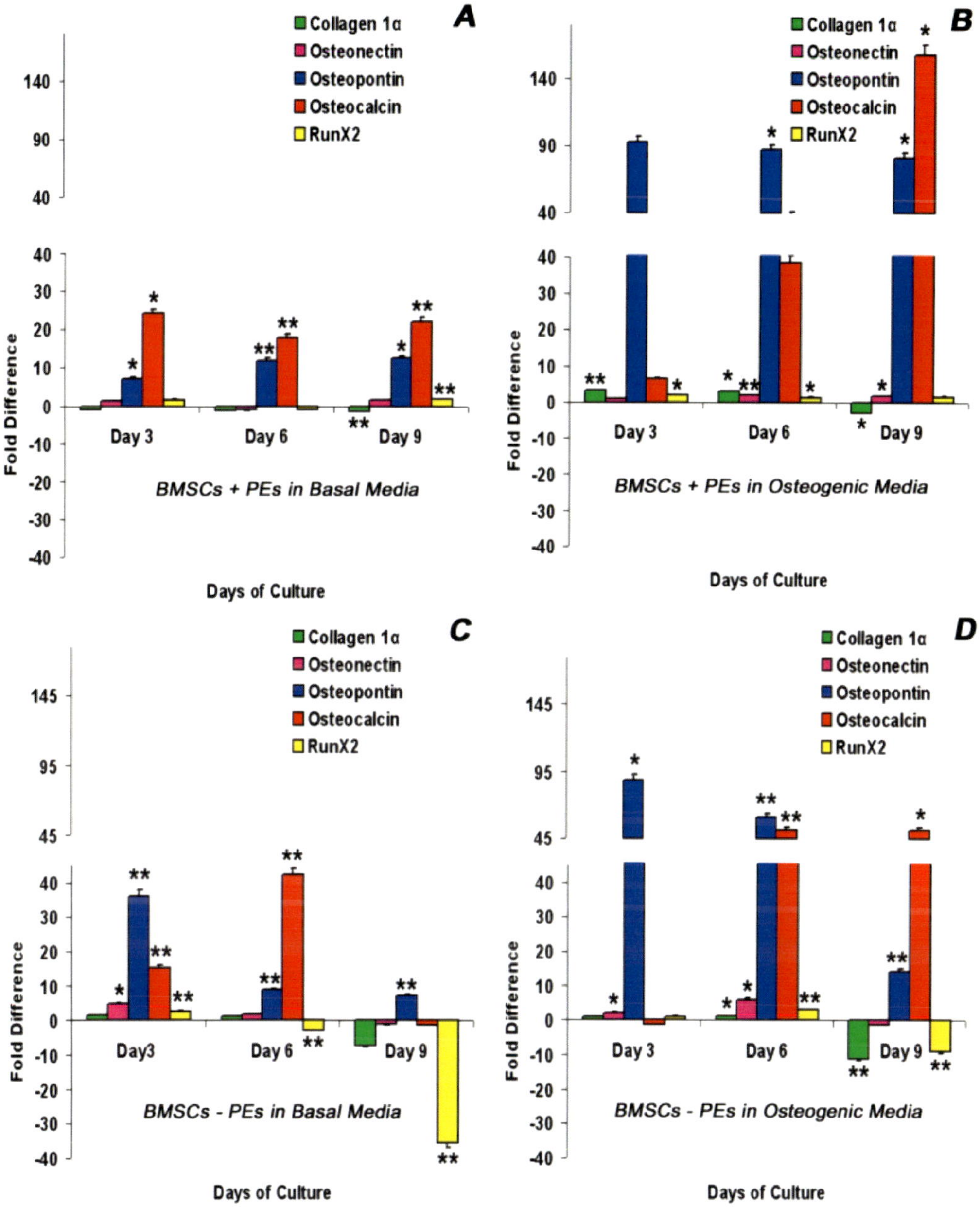

Figure 9. Quantitative real-time polymerase chain reaction (RT-qPCR) analysis of various key osteogenic markers, collagen 1α (Col1a1), osteonectin (Sparc), osteopontin (Spp1), osteocalcin (Bglap2) and runx2 (Runx2) as a function of time. BMSCs and BMSCs/PEs were cultured and maintained as described in the Research Methods section and harvested at the time points indicated on the X-axis. BMSCs and PEs co-cultured on tubular scaffold in basal media (A) and in osteogenic media (B). BMSCs cultured on the tubular scaffold in basal media (C) and in osteogenic media (D). The C_T (threshold cycle) values were calculated as the average of three replicate measurements for each sample analyzed. The expression ratio was calculated using the REST-XL version 2 software. The values are mean ± SE for three cultures (n=3), *p < 0.05; **p < 0.001. Adapted from Valarmathi et al., 2008b.

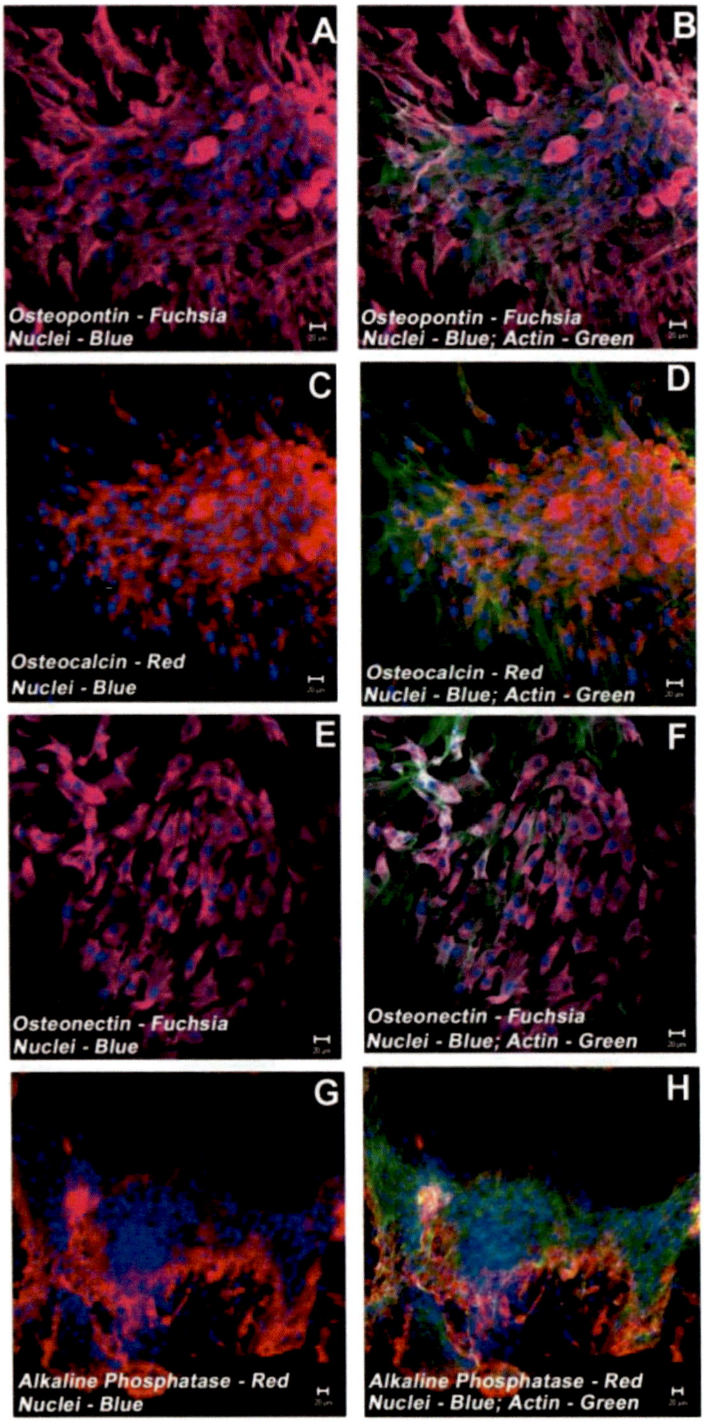

Figure 10. Expression pattern of various osteogenic markers in tubular scaffold by confocal microscopy. Immunostaining of osteogenic tube co-cultures revealed areas of cellular clustering and aggregation of mature osteoblasts represented by their distinct morphology and phenotypic expression (A-H). Localization of key osteoblastic phenotypic markers of day 9 osteoinductive co-culture tube sections demonstrated the expression of osteopontin (fuchsia, A-B), osteocalcin (red, C-D), osteonectin (fuchsia, E-F), and alkaline phosphatase (red, G-H). Cells were also stained for nuclei (blue, DAPI) and fibrillar actin (green, Alexa 488 phalloidin). Merged images A-H (A-H, Scale bar 20 μm). Adapted from Valarmathi et al., 2008b.

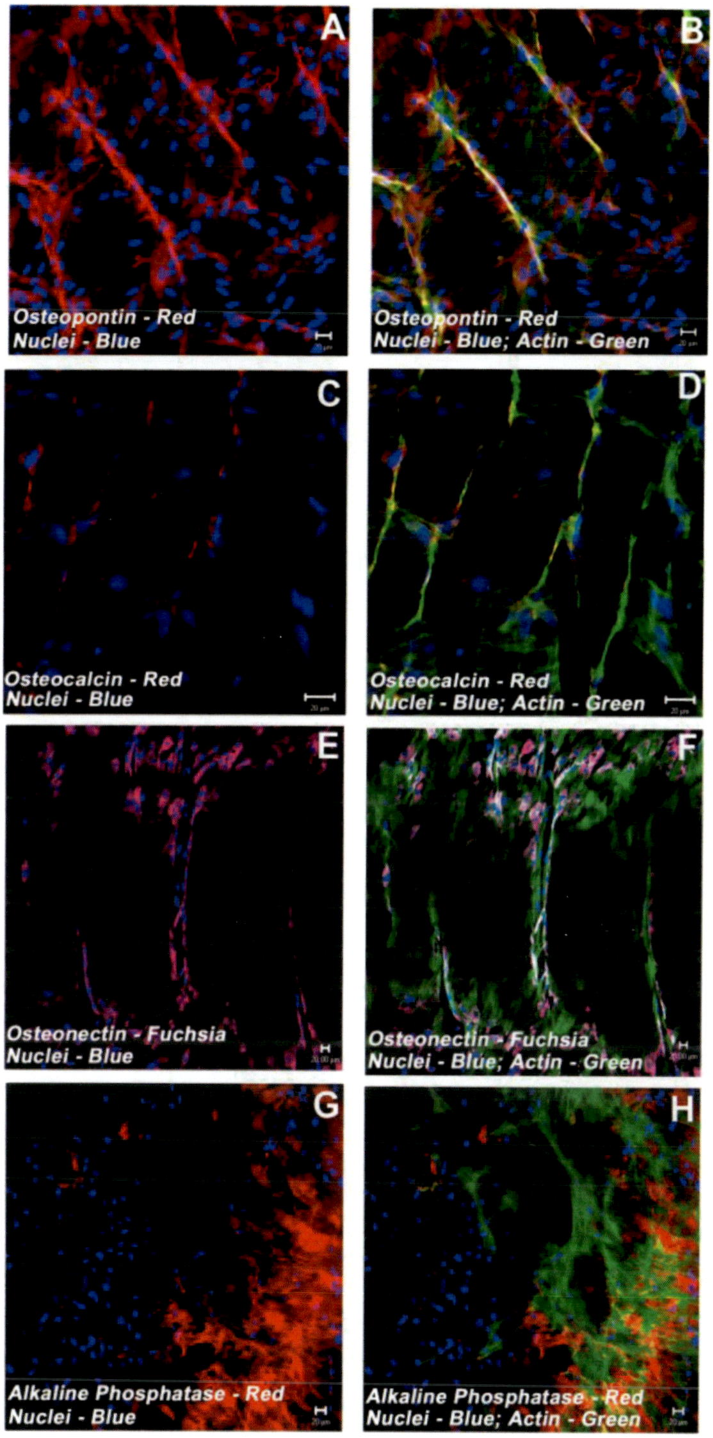

Figure 11. Expression pattern of various osteogenic markers in tubular scaffold by confocal microscopy. Immunostaining of non-osteogenic tube co-cultures revealed areas of interlacing fascicles of elongated cells with little evidence of cellular aggregation amidst the developing vessel-like structures (A-H, controls). Localization of osteoblastic phenotypic markers of day 9 basal tube co-culture sections demonstrated the expression pattern of osteopontin (red, A-B), osteocalcin (red, C-D), osteonectin (fuchsia, E-F), and alkaline phosphatase (red, G-H). Cells were also stained for nuclei (blue, DAPI) and fibrillar actin (green, Alexa 488 phalloidin). Merged images A-H (A-H, Scale bar 20 μm). Adapted from Valarmathi et al., 2008b.

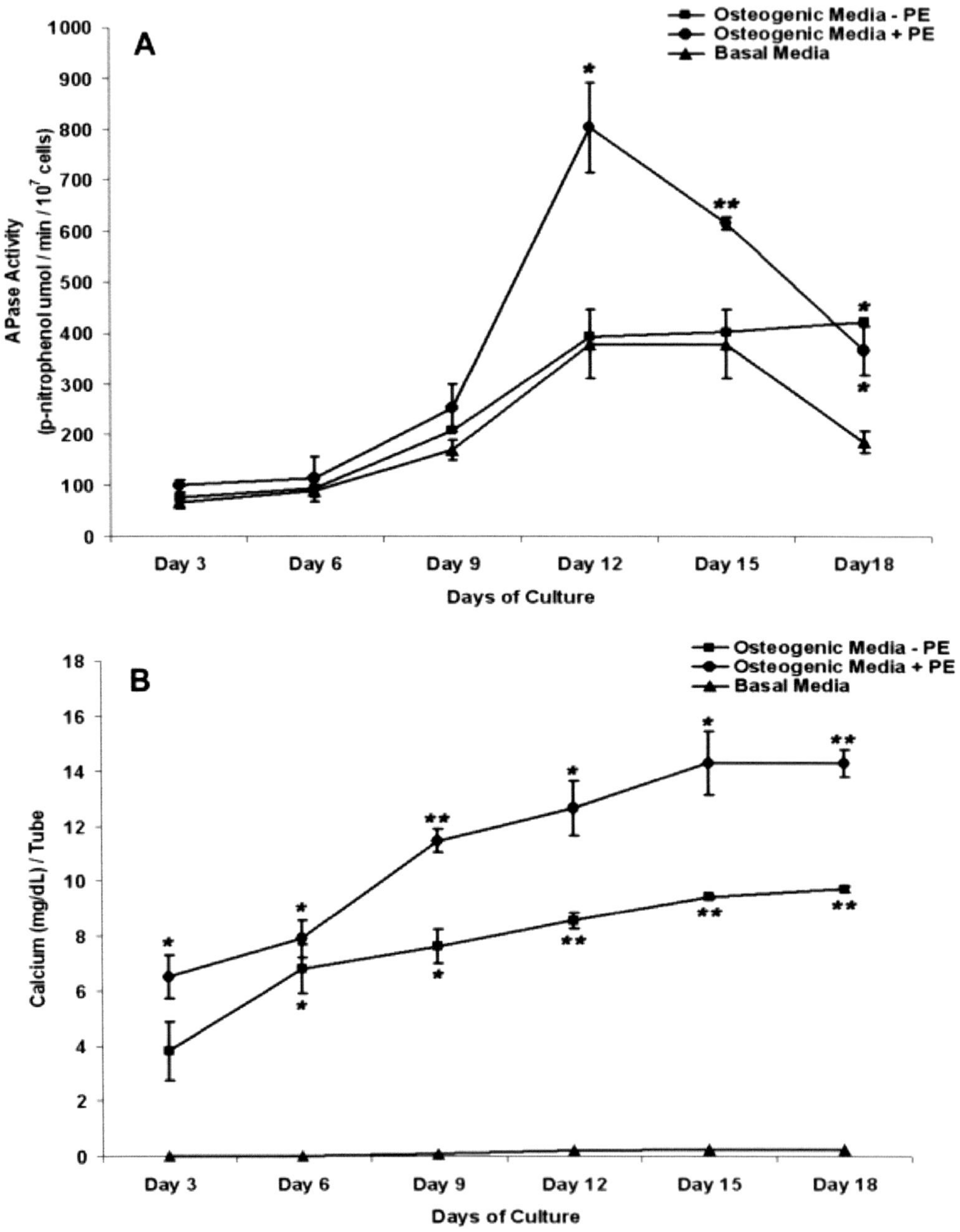

Figure 12. Osteogenic differentiation of BMSCs/PECs co-culture in 3-D collagen-gel tubular scaffolds. Osteogenic differentiation of BMSCs over a period of 18 days was demonstrated by the increase in alkaline phosphatase and the deposition of minerals. (A) The quantification of alkaline phosphatase demonstrated an increase in activity over 18 days. * $p < 0.05$; ** $p < 0.01$ (compared to the basal medium values). The data represent the mean ± SEM of duplicate cultures (n=2). (B) The quantification of calcium indicated that the accumulation continued beyond 14 days. * $p < 0.05$; ** $p < 0.01$ (compared to the basal medium values). The data represent the mean ± SEM of duplicate cultures (n=2). Adapted from Valarmathi et al., 2008b.

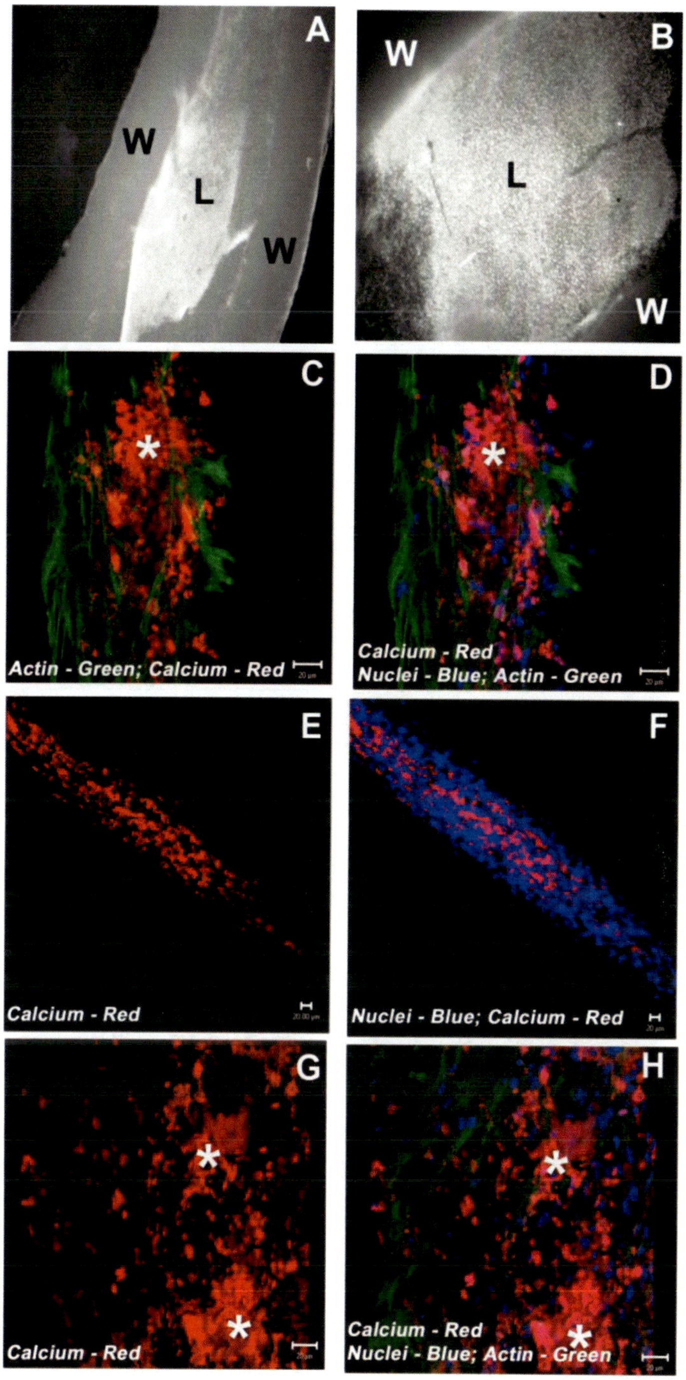

Figure 13. Pattern of mineralization and nodule formation. Longitudinal sections of the osteogenic (BMSCs/PEs) co-culture tubes showing areas of extensive mineralization on the luminal surfaces (A-B) (L, lumen; W, wall). Confocal scanning laser microscopic analysis of mineralized matrix by Alizarin red staining for calcium demonstrated extensive areas of diffuse and nodular (C, G, white asterisks) mineralization of the collagen-gel tubular scaffolds. Sections of day 9 osteoinductive co-culture tubes were stained for calcium (red, Alizarin red) (C), (E), (G) revealing the mineralized extracellular matrix materials. Cells were also stained for nuclei (blue, DAPI) and fibrillar actin (green, Alexa 488 phalloidin). Figures E and F were projections representing 64 sections collected at 4.96 μm intervals. Figures G and H were projections representing 20 sections collected at 5 μm intervals. Merged images (C-D, F, H). (C-H, Scale bar 20 μm). Adapted from Valarmathi et al., 2008b.

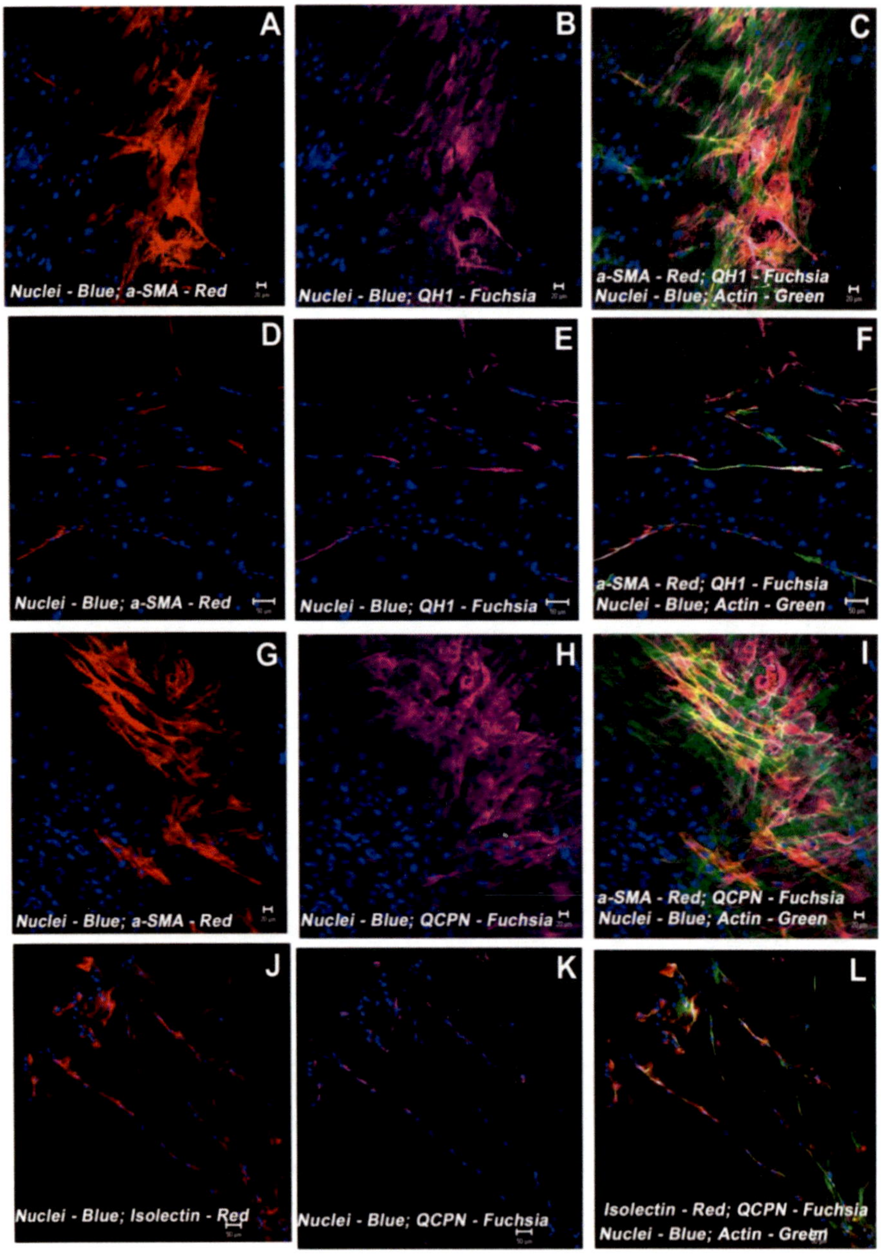

Figure 14. Expression pattern of various vasculogenic markers in tubular scaffold by confocal microscopy. Immunostaining revealed areas of abundant interlacing fascicles of QCPN, QH1, Isolectin and α-smooth muscle actin (α-SMA) positive cells in osteogenic tube (BMSCs/PEs) co-cultures (A-L). In addition, extensive arborizations of nascent capillary-like structures were also seen amidst the developing cellular aggregates. Localization of key vasculogenic phenotypic markers of day 9 osteoinductive co-culture tube sections demonstrated the expression of α-SMA (red, A, D, G), QH1 (fuchsia, B, E), QCPN (fuchsia, H, K) and Isolectin (red, J). The merged images showing the actin cytoskeleton (green) are shown in panels C, F, I and L. Sections of a day 9 osteogenic tube culture demonstrated nascent capillary-like structures positive for α-SMA (red, D) and QH1 (fuchsia, E). These elongated cord-like structures showed colocalization of α-SMA, QH1 and actin (merged, F). In the tubes nuclei appeared aligned (blue, DAPI). Similar sections of osteogenic (BMSCs\PEs) co-cultured tubes illustrate the sprouting and branching tube-like structures positive for the endothelial marker isolectin (red, J) and QCPN (fuchsia, K). This plexus contained arborising capillary-like vessels lined with quail endothelial cells and showed colocalization of isolectin, QCPN and actin (merged, L). Cells were also stained for nuclei (blue, DAPI) and fibrillar actin (green, Alexa 488 phalloidin). Merged images A-L (A-C, G-I, Scale bar 20 μm; D-F, J-L, Scale bar 50μm). Adapted from Valarmathi et al., 2008b.

PEs derived vessel formation is a combination of vasculogenesis, de novo endothelial tube formation, and angiogenesis, sprouting from existing endothelial tubes [Wada et al., 2003]. Blood vessels are stabilized by association with pericytes or smooth muscle cells [Koike et al., 2004; Carmeliet, 2003]. In this study, we have demonstrated that the isolated PEs were able to adhere and proliferate in the tubular scaffold in osteogenic conditions and continue their development to undergo vessel-like formation (Figure 14). Definitive endothelial cells were identified using the QH1 antibody, which identifies quail endothelial cells [Pardanaud et al., 1987], and the isolectin, another marker for endothelial cells which was found closely associated with QH-1 staining. These two endothelial-specific markers localized to capillary-like structures present on and within the scaffold. This suggests that PE-derived endothelial cells coalesced into endothelial tube-like structures and began the process of vasculogenesis, consistent with our previous study [Nesbitt et al., 2007]. The PE-derived cells and vessel-like structures expressed α-SMA. These α-SMA positive cells were recruited in juxtaposition to the aligned endothelial cells and they wrapped around the endothelium in an orientation that resembles the formation of in vivo vessel-like structures. Further work is in progress to elucidate the vessel maturation and utilization of mammalian derived PEs.

Taken together, our molecular, biochemical, immunocytochemical and histo-morphological data indicate that the specific geometric configuration of the 3-D collagen-gel tubular scaffold in the form of aligned fibers may comprise the principle matrix microenvironment, which is conducive and inductive to the sequence of maturation and differentiation events culminating into vascularized, mineralized bone-like elements.

CONCLUSION

Here we report the development of various novel 3-D model systems that recapitulate many aspects of osteogenesis. Since BMSCs alone underwent differentiation into osteoblastic and vascular cell lineages as well the BMSCs/PEs synergetically differentiated into both osteoblastic and vascular cell lineages, these in vitro model systems provide a platform for investigating the functional role and interplay of neo-vascularization in the maturation and differentiation of BMSCs derived osteoblasts as well as to study the factors that regulate vasculogenesis, angiogenesis and vessel maturation. Besides, in vitro engineering of vascularized bone as replacement tissue for variously sized segmental bone defects in regenerative medicine.

ACKNOWLEDGMENTS

"This work was supported by an award from the American Heart Association." – National Scientist Development Grant (11SDG5280022) as well "This material is based upon work supported by the National Science Foundation/EPSCoR under Grant No. (EPS – 0903795)." – The South Carolina Project for Organ Biofabrication, for Valarmathi Thiruvanamalai.

References

Aggarwal S, Pittenger MF. Human mesenchymal stem cells modulate allogeneic immune cell responses. *Blood* 2005;105:1815-22.

Antin P, Fallon JF, Schoenwolf GC. The chick embryo rules (still)! *Dev Dyn* 2004;229:413.

Bianco P, Kuznetsov SA, Riminucci M, Robey PG. Postnatal Skeletal Stem Cells. *Methods in Enzymology* 2006;419:117-48.

Bianco P, Riminucci M, Gronthos S, Robey PG. Bone marrow stromal stem cells: nature, biology, and potential applications. *Stem Cells* 2001;19:180-92.

Bianco P, Robey PG. Stem cells in tissue engineering. *Nature* 2001;414:118-21.

Byers RJ, Brown J, Brandwood C, Wood P, Staley W, Hainey L, et al. Osteoblastic differentiation and mRNA analysis of STRO-1-positive human bone marrow stromal cells using primary in vitro culture and poly(A) PCR. *J Pathol* 1999;187:374-81.

Carano RA, Filvaroff EH. Angiogenesis and bone repair. *Drug Discov Today* 2003;8:980-89.

Carlson BM. Tissue engineering and regeneration In: ed. *Principles of regenerative biology*. Amsterdam: Elsevier, 2007;pp259-78.

Carmeliet P, Luttun A. The emerging role of the bone marrow-derived stem cells in (therapeutic) angiogenesis. *Thromb Haemost* 2001;86:289-97.

Carmeliet P. Angiogenesis in health and disease. *Nat Med* 2003;9:653-60.

Carvalho RS, Einhorn TA, Lehmann W, Edgar C, Al-Yamani A, Apazidis A, et al. The role of angiogenesis in a murine tibial model of distraction osteogenesis. *J Artif Organs* 2004;34:849-61.

Cheng SL, Yang JW, Rifas L, Zhang SF, Avioli LV. Differentiation of human bone marrow osteogenic stromal cells in vitro: Induction of the osteoblast phenotype by dexamethasone. *Endocrinology* 1994;134:277-86.

Chung CH, Golub EE, Forbes E, Tokuoka T, Shapiro IM. Mechanism of action of beta-glycerophosphate on bone cell mineralization. *Calcif Tissue Int 1*992;51:305-11.

Dominici M, Le Blanc K, Mueller I, Slaper-Cortenback I, Marini F, Krause D, et al. Minimal criteria for defining multipotent mesenchymal stromal cells. The International Society For Cellular Therapy position statement. *Cytotherapy* 2006;8:315-7.

Finkenzeller G, Torio-Padron N, Momeni A, Mehlhorn AT, Bjorn Stark G. In vitro angiogenesis properties of endothelial progenitor cells: A promising tool for vascularization of ex vivo engineered tissues. *Tissue Eng* 2007;13:1413-20.

Franceschi RT, Xiao G, Jiang D, Gopalakrishnan R, Yang S, Reith E. Multiple signaling pathways converge on the Cbfal/Runx2 transcription factor to regulate osteoblast differentiation. *Connect Tissue Res* 2003;44(Suppl 1):109-16.

Fuseler JW, Valarmathi MT. Modulation of the migration and differentiation potential of adult bone marrow stromal stem cells by nitric oxide. *Biomaterials* 2012;33:1032-43.

Hamburger V, Hamilton HL. A series of normal stages in the development of the chick embryo. *J Morphol* 1951;88:49-92.

Heng BC, Cao T, Stanton LW, Robson P, Olsen B. Strategies for directing the differentiation of stem cells into the osteogenic lineage in vitro. *J Bone Miner Res* 2004;19:1379-94.

Koike N, Fukumura D, Gralla O, Au P, Schechner JS, Jain RK. Tissue Engineering: creation of long-lasting blood vessels. *Nature* 2004;428:138-9.

Krause DS, Theise ND, Collector MI, Henegariu O, Hwang S, Gardner R, et al. Multi-organ, multi-lineage engraftment by a single bone marrow-derived stem cell. *Cell* 2001;105:369-77.

Lagasse E, Connors H, Al-Dhalimy M, Reitsma M, Dohse M, Osborne L, et al. Purified hematopoietic stem cells can differentiate into hepatocytes in vivo. *Nat Med* 2000;6:1229-34.

Lan CW, Wang YJ. Collagen as an immobilization vehicle for bone marrow stromal cells enriched with osteogenic potential. *Artif Cells Blood Substit Immobil Biotechnol* 2003;31:59-68.

Lanza RP, Langer R, Vacanti J. *Principles of tissue engineering. Academic Press*, San Diego, California, CA, USA, 2000.

Levenber S, Rouwkema J, Macdonald M, Garfein ES, Kohane DS, Darland DC, et al. Engineering vascularized skeletal muscle tissue. *Nat Biotechnol* 2005;23:879-84.

Levenberg S. Engineering blood vessels from stem cells: recent advances and applications. *Curr Opin Biotechnol* 2005;16:516-23.

Lian JB, Stein GS, Owen TA, Tassinari MS, Aronow M, Collart D, et al. Gene expression during development of the osteoblast phenotype: An integrated relationship of cell growth to differentiation. In G. S. Stein and J. B. Lian, eds. *Molecular and Cellular Approaches to the Control of Proliferation and Differentiation.* Academic Press, San Diego, pp. 165-223, 1992.

Linsenmayer TF. Collagen. Cell Biology of Extracellular Matrix, 2nd Edition, Edited by Elizabeth D. Hay, Plenum Press, New York, 1991.

Majesky MW. Development of coronary vessels. *Curr Top Dev Biol* 2004;62:225-59.

Malaval L, Modrowski D, Gupta AK, Aubin JE. Cellular expression of bone-related proteins during in vitro osteogenesis in rat bone marrow stromal cell cultures. *J Cell Physiol* 1994;158:555-72.

Maniatopoulos C, Sodek J, Melcher AH. Bone formation in vitro by stromal cells obtained from bone marrow of young adult rats. *Cell tissue Res* 1988;254:317-30.

Moore MA. "Turning brain into blood": clinical applications of stem-cell research in neurobiology and hematology. *N Engl J Med* 1999;341:605-7.

Nesbitt TL, Patel PA, Yost MJ, Goodwin RL, Potts JD. A 3-D model of coronary vessel development. In *Vitro Cell Dev Biol Anim* 2007;43:10-16.

Orlic D, Kaistura J, Chimenti S, Jakoniuk I, Anderson SM, Li B, et al. Bone marrow cells regenerate infarcted myocardium. *Nature* 2001;410;701-5.

Pardanaud L, Altman C, Kitos P, Dieterlen-Lievre F, Buck CA. Vasculogenesis in the early quail blastodisc as studied with a monoclonal antibody recognizing endothelial cells. *Development* 1987;100:339-49.

Pera MF. Stem cells: The dark side of induced pluripotency. *Nature* 2011;471:46-7.

Perez-Pomares JM, Carmona R, Gonzalez-Iriarte M, Atencia G, Wessels A, Munoz-Chapuli R. Origin of coronary endothelial cells from epicardial mesothelium in avian embryos. *Int J Dev Biol* 2002;46:1005-13.

Perez-Pomares JM, Mironov V, Guadix JA, Macias D, Markwald RR, Munoz-Chapuli R. In vitro self-assembly of proepicardial cell aggregates: an embryonic vasculogenic model for vascular tissue engineering. *Anat Rec A Discov Mol Cell Evol Biol* 2006;288:700-13.

Poole TJ, Coffin JD. Vasculogenesis and angiogenesis: two distinct morphogenetic mechanisms establish embryonic vascular pattern. *J Exp Zool* 1989;251:24.

Reddi AH. Role of morphogenetic proteins in skeletal tissue engineering and regeneration. *Nat Biotechnol* 1998;16:247-52.

Reyes M, Dudek A, Jahagirdar B, Koodie L, Marker PH, Verfaillie CM. Origin of endothelial progenitors in human postnatal bone marrow. *J Clin Invest* 2002;109:337-46.

Rickard DJ, Kassem M, Hefferan TE, Sarkar G, Spelsberg TC, Riggs BL. Isolation and characterization of osteoblast precursor cells from human bone marrow. *J Bone Miner Res* 1996;11:312-24.

Ripamonti U, Ramoshebi LN, Patton J, Matsaba T, Teare J, Renton L. Soluble Signals and Insoluble Substrata: Novel Molecular Cues Instructing the Induction of Bone. In: Massaro EJ, Rogers JM eds., *The Skeleton.* Humana Press. Totowa, New Jersey, NJ, USA, pp. 217-227, 2004.

Ripamonti U. Soluble, insoluble and geometric signals sculpt the architecture of mineralized tissues. *J Cell Mol Med* 2004;8:169-80.

Robey PG. Vertebrate mineralized matrix proteins: structure and function. *Connect Tissue Res* 1996;35:131-6.

Runyan RB, Potts JD, Sharma RV, Loeder CP, Chiang JJ, Bhalla RC. Signal transduction of a tissue interaction during embryonic heart development. *Cell Regul* 1990;1:301-13.

Shi S, Kirk M, Kahn AJ. The role of type I collagen in the regulation of the osteoblast phenotype. *J Bone Miner Res* 1996;11:1139-45.

Stein GS, Lian JB, Owen TA, Holthuis J, Bortell R, van Wijnen AJ. Molecular mechanisms that mediate a functional relationship between proliferation and differentiation. In G. S. Stein and J. B. Lian, eds. *Molecular and Cellular Approaches to the Control of Proliferation and Differentiation.* Academic Press, San Diego, pp. 299-341, 1992.

Taipale J, Keski-Oja J. Growth factors in the extracellular matrix. *FASEB J* 1997;11:51-9.

Taira M, Toyosawa S, Ijyuin N, Takahashi J, Araki Y. Studies on osteogenic differentiation of rat bone marrow stromal cells cultured in type I collagen gel by RT-PCR analysis. *J Oral Rehabil* 2003;30:802-7.

Taub M, Wag Y, Szczesny TM, Edelman GM. Asymmetric expression in somites of cytotactin and its proteoglycan ligand is correlated with neural crest cell distribution. *Proc Natl Acad Sci USA* 1990;87:4002-6.

Tomanek RJ. Formation of the coronary vasculature during development. *Angiogenesis* 2005;8:273-84.

Valarmathi MT, Davis JM, Yost MJ, Goodwin RL, Potts JD. A three-dimensional model of vasculogenesis. *Biomaterials* 2009;30:1098-112.

Valarmathi MT, Fuseler JW, Goodwin RL, Davis JM, Potts JD. The mechanical coupling of adult marrow stromal stem cells during cardiac regeneration assessed in a 2-D co-culture model. *Biomaterials* 2011;32:2834-50.

Valarmathi MT, Goodwin RL, Fuseler JW, Davis JM, Yost MJ, Potts JD. A 3-D cardiac muscle construct for exploring adult marrow stem cell based myocardial regeneration. *Biomaterials* 2010;31:3185-200.

Valarmathi MT, Yost MJ, Goodwin RL, Potts JD. A three-dimensional tubular scaffold that modulates the osteogenic and vasculogenic differentiation of rat bone marrow stromal cells. *Tissue Eng* 2008a;14:491-504.

Valarmathi MT, Yost MJ, Goodwin RL, Potts JD. The influence of proepicardial cells on the osteogenic potential of marrow stromal cells in a three-dimensional tubular scaffold. *Biomaterials* 2008b;29:2203-16.

Villanueva JE, Nimni ME. Promotion of calvarial cell osteogenesis by endothelial cells. *J Bone Miner Res* 1990;5:733-39.

Vukicevic S, Kleinman HK, Luyten FP, Roberts AB, Roche NS, Reddi AH. Identification of multiple active growth factors in basement membrane Matrigel suggests caution in interpretation of cellular activity related to extracellular matrix components. *Exp Cell Res* 1992;202:1-8.

Wada AM, Smith TK, Osler ME, Reese DE, Bader DM. Epicardial/Mesothelial cell line retains vasculogenic potential of embryonic epicardium. *Circ Res* 2003;92:525-31.

Wessels A, Perez-Pomares JM. The epicardium and epicardially derived cells (EPDCs) as cardiac stem cells. *Anat Rec A Discov Mol Cell Evol Biol* 2004;276:43-57.

Yoshikawa H, Myoui A. Bone tissue engineering with porous hydroxyapatite ceramics. *J Artif Organs* 2005;8:131-36.

Yost MJ, Baicu CF, Stonerock CE, Goodwin RL, Price RL, Davis JM, et al. A novel tubular scaffold for cardiovascular tissue engineering. *Tissue Eng* 2004;10:273-84.

Young MF, Kerr JM, Ibaraki K, Heegaard AM, Robey PG. Structure, expression, and regulation of the major noncollagenous matrix proteins of bone. *Clin Orthop Relat Res* 1992;281:275-94.

Zelzer E, Glotzer DJ, Hartmann C, Thomas D, Fukai N, Soker S, et al. Tissue specific regulation of VEGF expression during bone development requires Cbfa1/Runx2. *Mech Dev* 2001;106:97-106.

In: Type I Collagen
Editors: Maria Eduarda Henriques and Marcio Pinto
ISBN: 978-1-62257-625-8

Chapter V

COLLAGEN I SYNTHESIS, BIOLOGICAL FUNCTIONS AND MEDICAL APPLICATIONS DURING SYSTEMIC INFLAMMATION

Ricardo Costa Petroni, Ester Correia Sarmento Rios and Francisco Garcia Soriano
Department of Emergency Medicine,
University of São Paulo Medicine School, Brazil

ABSTRACT

Type I collagen is an important component in the wound-healing process and large quantities is found in scar tissue associated with a variety of pathological conditions. The equilibrium between synthesis and degradation of collagen has been targeted as therapeutic goal in chronic diseases. However, acute inflammation activated both fibrogenesis and degradation, which causes the release of activated extracellular matrix components causing a vicious cycle that would in turn contribute to the progression of the inflammatory process. The functional compromising of the organ by the collagen accumulation could aggravate the systemic inflammation. Consequently, type I collagen deposition have been investigated as an attractive target for anti-fibrotic therapies, marker of disease severity, as hemostatic sponges and implants to repair wounds and tissue engineering applications as scaffolds.

The studies of biogenesis of collagen and the extracellular matrix components are crucial to determinate new therapeutic alternatives as medical application.

INTRODUCTION

The inappropriately severe systemic inflammation is suggested to disturb wound healing. Therefore, pro inflammatory cytokines and mediators of systemic inflammation have an important role in regulating collagen metabolism in fibroblasts [1]. In most organs, tissue injury is followed by cycles of inflammation and repair. When injury is repetitive or larger in magnitude, the result is fibrosis (Figure 1).

Collagen synthesis has been shown to be pathologically increased in acute respiratory distress syndrome, liver diseases, myocardial infarction and acute kidney diseases. Taken together these results suggested that progressive fibrosis is a central mechanism of organ failure. Systemic inflammation leads to tissue injury. Following tissue injury, inflammatory cells secrete mediators that initiate a tissue regenerative process. This is followed by a proliferative phase, when leukocytes are recruited and then activated. The leukocytes release profibrotic cytokines. The epithelial cells and myofibroblasts also produce metalloproteinases, MMPs, which disrupt the basement membrane, and additional cytokines that recruit cells required to reparative process. After the initial inflammatory phase, myofibroblasts produce ECM components, such as collagen, and endothelial cells form new blood vessels.

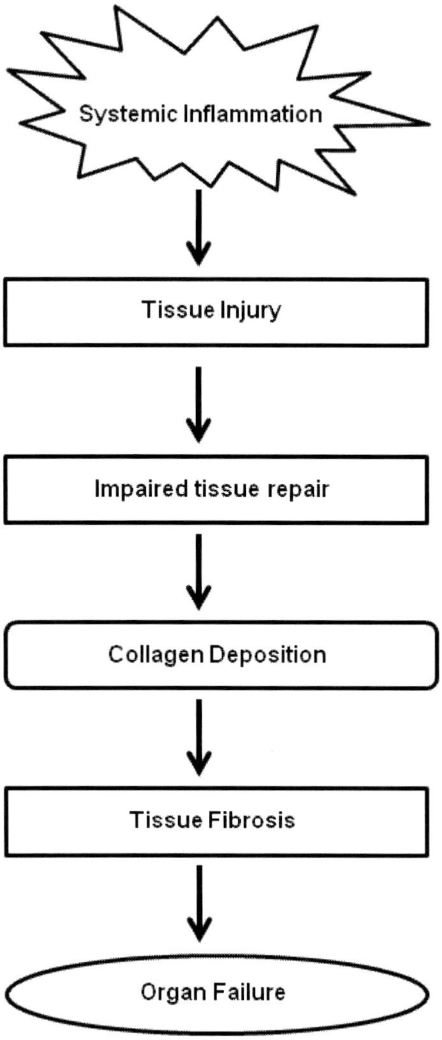

Figure 1. Fibrosis pathway in systemic inflammation.

In the remodeling phase, the activated myofibroblasts stimulate wound contraction and extracellular matrix production. Collagen fibers become more organized, blood vessels are restored to normal, and scar tissue is eliminated and epithelial cells restoring the injured tissue to its normal appearance. However, in the case of systemic inflammation, the normal healing process is disrupted. Persistent inflammation, tissue necrosis, and infection lead to chronic myofibroblast activation and excessive accumulation of ECM components, which promotes the formation of fibrosis and consequently organ failure.

There are several pathways implicated in the systemic inflammation. Activation of inflammatory cells and alteration of redox state are known to lead alteration in the extracellular matrix. Inflammation activated both fibrogenesis and degradation, which causes the release of activated extracellular matrix components causing a vicious cycle that would in turn contribute to the progression of the inflammatory process [2]. The functional compromising of the organ by the collagen accumulation could aggravate the systemic inflammation. An enhanced collagen production associated to increased expression of collagen chaperon HSP47 was demonstrated in a very early phase of acute pancreatitis. Different studies of other diseases that deflagrate systemic inflammation correlated the cell death with the increase in the proinflammatory cytokines production. Cell death, mainly by necrosis, is a stimulus to healing by fibrogenesis [3]. Type I collagen is an important component in the wound-healing process and is found in large quantities in scar tissue associated with a variety of pathological conditions. Type I collagen is fibrous and is synthesized predominantly by fibroblast, myofibroblast, and other reparative cells during systemic inflammation [4].

Many fragments derived from collagen metabolisms that are detected in the serum after extracellular matrix remodeling is generated from newly synthesized collagen or degraded mature collagen. The characterization of these fragments and the development of assays form the basis of a new area in matrix extracellular turnover evaluation in conditions such systemic inflammation [5]. In patients with acute respiratory distress syndrome type I collagen has been showed elevated in plasma and bronchoalveolar lavage fluids during the first days of disease and is associated with increased risk of death. Both cardiac and hepatic fibrosis in inflammatory diseases show increased type I collagen synthesis. Patients with sepsis showed increased levels of procollagen type I aminoterminal propeptides and this increase was associated with disease severity and mortality. Thus, irreversible end-stage organ failure due to fibrotic diseases is a major cause of morbidity and mortality, and treating these progressive fatal diseases is a major challenge in modern medicine.

The equilibrium between synthesis and degradation of collagen has been targeted as therapeutic goal in chronic diseases. Consequently, type I collagen deposition have been investigated as an attractive target for anti-fibrotic therapies, marker of disease severity, as hemostatic sponges and implants to repair wounds and tissue engineering applications as scaffolds. Therapies to limit pro-fibrotic mediators, have produced promising results, attempts to reduce accumulated type I collagen through metalloproteinases-mediated fibrinolysis has generated attractive results in animal models, however, their efficacy has yet to be tested in human trials. Also, Type I collagen is the most favorable for tissue engineering because it is a major extracellular matrix protein and has been extensively used for this purpose [6]. There are several inflammatory diseases where the study of collagen has been showed its relevance as a marker of severity. The study of biogenesis of collagen and extracellular matrix components raise new therapeutic alternative for medical application. We sought to study the role of collagen type I in some of these inflammatory diseases described below.

Acute Respiratory Distress Syndrome (ARDS)

Inflammation is a complex pathophysiological state, adopted primarily by innate immune cells in response to infection and/or tissue damage. Inability to control this augmented inflammatory response leads to tissue injury, organ dysfunction, and consequently death. Organ dysfunction and damage are frequent events in acute lung injury (ALI) induced by systemic inflammation. Lung is one of the most frequent organs affected in these cases [4]. The predisposing insult is thought to induce an inflammatory cascade that subsequently leads to lung injury. Pulmonary fibrosis is a well-recognized event in this inflammatory response, which contributes to the respiratory failure and death in a significant proportion of patients with ALI [7].

The lung parenchyma contains mostly types I and III collagens which provide the structural framework for the alveolar wall. Their turnover is a dynamic process that is necessary for the maintenance of the normal lung architecture. Ultimately, collagen accumulation depends not only on its synthesis, but also on its degradation. In patients with ALI who survive after disease, content more than double pulmonary collagen. The analysis of lung tissue from these patients showed an abundance of type I and III collagen [7]. Some studies showed that during ALI, type III collagen, characterized by elastic properties, is replaced by type I collagen, more resistant, leading to decreased pulmonary elasticity and consequently loss of function. Type I collagen deposition is a precocious event during systemic inflammation and are often related to severity of disease [8].

Type I collagen is the most fibrous form and comprises approximately 84% of the collagen synthesized by fibroblasts. Therefore, the large deposition of Type I collagen leads to internal organ fibrosis. Fibrosis of soft internal organs such as lung leads to loss of function and ultimately organ failure and death. The type I collagen is degraded by the activity of collagenases in fragments. These fragments can be detected by a specific antibody and measured by immunoassay, consequently could be used as an important and fast diagnosis [9]. The importance of type I collagen in ALI have been described by several authors. Type I collagen fragments have been showed elevated in plasma and bronchoalveolar lavage fluid in patients with ALI during the first days of disease and are associated with increased risk of death. Further evidence for early fibroproliferation is provided by many studies, which has shown upregulation of type I collagen mRNA expression in biopsy specimens of patients with diseases resulting from inflammatory process, a common predisposing risk factor for the development of ALI [9]. These data indicate the important role of type I collagen on pulmonary disorders induced by systemic inflammation.

Renal Fibrosis

Fibrosis is a hallmark that determines the prognosis of any kind of progressive kidney failure. Renal fibrosis is caused by the intense and prolonged injury and deregulation of repair processes, and by an excess deposition of extracellular matrices, such as collagen [10]. Kidney fibrosis is a major cause of end-stage renal disease (ESRD), a progressive loss in renal function that occurs over a period of months or years, is characterized by a decreased capacity of the kidneys to excrete waste products. The renal fibrosis exhibit increased proinflammatory and fibrogenic cytokines, thereby inducing macrophage infiltration and interstitial fibrosis [11]. Renal fibrosis is common among patients with kidney diseases, regardless of the initial disease. It is characterized by accumulation of extracellular matrix proteins in the interstitial space between nephrons including type I collagen and type III collagen and is both strongly associated with and a predictor of declined kidney function [12].

Different authors showed an increase in type I collagen fragments, associated with renal failure post inflammatory process. Interstitial collagens I and III and fibronectin predominate in renal fibrosis and these extracellular matrix proteins do not support the survival of mesangial cells promoting renal failure and consequently leads to hemodialysis necessity [13]. Hemodialytic patients can develop renal osteodystrophy, a major complication in these processes, characterized as a bone disease that occurs when the kidneys fail to maintain the proper levels of calcium and phosphorus in the blood. There are many studies suggesting that the C-terminal telopeptide of type I collagen is an important marker of osteodystrophy in these patients, increasing the early prognosis and treatment [14].

Heart Fibrosis

Cardiac inflammation, or myocarditis, usually results from infections, and it is often associated with autoimmune responses against heart antigens. Myocarditis of different etiology can progress to a characteristic final pathway of ventricular dilation, fibrosis, and heart failure in some affected individuals [15].

Enhanced fibrosis is characterized by a disproportionate accumulation of fibrillar (mainly type I) collagen, leading to stiffening of the ventricular and impaired diastolic filling. Cardiac inflammatory cells induced extracellular remodeling with increased accumulation of collagen, mainly type I collagen. Cardiac fibrosis was observed in endomyocardial biopsy samples from patients with cardiac inflammation [16]. Cardiac type I collagen is a stable protein with low turnover, but its balance can be disrupted in pathological conditions, such inflammatory diseases [18]. The aminoterminal propeptide levels of type I collagen are released during collagen synthesis and can be used as markers of rapidly increased collagen turnover and myocardial fibrosis after acute myocardial infarction. Moreover, the changes in the levels of serum collagen markers seem to be related to left ventricular remodeling and is not only used as a prognosis after acute myocardial infarction, but also in non-ischemic cardiomyopathy and hypertension.

Consequently, it has been concluded that measuring serum concentration of procollagen peptides can be used as markers of myocardial fibrosis formation or collagen degradation, indicating tissue injury [16]. Some data showed an increase of type I collagen in cardiac inflammatory disease and also a change in the collagen type I to III ratio in favor of the collagen type I. The increase in type I collagen deposition confer resistance to cardiac tissue and can explain the decreasing heart function showed in patients with systemic inflammatory diseases [16, 17].

Gastrointestinal Dysfunctions

It has been known that pancreatitis is strongly correlated with liver injury which involves modulation of metalloproteinases activity and matrix extracellular remodeling [19]. Changes in the extracellular matrix have direct effect on liver function. In the acute phases of liver injury, there is increased expression of metalloproteinases mediating the degradation of fibrillar collagens [19]. The 47 kDa heat shock protein (HSP47) interacts transiently with procollagen during its folding assembly and transport from the endoplasmic reticulum [20]. It is interesting to note that HSPs participate of the inflammatory process and have cytoprotective effects [20, 21, 22]. Unbalance of the enzymatic machinery involved in extracellular matrix damage may be an important contributing factor to the pathogenesis of many hepatic and pancreatic diseases [23].

The main component of the extracellular matrix in normal liver is collagen, principally the collagen type I. In the liver, hepatic stellate cells (HSCs) produce extracellular matrix proteins and are responsible for the expression of HSP47, which is an intracellular chaperone protein capable to binding to gelatin, as well as to native Type 1 collagen. Moreover, HSP47 plays an important role in liver protein synthesis and regeneration. The preferential expression of HSP47 in hepatic stellate cells seems to be related with their ability to collagens. In fact, it was demonstrated a strong relation between the hepatic production of collagen I and the expression of HSP47 during pancreatitis.

The inflammatory mediator such as cytokines released by the injured pancreatic tissue during pancreatitis stimulate inflammatory infiltrate and the resident liver macrophages (Kupffer Cells) to produce reactive species derivative from oxygen and nitrogen, leading to redox state. The oxidative stress might directly activate the HSCs to produce collagen Type I or indirectly by the tissue repair required after cell death [19] (Figure 2).

Besides the indirect effect of the pancreatitis in the hepatic collagen Type I production, there is a significant pancreatic collagen deposition activated by the pancreatic stellate cells (PSCs) [24, 25]. This event has been studied in the alcoholic pancreatitis that it is characterized as an inflammation causing necrosis and scarring. The activation of the immunologic system, primary the activation of macrophages and mononuclear cells with the consequent activation on release of cytokines, chemokines and inflammatoy factors activates the PSCs that are responsible to stimulate fibrosis through the collagen I synthesis. In a different model of pancreatitis, with a persistent fibrosis, it was demonstrated that the collagen type I expression was correlated with inflammatory cell infiltration [22]. Chronic pancreatitis is an inflammatory disease that is accompanied by damage of the pancreas, infiltration of inflammatory cells and accumulation of extracellular matrix proteins. In this disease also it was demonstrated that there is a relation among modulation of mononuclear cells, activation of PSCs, release of proinflammatory mediators and production of extracellular matrix components, mainly collagen Type I [26]. During pancreatic cancer, hypoxia is strongly associated to PSCs activation and consequent increase of collagen Type I production [27].

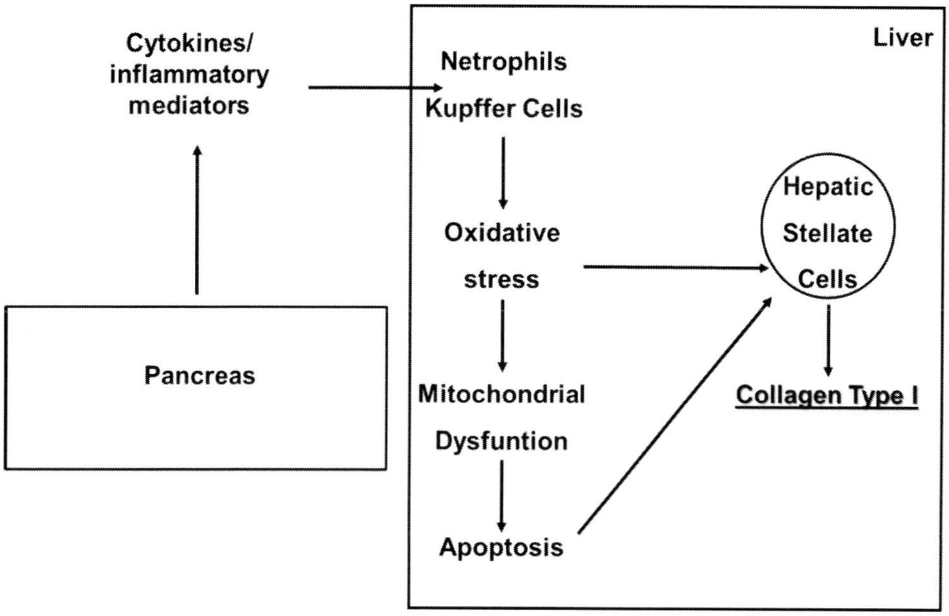

Figure 2. Hepatic Collagen 1 production during pancreatitis.

In a similar pathway, liver injury leads to a persistent hepatocyte hypoxia and to an excessive collagen Type I expression by hepatic stellate cells. This collagen production is associated to an inflammatory mechanism, once the hypoxia causes damage in the respiratory cell function due to reduction of mitochondrial capacity for oxidative phosphorylation, modulating the cytokine production and consequently activating stellate cells [28]. Equally, the injured acinar cells after pancreatitis produce cytokines and other inflammatory factors that activate the PSCs. In this case, the oxidative stress act as a potential enhancer of the activation, leading to the exacerbated collagen production [29].

A study of chronic pancreatitis confirmed the role of oxidative stress and the activation of PSCs with the subsequent increase of the collagen deposition [30]. In fact, both PSCs (pancreas) and HSCs (liver) modulate the balance of extracellular matrix secretion and digestion by producing collagen and metalloproteinases together with their corresponding inhibitors (TIMPs – tissue inhibitors of metalloproteinases) [31, 32]. The PSCs and HSCs play and important role in fibrogenesis, an imperative component of chronic inflammatory diseases. Recent evidences suggest that gastrointestinal diseases that stimulate the release of colecistokynin (CCK) also promote the collagen I production in different organs, once that many tissues express receptor to this hormone. In the pancreas, for example, CCK can activate PSCs to produce collagen Type I concomitantly to inhibition of the PSCs proliferation [33]. Acute pancreatic inflammation also results in PSC activation and deposition of collagen types I, III and IV as well as fibronectin and laminin in the same area [34]. Some authors believe that the deposition of collagen in the pancreas resolve after acute pancreatic injury while others accept that induction of repetitive episodes of acute pancreatitis culminate in a persistent fibrosis [35, 36]. The Stellate Cells from pancreas or liver are responsible by the collagen deposition after an acute injury, by generating increased fibrosis. Understanding of the fibrosis mechanism triggered by acute inflammation has a key role, once many acute inflammatory diseases are worsened with the collagen deposition. In steatohepatitis, for instance, inflammatory cytokines trigger a molecular pathway in different hepatic cells, leading to HSC activation and collagen deposition.

The activation of essential genes to avoid delayed liver repair is a consequence of the inflammatory pathway, suggesting the significant matter of inflammation in the progress of the collagen production. Liver fibrosis, especially by deposition of collagen Type I, is an important complication during the sepsis, when the systemic inflammation perpetuates the fibrosis due to the persistent activation of stellate cells. HSC activated presented a different morphology and changes in the gene expression profile [37, 38]. It has been known that HSCs are involved in the hepatic immune response through increased toll-like 4 receptor signaling. The TLR signaling mediates the upregulation of NF-kβ, the overexpression of adhesion molecules and cytokines promoting both inflammatory response and perpetuation of fibrosis through activation of TGF-β. On the other hand, the suppression of c-JUN-N-terminal kinases signal (which phosphorylation culminates in the translocation of NF-kβ) decreases the mRNA expression of profibrogenic and procollagen genes [39, 40, 41]. The rapid progress of an acute inflammatory disease to collagen deposition could be explained by the existence of a subset of the HSC population that serves as primers for healing response activation of an injured liver [42, 43]. These cells are preactivated, i.e., they are not fully activated, but they present some characteristics that became possible the quick transition from a quiescent HSC to a myofibroblastic cell [44, 38]. In the liver, there is a tight relation between inflammation and fibrosis [45]. Hepatocyte apoptosis promotes hepatic collagen production via HSC activation. However, Kupffer cells and HSCs produce inflammatory cytokines after engulf the apoptotic bodies, amplifying the profibrotic response [46]. On the other hand, the apoptotic and inflammatory pathway are not the only events involved in the HSC activation and it is not a “one-handed” pathway.

Indeed, Interferon gamma (IFNγ) has been recognized as a potent antifibrotic cytokine [47]. Reiterating, HSC are considered central ECM-producing cells, playing a significant role in Collagen-I deposition. It is interesting to note that these cells are susceptible to cytokine modulation [48]. However, the osteopontin, an extracellular matrix cytokine is expressed in HSC at the same time that could orientate fibrogenesis by modulating the HSC phenotype to Collagen Type I deposition [49]. Activated platelets are other important event participating to inflammation and tissue regeneration, in particular during liver and gastrointestinal diseases [50]. Besides platelets are protagonists of inflammation, extracellular matrix components can activate platelets. Collagen induces the release of activated microparticles derivative from platelets that, on the other hand, stimulate the secretion of cytokines by fibroblast through am IL-1-dependent mechanism [51]. During acute liver damage, inflammatory mediators such as TNF-α, IL-1β, nitric oxide play key role in the induction and maintenance of inflammation in macrophages [43, 52]. The expression of these mediators occurs in a NF-κβ activation-dependent mechanism and has a positive correlation with the alanine aminotransferase (ALT) release, which indicates liver damage. ALT release and activation of antioxidant system are correlated to expression of collagen type I in different hepatic diseases. It is possible that the oxidative burst trigger premature profibrogenic gene expression, contributing to accelerate liver fibrosis [53, 54].

In fact, during hepatocellular carcinoma pro-inflammatory cytokines are associated to acceleration of liver fibrosis due to mitogenic signalization that lead to phosphorylation of specific sites [31]. The strong association between some pro-inflammatory cytokines and fibrosis suggest the monitoring of the cytokines and some active particles of extracellular matrix as a new insight in the diagnosis of the fibrosis evolution [46]. Considering that in hepatic stellate cells TNF- α and IL-6 induce cellular differentiation and activation resulting in secretion of pro-fibrotic factors, different studies propose the inhibition of the inflammation state of HSC as an alternative control of the collagen-I deposition. Although the unsuccessful experience with TNF-α blocker in the control of systemic inflammation, some studies have shown its efficacy in the treatment of collagen vascular diseases corroborating the tight relation between collagen synthesis and cytokine production. Alternative therapies with phytotherapics also demonstrated a reduction of cytokine production concomitantly to diminished liver fibrosis [55]. The study of collagen deposition after different gastrointestinal surgeries demonstrated significant higher subcutaneous collagen amount after surgical wound [56]. Minor surgery as groin hernia repair did not induced significant subcutaneous deposition of collagen. However, patients submitted to major general surgery showed a decline of this measurement of collagen during postoperative phase and an important decline in cases with infectious complications. This is a simple model of assessment of the matrix deposition during wound healing that shows the influence of the inflammation in the collagen deposition [57].

A set of gastrointestinal inflammation have become recognized by subsurface collagen deposition [58, 59]. Collagenous gastritis, collagenous ileitis and collagenous colitis are important examples of gastrointestinal diseases characterized by the deposition of a subepithelial collagen band accompanying inflammatory infiltrate [60, 61]. Considering that mucosal tissue are submitted to contraction and relaxation on a continuous basis, inflammatory diseases in this tissue can become stiff and fibrotic culminate in the losing of normal motility. Besides this importance, the wound healing, scar formation and tissue remodeling during these disease are not well clarified. The physiological and pathological mechanisms that alter the contraction dynamic involve both intracellular and extracellular events.

The gastrointestinal tract is formed by several cells, including fibroblasts, and extracellular matrix, including collagen. The interaction among cells and extracellular matrix molecules provide a consistent manner of contraction supported by the cell-populated collagen matrix. Remained in the study of cell and collagen interaction in the gastrointestinal tract, it is important to consider that the proteolytic degradation of the extracellular matrix also contributes to the complication of intestinal inflammation. In general, the degradation of extracellular matrix component is resulted of the metalloproteinases activation. The enzymes are responsible by the digestion of collagen, proteoglycan, fibronectin, elastin and laminin. However, some metalloproteinases are involved in the degradation of nomatrix proteins such as cytokines and chemokines, which gives them as important inflammatory role. In the gut area we have to consider the microbial-derived proteolytic activity and its influence in the mucosal homeostasis, principally during inflammatory diseases that alter the collagen dynamic. Indeed, an important study confirmed the contribution of human gut microbiota in host matrix degradation through proteolytic activity and its implication during diseases, in particular with changes of the bacterial flora [62]. Several bacteria present in the gut tract produce an enterotoxin that contains a zinc site of metalloprotease capable to cleave collagen type I.

The interaction between certain protease from bacteria and intestinal epithelial cells increases unbalance of gut barrier and bacterial translocation due the degradation of basement membrane components. The systemic infection deflagrates systemic inflammation, production of cytokines, extracellular matrix degradation or collagen deposition in distant organs.

MEDICAL APPLICATION OF TYPE I COLLAGEN IN SYSTEMIC INFLAMMATION

The use of Type I collagen in medical applications is extensively studied by several authors. Type I collagen is the most favorable for tissue engineering, mainly for vascular tissue, because it is a major extracellular matrix protein, present in large amounts in most tissues [63]. Type I collagen is relatively easily shaped into tubular configurations, like vessels, or others shapes for different tissues. Therefore it has been extensively used in tissue engineering [64]. Another important use of type I collagen is related to its potential as an indicator of severity of inflammatory diseases and organ injury. Clinical studies showed that high levels of carboxy-terminal telopeptide of collagen type I (CITP), a marker of collagen degradation, are associated with hospital death, heart failure, and renal failure in systemic inflammatory diseases [65]. Recent studies have shown that biomarker of type I collagen synthesis, are increased in hypertension and predict cardiac death or hard failure following inflammatory diseases. Patients with severe sepsis showed increased serum levels of procollagen type I aminoterminal propeptides demonstrating its potential as markers of disease severity and outcome [66].

The increase in type I collagen deposition had been showed in acute lung injury. Patients with respiratory failure present increased amount of type I collagen deposition compared with type III collagen, indicating a decrease in pulmonary compliance and consequently increased resistance. What can explain the decreased of gas exchange. Attempts to reduce accumulated type I collagen through metalloproteinase mediated fibrinolysis has generated attractive results in animal models, however, their efficacy has yet to be tested in humans trials. Thus, type I collagen showed an important target to control inflammation conditions in different injuries process [7,8,9]. Continued investigation into molecular mechanisms of type I collagen synthesis in inflammatory diseases should be performed to produce ant-fibrotic therapy in humans.

REFERENCES

[1] Wynn TA. Cellular and molecular mechanisms of fibrosis. *J. Pathol.* 2008 Jan 214(2):199-210.

[2] Sweeney SM, Orgel JP, Fertala A, McAuliffe JD, Turner KR, Di Lullo GA, Chen S, Antipova O, Perumal S, Marini JC, San Antonio JD. Candidate cell and matrix interaction domains on the collagen fibril, the predominant protein of vertebrates. *J. Biological Chemistry*. 2008 July 25; 283(30):21187-21197.

[3] Kadler KE, Hill A, Canty-Laird. Collagen fibrillogenesis: fibronectin, integrins, and minor collagens as organizers and nucleators. *Curr. Opin. Cell Biol.* 2008. Oct 15; 20(5-24): 495-501.

[4] Hagiwara S, Iwasaka H, Matsumoto S, Nogushi T, Yoshioka H. Coexpression of HSP47 gene and type I and type III collagen genes in LPS-induced pulmonary fibrosis in rats. *Lung*. 2007 November 13; 185(5):31-37.

[5] 5. Gaddnas FP, Koskela M, Koivukangas V, Laurila J, Saarnio J, Risteli J, Oikarinen A, Ala-Kokko T. Skin collagen synthesis is depressed in patients with severe sepsis. *J. anesthesiaandanalgesia*. 2010 July 111(1): 156-163.

[6] 6. Sime PJ, O'Reilly KMA. Fibrosis of the lung and other tissues: new concepts in pathogenisis and treatment. *Clinical Immunology*. 2001 June 21; 99(3): 306-319.

[7] 7. Petroni RC, Teodoro WR, Guido MC, Barbeiro HV, Abatepaulo F, Theobaldo MC, Biselli PC, Soriano FG. Role of focal adhesion kinase in lung remodeling of endotoxemic rats. *Shock*. 2012 January 23; 37(5): 524-530.

[8] 8. Knight D, Mutsaers SE, Prêle CM. STAT3 in tissue fibrosis: Is there a role in the lung?. *Pulmonary Pharmacology and Therapeutcs*. 2010 Oct 8; 24(6): 193-198.

[9] 9. Anders HJ, Ryu M. Renal microenvironments and macrophage phenotypes determine progression or resolution of renal inflammation and fibrosis. *Kidney International*. 2011 August 2011; 80(3): 915-925.

[10] 10. Omori H, Kawada N, Inoue K, Ueda Y, Yamamoto R, Matsui I, Kaimori J, Takabatake Y, Moriyama T, Isaka Y, Rakugi H. Use of xanthine oxidase inhibitor febuxostat inhibits renal interstitial inflammation and fibrosis in unilateral ureteral obstructive nephropathy. *Clin. Exp. Nephrol*. 2012 January 29; Epub already.

[11] 11. Tsuchida T, Ishimura E, Miki T, Matsumoto N, Naka H, Jono S, Inaba M, Nishizawa Y. The clinical significance of serum osteocalcin and N-terminal propeptide of type I collagen in predialysis patients with chronic renal failure. *Osteoporos. Int*. 2005 May 26; 16(2); 172-179.

[12] 12. Wada T, Sakai N, Sakai Y, Matsishima K, Kaneko S, Furuichi K. Involvement of bone-marrow-derived cells in kidney fibrosis. *Clin. Exp. Nephrol*. 2011. January 12; 15(1): 8-13.

[13] 13. Okuno S, Inaba M, Kitatani K, Ishimura E, Yamakawa T, Nishizawa Y. Serum levels of C-terminal telopeptide of type I collagen: a useful new marker of cortical bonė loss in hemodialysis patients. *Osteoporos Int*. 2005. August 11; 16(2): 501-509.

[14] 14. Zanotti-Cavazzoni SL, Hollenberg SM. Cardiac dysfunction in severe sepsis and septic shock. *Curr. Opin. Crit. Care*. 2009. 15(2):392-397.

[15] 15. Barthélémy O, Beygui F, Vicaut E, Rouanet S, Van Belle E, Baulac C, Degrandsart A, Dallongeville J, Montalescot G. Relation of high concentration of plasma carboxy-termiinal telopeptide of collagen type I with outcome in acute myocardial infarction. *Am. J. Cardiol*. 2009.104(6):904-909.

[16] 16. Rudiger A, Singer M. Mechanisms of sepsis-induced cardiac dysfunction. *Crit. Care Med*. 2007. 35(6):1599-1606.

[17] 17. Guido MC, Clemente CF, Moretti AI, Barbeiro HV, Debbas V, Caldini KG, Franchini KG, Soriano FG. Small interfering RNA targeting focal adhesion kinase prevents cardiac dysfunction in endotoxemia. *Shock*. 2012 Jan; 37(1):77-84.

[18] 18. Yannas IV, Tzeranis DS, Harley BA, So TC. Biologically active collagen-based scaffolds: advances in progressing and characterization. *Phil. Trans. R. Soc*. 2010. 368, 2123-2139.

[19] Rios EC, Moretti AS, Velasco IT, Souza HP, Abatepaulo F, Soriano F. Hypertonic saline and reduced peroxynitrite formation in experimental pancreatitis. *Clinics* (Sao Paulo). 2011; 66(3):469-76.
[20] Rios EC, Moretti AI, de Souza HP, Velasco IT, Soriano FG. Hypertonic saline reduces metalloproteinase expression in liver during pancreatitis. *Clin. Exp. Pharmacol. Physiol.* 2010 Jan; 37(1):35-9.
[21] Tsan MF, Gao B. Cytokine function of heat shock proteins. Am. J. Physiol. Cell Physiol. 2004; 286: C739–44.
[22] Snoeckx LH, Cornelussen RN, Van Nieuwenhoven FA, Reneman RS, Van Der Vusse GJ. Heat shock proteins and cardiovascular pathophysiology. *Physiol. Rev.* 2001; 81: 1461–97.
[23] Ulmasov B, Xu Z, Tetri LH, Inagami T, Neuschwander-Tetri BA. Protective role of angiotensin II type 2 receptor signaling in mouse model of pancreatic fibrosis. *Am J Physiol Gastrointest Liver Physiol.* 2009 Feb; 296(2):G284-94.
[24] Ciesla DJ, Moore EE, Biffl WL, Gonzalez RJ, Moore HB, Silliman CC. Hypertonic saline activation of p38 MAPK primes the PMN respiratory burst. *Shock* 2001; 16: 285–9.
[25] Ceyhan GO, Deucker S, Demir IE, Erkan M, Schmelz M, Bergmann F, Müller MW, Giese T, Büchler MW, Giese NA, Friess H. Neural fractalkine expression is closely linked to pain and pancreatic neuritis in human chronic pancreatitis. *Lab Invest.* 2009 Mar; 89(3):347-61.
[26] Charrier AL, Brigstock DR. Connective tissue growth factor production by activated pancreatic stellate cells in mouse alcoholic chronic pancreatitis. *Lab Invest.* 2010 Aug; 90(8):1179-88.
[27] Yang L, Shen J, He S, Hu G, Shen J, Wang F, Xu L, Dai W, Xiong J, Ni J, Guo C, Wan R, Wang X. L-cysteine administration attenuates pancreatic fibrosis induced by TNBS in rats by inhibiting the activation of pancreatic stellate cell. *PLoS One.* 2012; 7(2):e31807.
[28] Masamune A, Kikuta K, Watanabe T, Satoh K, Hirota M, Shimosegawa T. Hypoxia stimulates pancreatic stellate cell to induce fibrosis and angiogenesis in pancreatic cancer. *Am. J. Physiol. Gastrointest. Liver Physiol.* 2008 Oct; 295(4):G709-17.
[29] Erkan M, Reiser-Erkan C, Michalski CW, Deucker S, Sauliunaite D, Streit S, Esposito I, Friess H, Kleeff J. Cancer-stellate cell interaction perpetuate the hypoxia fibrosis cycle in pancreatic ductal adenocarcinoma. *Neoplasia.* 2009 May; 11(5):497-508.
[30] Silva R de B, Ramalho FS, Ramalho LZ. The effect of anti-hypertensive drugs on the obstructive pancreatitis in rats. *Acta. Cir. Bras.* 2010 Oct; 25(5):396-400.
[31] Weylandt KH, Nadolny A, Kahlke L, Köhnke T, Schmöcker C, Wang J, Lauwers GY, Glickman JN, Kang JX. Reduction of inflammation and chronic tissue damage by omega-3 fatty acids in fat-1 transgenic mice with pancreatitis. *Biochim. Biophys. Acta.* 2008 Nov; 1782(11):634-41.
[32] Erkan M, Weis N, Pan Z, Schwager C, Samkharadze T, Jiang X, Wirkner U, Giese NA, Ansorge W, Debus J, Huber PE, Friess H, Abdollahi A, Kleeff J. Organ inflammation and cancer specific transcriptional fingerprints of pancreatic and hepatic stellate cells. *Mol. Cancer.* 2010 Apr 23; 9: 88.

[33] Yokota T, Denham W, Murayama K, Pelham C, Joehl R, Bell RH Jr. Pancreatic stellate cell activation and MMP production in experiemental pancreatic fibrosis. *J. Surg. Res.* 2002 May 15; 104(2):106-11.

[34] Berna MJ, Seiz O, Nast JF, Benten D, Bläker M, Koch J, Lohse AW, Pace A. CCK1 and CCK2 receptors are expressed on pancreatic stellate cells and induce collage production. *J. Biol. Chem.* 2010 Dec 10; 285(50):38905-14.

[35] Bombardelli L, Carpenter ES, Wu AP, Alston N, DelGiorno KE, Crawford HC. Pancreas-specific ablation of beta 1 integrin induces tissue degeneration by disrupting acinar cell polarity. *Gastroenterology*. 2010 Jun; 138(7):2531-40, 2540.e1-4.

[36] Nathan JD, Romac J, Peng RY, Peyton M, Rockey DC, Liddle RA. Protection against chronic pancreatitis and pancreatic fibrosis in mice overexpressing pancreatic secretory trypsin inhibitor. *Pancreas*. 2010 Jan; 39(1):e24-30.

[37] Shimizu K. Mechanisms of pancreatic fibrosis and applications to the treatment of chronic pancreatitis. *J. Gastroenterol.* 2008; 43:823–832.

[38] Gonnert FA, Kunisch E, Gajda M, Lambeck S, Weber M, Claus RA, Bauer M, Kinne RW. Hepatic Fibrosis in a Long-term murine model of sepsis. *Shock*. 2012 Apr; 37(4):399-407.

[39] Matsuzaki K. Smad phosphoisoform signals in acute and chronic liver injury: similarities and differences between epithelial and mesenchymal cells. *Cell Tissue Res.* 2012 Jan; 347(1):225-43.

[40] Ye Y, Dan Z. All-trans retinoic acid diminishes collage production in a hepatic stellate cell line via suppression of active protein-1 and c-Jun-N-terminal kinase signal. *J. Huazhong Univ. Sci. Technolog. Med. Sci.* 2010 Dec; 30(6):726-33.

[41] Neuman MG, Schmilovitz-Weiss H, Hilzenrat N, Bourliere M, Marcellin P, Trepo C, Mazulli T, Moussa G, Patel A, Baig AA, Cohen L. Markers of inflammation and fibrosis in alcoholic hepatitis and viral hepatitis C. *Int. J. Hepatol.* 2012; 347(1):225-43.

[42] Shigekawa M, Takehara T, Kodama T, Hikita H, Shimizu S, Li W, Miyagi T, Hosui A, Tatsumi T, Ishida H, Kanto T, Hiramatsu N, Hayashi N. Involvement of STAT3 regulated hepatic soluble in attenuation of stellate cell activity and liver fibrogenesis in mice. *Biochem. Biophys. Res. Commun.* 2011 Mar 25; 406(4):614-20.

[43] D'Ambrosio DN, Walewski JL, Clugston RD, Berk PD, Rippe RA, Blaner WS. Distinct population of hepatic stellate cells in mouse liver have different capacities for retinoid and lipid storage. *PLoS One*. 2011; 6(9):e24993.

[44] Day SA, Lakner AM, Moore CC, Yen MH, Clemens MG, Wu ES, Schrum LW.Opioidlike compound exerts antifibrotic activity via decreased hepatic stellate cell activation andinflammation. *Biochem Pharmacol*. 2011 Apr 15; 81(8):996-1003.

[45] Chen ZZ, Wang ZL, Deng CY, Zheng H, Wang XH, Ma L, Ye X, Ma YH, Xie CF, Chen LJ, Wei YQ. (Z)-5-(4-methoxybenzylidene) thiazolidine-2-4-dione protects rats from carbon tetrachloride induced liver injury and fibrogenesis. *World J. Gastroenterol.* 2012 Feb 21; 18(7):654-61.

[46] Moriya K, Sakai K, Yan MH, Sakai T. Fibronectin is essential for survival but is dispensable for proliferation of hepatocytes in acute liver injury. *Hepatology*, 2012. Epub already.

[47] Olaso E, Arteta B, Benedicto A, Crende O, Friedman SL. Loss of discoidin domain receptor 2 promotes hepatic fibrosis after chronic carbon tetrachloridethrough altered

paracrine interactions between hepatic stellate cells and liver-associated macrophages. *Am. J. Pathol.* 2011 Dec; 179(6):2894-904.

[48] Bansal R, Prakash J, de Ruijter M, Beljaars L, Poelstra K. Peptide-modified albumin carrier explored as a novel strategy for a cell-specific delivery of interferon gamma to treat liver fibrosis. *Mol. Pharm.* 2011 Oct 3; 8(5):1899-909.

[49] Fourcot A, Couchie D, Chobert MN, Zafrani ES, Mavier P, Laperche Y, Brouillet A. Gas 6 deficiency prevents liver inflammation, steatohepatitis and fibrosis in mice. *Am. J. Physiol. Gastrointest. Liver Physiol.* 2011 Jun; 300(6):G1043-53.

[50] Urtasun R, Lopategi A, George J, Leung TM, Lu Y, Wang X, Ge X, Fiel MI, Nieto N. Osteopontin, an oxidant stress sensitive cytokine, up-regulates collagen-I via integrin α(V)β(3) engagement and PI3K/pAkt/NFκB signaling. *Hepatology.* 2012 Feb; 55(2):594-608.

[51] Ripoche J. Blood platelets and inflammation: their relationship with liver and digestive diseases. *Clin. Res. Hepatol. Gastroenterol.* 2011 May; 35(5):353-7.

[52] Pratap A, Panakanti R, Yang N, Lakshmi R, Modanlou KA, Eason JD, Mahato RI. Cyclopamine attenuates acute warm ischemia reperfusion injury in cholestatic rat liver: hope for marginal livers. *Mol. Pharm.* 2011 Jun 6; 8(3):958-68.

[53] Dorn C, Heilmann J, Hellerbrand C. Protective effect of xanthohumol on toxin-induced liver inflammation and fibrosis. *Int. J. Clin. Exp. Pathol.* 2012; 5(1):29-36.

[54] Corpechot C, Barbu V, Wendum D, Kinnman N, Rey C, Poupon R, Housset C, Rosmorduc O. Hypoxia induced VEGF and collagen I expressions are associated with angiogenesis and fibrogenesis in experimental cirrhosis. *Hepatology.* 2002 May; 35(5):1010-21.

[55] Sebastiani G, Gkouvatsos K, Maffettone C, Busatto G, Guido M, Pantopoulos K. Accelerated CCl4-induced liver fibrosis in Hjc-/-mice, associated with an oxidative burst and precocious profibrogenic gene expression. *PLoS One.* 2011; 6(9):e25138.

[56] Manger K, Manger B. TNF alpha-antagonists in collagen vascular disease. *Z Rheumatol.* 2003 Jun; 62(3):240-5.

[57] Gopal P, McKenna BJ. The collagenous gastroenteritides: similarities and differences. *Arch. Pathol. Lab Med.* 2010 Oct; 134(10):1485-9.

[58] Jørgensen LN. Collagen deposition in the subcutaneous tissue during wound healing in humans: a model evaluation. *APMIS Suppl.* 2003; (115):1-56.

[59] Cacoub P, Sbaï A, Toan SV, Bellanger J, Hoang C, Godeau P, Piette JC. Collagenous colitis. A study of 11 cases. *Ann. Med. Interne.* 2001 Sep; 152(5):299-303.

[60] Ngo P, Ramalingam P, Phillips JA, Furuta GT. Collagen gel contraction assay. *Methods Mol. Biol.* 2006; 341: 103-9.

[61] Leung ST, Chandan VS, Murray JA, Wu TT. Collagenous gastritis: histophatologic features and association with other gastrointestinal diseases. *Am. J. Surg. Pathol.* 2009 May; 33(5):788-98.

[62] O'Brien BH, McClymont K, Brown I. Collagenous ileitis: a study of 13 cases. *Am. J. Surg. Pathol.* 2011 Aug; 35(8):1151-7.

[63] Pruteanu M, Hyland NP, Clarke DJ, Kiely B, Shanahan F. Degradation of the extracellular matrix components by bacterial-derived metalloproteases: implication of inflammatory bowel diseases. *Inflamm. Bowel Dis.* 2011 May; 17(5):1189-200.

[64] Thompson KJ, McKillop IH, Schrum LW. Targeting collagen expression in alcoholic liver disease. *World J. Gastroenterol.* 2011. May 28, 17(20):2473-2481.

[65] Pang Y, Greisler H. Using a type I collagen based system to understand cell-scaffold interactions and to deliver chimeric collagen binding growth factors for vascular tissue engineering. *J. Investing. Med.* 2010. October 1, 58(7): 845-848.

[66] Gaddnas F, Koskela M, Koivukangas V, Risteli J, Oikarinen, Laurila J, Saarnio J, Ala-Kokko T. Markers of collagen synthesis and degradation are increased in serum in severe sepsis: a longitudinal study of 44 patients. *Critical Care.* 2009. April 9, 13(2):R53.

In: Type I Collagen
Editors: Maria Eduarda Henriques and Marcio Pinto
ISBN: 978-1-62257-625-8

Chapter VI

Collagen Scaffolds: Tissue Engineering and Repair

Eman Allam,[1] Marco C. Bottino,[2] Nouf Al-Shibani[1] and L. Jack Windsor[1*]

[1]Department of Oral Biology, Indiana University School of Dentistry, Indianapolis, IN, US
[2]Department of Restorative Dentistry, Indiana University School of Dentistry, Indianapolis, IN, US

Abstract

Tissue engineering is an emerging field that includes the development of structures that replace, repair, and maintain tissue functions. Tissue engineering is an attractive and cost-effective strategy when compared to conventional or surgical therapies. The technique involves in vitro seeding and attachment of human cells onto a scaffold. These cells then proliferate, migrate, and differentiate, as well as secrete extracellular matrix components in order to form and repair tissues. The type of scaffold and its components are therefore crucial for controlling the behavior of the cells and for the success of the therapy. Among the many scaffold materials that have been developed, the collagen-based scaffolds offer many advantageous features, as well as some limitations. The aim of this chapter is to describe the use of collagen-based scaffolds in tissue engineering and repair.

* Corresponding author: L. Jack Windsor, Ph.D. Office Address: Indiana University School of Dentistry, Department of Oral Biology, 1121 W. Michigan Street, Room 271, Indianapolis, Indiana 46202. Position/title: Associate Professor of Oral Biology, Adjunct Associate Professor of Anatomy and Cell Biology, and Director Tobacco Cessation and Biobehavioral Group. Phone: (317) 274-1448, Fax: (317) 278-1411, E-Mail: ljwindso@iupui.edu.

TISSUE ENGINEERING AND CONNECTIVE TISSUE REPAIR

The loss or malfunction of tissues and organs as a result of a primary disease or the subsequent surgical intervention is a common medical problem that significantly affects the patient's health and quality of life. The restoration of the lost tissues or its function is traditionally done by tissue or organ transplantation, a technique that is frequently hindered by major problems and complications such as the donor shortage, immune rejection, and infection.

Tissue engineering is an emerging field that includes the development of structures that replace, repair, and maintain tissue functions. The technique involves the interaction of cells, scaffolds, biological signaling molecules and bioreactors. Tissue engineering is a topic of intensive investigation in both the scientific community and the health care field in general. It is a multidisciplinary approach that represents an attractive and cost-effective strategy when compared to conventional, transplantation, or surgical therapies. [1,2]

The technique is comprised of in vitro seeding and attachment of human cells onto a scaffold. These cells then proliferate, migrate, and differentiate, as well as secrete extracellular matrix (ECM) components in order to form and repair tissues. The type of the scaffold and its components are therefore crucial for controlling the behavior of the cells and for the success of the therapy. This approach represents a unique model for the interactions of cells with the environmental factors and the matrices. Therefore, the key factor in the success and the future of tissue engineering is increasing scientific knowledge regarding the interactions of cells with matrices and cellular responses to these interactions. [3]

Biological signals play an active role in tissue engineering. They activate the pathways which initiate cascade that result in ECM protein production to regenerate the native tissues. Growth factors are the most common biological signals utilized in tissue engineering. Sometimes other chemicals may also be used as signals such as ascorbic acid, proline, and glutamine. Recently, gene therapy has been used to express these and other therapeutic agents within the cells. Physical stimuli or mechanical forces may also be applied during the culturing process to produce a phenotypically correct tissue with proper ECM alignment, which is often obtained through the use of bioreactors. [4]

SCAFFOLDS FOR TISSUE ENGINEERING

The principal function of the scaffolds is to provide the suitable architecture and environment that allows cellular attachment, proliferation, migration, and differentiation (tissue conduction). The scaffold material should basically be constructed from materials that permit the cells to maintain their phenotype and secrete the necessary extracellular proteins. Some scaffolds also releases bioactive materials at a controlled rate, which directly influences the behavior of the integrated cells. [5] Scaffolds in tissue engineering act as templates for tissue formation. The technique includes typically seeding the cells, adding growth factors and then exposing it to biophysical stimuli in the form of a bioreactor, which is a device or system that applies different types of mechanical or chemical stimuli to cells. The cell-seeded scaffolds are then either cultured in vitro to synthesize tissues which can then be implanted into an injured site or are implanted directly into the injured site using the body's own systems, where regeneration of tissues or organs is induced in vivo. [6] This combination of signals, cells and scaffolds is frequently referred to as the tissue engineering triad (Figure 1). The concept of tissue engineering has been applied towards the regeneration of a wide variety of human tissues and organs including oral-maxillofacial structures, bone and cartilage tissue engineering, facial soft tissue augmentation, skin and cardiovascular applications (Figure 1). Characteristics required for scaffolds include biocompatibility, biodegradability, and proper physical properties such as high porosity, structural strength, and high surface area. Biocompatibility is essential to prevent unwanted immune reactions, while the biodegradability is essential to allow the eventual replacement of the implanted scaffold with the body's own products. High porosity provides the scaffolds with the channels that allow entry and exchange of molecules between the cells and blood. It also results in increased surface area for cell attachment and cellular interactions. The scaffold architecture is another critical requirement. Scaffolds should have an interconnected pore structure and high porosity to ensure cellular penetration, and sufficient diffusion of nutrients to the cells inside and diffusion of waste products out of the scaffold. The mechanical properties of the scaffold should be consistent with the anatomical site into which it is to be used. [7-9]

Since the primary role of the scaffold is to serve as a temporary artificial ECM, it is useful to mimic certain characteristics of the native ECM while designing a perfect scaffold. The scaffold material should also meet the biological needs for a specific cell population involved in tissue formation. Several materials are currently used in the construction of scaffolds which can be broadly classified as biological matrices or synthetically derived.These biomaterial groups have their own advantages and disadvantages, which highlight the necessity of the use of composite scaffolds, comprised of different phases.

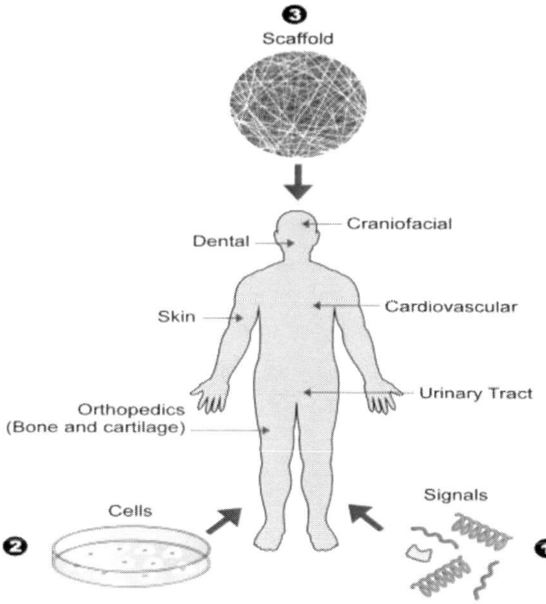

Figure 1. Schematic representation of the three major components involved in tissue engineering of major human tissues and organs: (1) signaling molecules (e.g., bone morphogenetic proteins and fibroblast growth factors), (2) progenitor/stem cells (e.g., dental pulp stem cells), and (3) extracellular-matrix mimicking scaffolds (e.g., natural and/or synthetic-based polymers).

Substances frequently used for scaffolds include natural polymeric materials, synthetic polymers or ceramics, biodegradable polymers, or polymers with adsorbed proteins. Naturally occurring matrices, in general, are more strategic because of their biocompatibility properties. The main ECM molecules of connective tissues are collagen, hyaluronan, and glycosaminoglycans. [10,11] Collagen is the most common protein in the body and provides strength and structuralstability to tissues in the body, which include the skin, blood vessels, tendon, cartilage and bone. Collagen scaffolds are not only used for tissue engineering but also as a neuro regeneration guide substrate, drug delivery systems, and for wound healing. Collagen Type I is most commonly used because of its biocompatibility and suitable physical and chemical properties,as well as its abundance and ubiquity. [12,13]

Collagen based scaffolds may be constructed using either the native form or the denatured form (gelatin). Gelatin, the natural polymer obtained from collagen by acidic or alkaline processing and thermal denaturation is widely used as a scaffold material because of its more favorable properties. It is characterized by being highly compatible, bioresorbable, non-immunogenic, and favorable functional properties. Studies [14-16] report that gelatin does not elicit any noticeable antigenic responses upon implantation, promotes cellular growth, and has low coagulation activity toward platelets. The physical and chemical properties of gelatin is relatively similar to collagen, but with better biological responses. Therefore, it is advantageous when used as a scaffolding material in tissue engineering applications.

Collagen Type I can be used intact or after proteolytic removal of the small non-helical telopeptides. Telopeptides removal significantly affects antigenicity. Native collagen can be used either as sparse fibers in a lattice-like organization or in the form of swollen hydrogels. The mechanical properties of collagen fibers depend principally on the intermolecular crosslinks within the fibers. Crosslinking prevent slippage under loading. Although collagen molecules self-assemble through enzymatic formation of intermolecular crosslinks which makes the head to tail network within the fiber, the density of this type of crosslinking is not sufficient for practical applications. [17-18]

Crosslinking collagen fibers can be achieved with different techniques such as dehydration or glutaraldehyde crosslinking. Dehydrative crosslinking is accomplished when water content by weight falls below approximately 1% and this causes the formation of interchain peptide bonds. Glutaraldehyde is the most common chemical crosslinking agent used for collagen. It induces covalent bonds between the collagen fibrils from aldehyde-amino reactions, as well as by aldol condensation. This results in a more tightly crosslinked network. Glutaraldehyde crosslinking is preferred particularly in cases involving copolymers of collagen Type I and chondroitin 6-sulfate. Problems with cytotoxicity and bio-incompatibility of some glutaraldehyde crosslinked collagens have been raised and limit their in vivo use. Cytotoxicity can be minimized by neutralization, by using lower concentrations of glutaraldehyde, or by substitution with other tanning agents such as hexamethylenediisocyanate. Ultraviolet irradiation has been used in some trials to stabilize the collagen fibrillar organization, as well as to decrease degradation and antigenicity. Uncrosslinked collagen scaffolds are more delicate and more biodegradable, which makes them more appropriate for guided tissue regeneration. [19-22]

Improving the mechanical properties of collagen scaffolds by crosslinking and fiber alignment are major determinants for the future of their use in tissue regeneration as most of the applications require that the scaffolds operate under mechanical stresses. Using a combined experimental and modeling approach, a study on the structure and function of Type I collagen gels with the effects of spatial fiber alignment and crosslinking was conducted. Aligned collagen scaffolds were created through the flow of magnetic particles enmeshed in collagen fibrils to mimic the anisotropy seen in native tissue. Inter- and intra-molecular crosslinking was modified chemically with Genipin to further improve the stiffness of the collagen scaffolds. The anisotropic mechanical properties of the collagen scaffolds were characterized using a planar biaxial tensile tester and parallel plate rheometer. It was reported that the stiffness of the collagen scaffolds increased significantly with the Genipin concentration and that the anisotropic behavior of the collagen scaffolds directly correlated with the presence of preferred collagen fiber alignment. The results of this study also demonstrated that crosslinking of the scaffolds can be used to tune the overall stiffness of the scaffolds without affecting the presence of anisotropy in the collagen matrix and that the movement of the interstitial fluid plays a significant role in determining the overall mechanical properties of a collagen gel. [23]

Collagen-Based Scaffolds for Oral-Maxillofacial, Bone, Cartilage, Skin, and Vascular Tissue Engineering

Collagen is the most commonly used naturally derived polymer in tissue engineering scaffolds. Since natural collagen is capable of provoking an immunogenic response when implanted, reconstituted collagen or purified collagen produced by biochemical processing for commercial use is more widely used.

Collagen Type I is a primary structural protein of the native ECM and has properties favorable for cellular growth; therefore it has been used in a variety of tissue-engineering applications including but not limited to oral-maxillofacial (e.g., periodontal regeneration), bone and cartilage tissue engineering, facial soft tissue augmentation, skin, and cardiovascular applications. [24]

Periodontitis affects the integrity of the periodontal tissues. The periodontium consists of periodontal ligament (PDL), the dentogingival junction, root cementum, and alveolar bone (Figure 2). The periodontium anchors teeth to both the maxilla and the mandible, preserves their position, and provides nourishment to the teeth.

In periodontal tissue engineering, the development of new cementum with PDL fibers connected to alveolar bone is the main goal. Periodontal disease can progressively destroy the periodontium and ultimately result in tooth loss. Loss of alveolar bone results in the formation of a periodontal pocket around the tooth that acts as a reservoir supporting the growth of anaerobic bacteria (e.g., *Porphyromonas gingivalis* and *Prevotella intermedia*). [25,26]

Succinctly, the distinct strategies of periodontal therapy target are to (1) reduce and/or eliminate inflamed tissues caused by bacterial plaque, (2) correct defects or anatomical problems due to the disease, and (3) regenerate new periodontal tissues.The use of an occlusive membrane made of synthetic (e.g., polylactic acid/PLA) or natural polymers (e.g., collagen) interfacing with gingival connective tissue/epithelium and a PDL/alveolar bone tissue to promote periodontal tissue regeneration is called GTR.

An occlusive membrane acts as a barrier when placed into the surgical site, preventing connective and epithelial tissue migration into the defect.

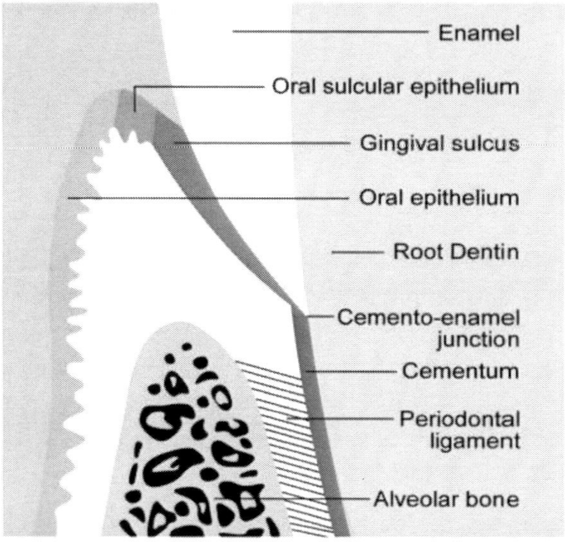

Figure 2. Schematic illustration showing a longitudinal section through dento-gingival part of a tooth and its periodontal tissue apparatus.

Progenitor cells located in the remaining periodontal ligament, adjacent alveolar bone, or blood are then able to recolonize the root area and differentiate into a new periodontal supporting apparatus with the formation of new bone, PDL, and cementum. [27-29]

To date, tissue-derived collagen-based membranes or scaffolds from human skin (Alloderm®, LifeCell, Branchburg, NJ, US), bovine Achilles tendon (Cytoplast® RTM Collagen, City, State, US) or porcine skin (Bio-Gide®, Osteohealth, Shirley, NY, US) are important alternatives to synthetic polymers in GTR/GBR procedures due to their excellent cell affinity and biocompatibility. [30-32] AlloDerm® is an acellular freeze-dried dermal matrix graft (Figure 3) composed mainly of Type I collagen derived from human cadaveric skin. [33-35] According to its manufacturer, this proprietary process does not cause damage to the critical biochemical structural cues needed to maintain the tissue's natural regenerative properties and leaves behind an extracellular collagenous matrix that provides the basis for tissue structure and guides cellular functions. [36]

Skin tissue engineering is one of the most common and practical applications of tissue engineering, especially in the treatment of burns and extensive dermal loss. In cases with deep second-degree or third-degree burns, tissue engineering is a relevant strategy to guarantee adequate coverage in reconstructive surgeries. [37] Several studies have reported the use of synthetic collagen sponges as scaffolds in skin grafts. [38-40] Collagen sponges inoculated with autologous epidermal basal cells and placed on a full-thickness guinea pig wound resulted in wound closure in less than 2 weeks and neodermis was reported in place of the collagen sponge in the first month. After 4 months, it was reported that the cell seeded sponge could not be differentiated from the autograft. Advantages of this cell inoculated collagen sponge are that it actively controls wound contraction, encourages the fibrovascular tissue ingrowth, and reduces scar formation. [38] Trials on patients with epidermolysis bullosa reported that the grafts were successful 7 months after surgery. [40]

A dermal equivalent was constructed from rat tail tendon collagen seeded with autologous fibroblasts and cultured with keratinocytes to mimic skin. [41] This model was reported to be easily contoured to the wound and produced in large enough quantities to treat extensive skin injuries. Within the first 3 months, it produced a woven vascularized dermal mat in rat wounds. After 13 months, a hairless, slightly thinner skin structure lacking sebaceous glands was reported. Several later studies utilized this graft design in humans for either the treatment of burns or in epidermolysis. [42,43]

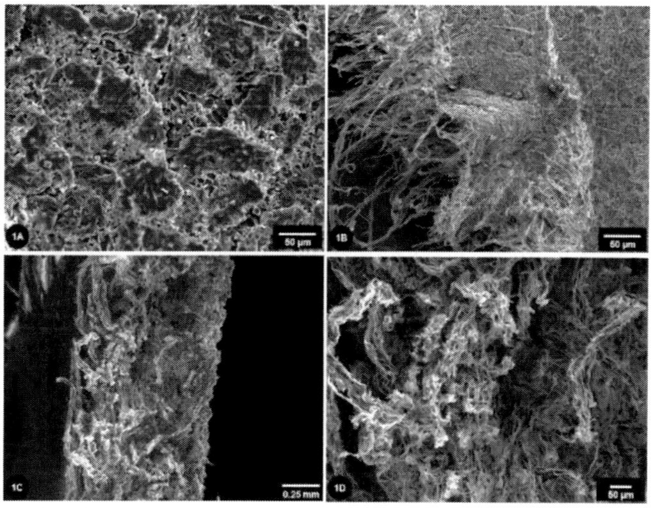

Figure 3. Morphology of the AlloDerm graft tissue. 1A) SEM image showing the webbed structure of the outer surface; 1B) SEM image showing the fibrous nature of the graft (cross-section); 1C and 1D) SEM images taken at different magnifications showing the highly porous graft morphology (cross-section).

Guerr et al. [44] reported another model for dermal tissue engineering utilizing collagen as a scaffold. They studied Apligraf, a bioengineered living skin, composed of a bovine collagen lattice containing living human fibroblasts overlaid with a fully differentiated epithelium made of human keratinocytes. Athymic mice were grafted with the lattice and progressive remodeling was investigated by studying the cellular and ECM components of the grafts from 0 to 365 days after grafting. Biopsies were analyzed using immunohistochemistry and electron microscopy techniques. They reported that this bioengineered tissue provided living and bioactive cells to the wound site up to 1 year after grafting. The graft was rapidly incorporated within the host tissue and the bovine collagen present in the graft was progressively replaced by human and mouse collagens.A normal healing process was observed and Type III collagen appeared transiently with Type I collagen at later stages of wound healing. New molecules, such as elastin, were produced by the living human cells contained within the graft. [44]

Because collagen is the major component of skeletal tissues, collagen-based scaffolds favor the attachment of bone and cartilage cells embedded within a collagen delivery device. Collagen scaffolds have been used extensively for decades for the in vitro characterization of osteoblasts, chondrocyte and stem cell behaviors. [45] Autogenous cells or tissue transplantation is one of the most promising techniques in bone and cartilage generation and orthopedic tissue engineering. It is considered superior to other alternatives as it overcomes the problems of donor site scarceness, unwanted immune reactions and trans-infections.

Mesenchymal stem cells, osteoblasts, and chondrocytes are taken from the patient's hard or soft tissues, expanded in culture and seeded onto a scaffold that will later degrade and resorb as the tissue structures grow in vivo. The scaffold offers the required support for cells to grow and differentiate, and its shape or architecture defines the ultimate shape of the new bone and cartilage. [46]

Collagen gels have been used as scaffolds for chondrocytes and bone-marrow-derived mesenchymal stem cells with encouraging results. Wakitani et al. [47] reported that mesenchymal stem cells in collagen gels resulted in significant repair in rabbit full-thickness defects. At 12 weeks, the subchondral bone had healed and the defects were filled in with hyaline-like cartilage but with a slight gap between the edges of the repair tissue and the surrounding articular cartilage. By 24 weeks, there was thinning of the repair tissue. There were areas of incomplete integration of the repair and host cartilage. The repair tissue was found to be less stiff and more compliant than normal cartilage.

Collagen scaffolds have been also used to deliver chondrocytes treated with gene therapy to wound sites with promising results, especially with collagen fiber scaffolds delivering chondrocytes and bone morphogenetic proteins in rabbit models. Chondrocytes in collagen fibers induced a hyaline-like repair that was mechanically and biochemically analogous to the natural tissue at 6 months. At 1 year, cell-free bone morphogenetic proteins-collagen implants resulted histologically in remarkable repair tissues. [48,49]

Crosslinking through either the physical or the chemical methods improves the compressive and tensile mechanical properties of collagen scaffolds and overcomes the problem of poor mechanical properties that limits the use of collagen, as well as all natural polymers, as the main constituent of a scaffold for orthopedic tissue engineering. A successful collagen-glycosaminoglycan scaffold with an improved composition, crosslinking density and pore size for bone regeneration was developed as the end result of a series of trials and studies. This collagen-glycosaminoglycan scaffold was established after the identification of the optimal composition for osteogenesis and optimal pore structure that facilitate bone tissue formation. Studies have demonstrated the ability of these scaffolds to heal bone defects in vivo in minimally loaded calvarial defects. [50-51]

For regions subjected to higher levels of loading, collagen based scaffolds strengthened by a ceramic phase was constructed. This produced a highly porous biomimetic collagen-hydroxyapatite (CHA) scaffold that is composed of the two primary components of bone. Studies that compared the CHA scaffolds to the collagen scaffolds indicated better healing responses with the CHA. The reasons for this enhanced healing were explained by the greater mechanical properties and permeability provided by the CHA scaffold, which allowed more cellular infiltration and vascularization and also due to the presence of calcium phosphate which triggered an osteoinductive response whereby its chemical composition enhanced the osteogenic potential of the host cells resulting in increased bone formation. [52-53]

For ligament tissue engineering, collagen gels have been also extensively investigated. The results were promising where cells cultured on or within these gels produced ECM, and showed longitudinal alignment with the long axis of the tissue mimicking normal cell alignment in ligaments in vivo. The disadvantage of this application is that the collagen gels do not have the required mechanical properties for functional ligament replacement. [54] Fibroblast-seeded collagen fiber scaffolds have been assessed as a better alternative because of their potentially superior mechanical strength in implantation studies and showed encouraging results. [55]

Vascular tissue engineering is one of the most vital fields because of the high clinical need for improved blood vessel substitutes, especially in small-diameter applications. [56] The blood vessel is a complex structure both structurally and functionally. Several approaches have been used to create engineered tissue that simulates the structure and function of blood vessels. The typical tissue engineering approach that is currently applied clinically is the use a degradable synthetic scaffold seeded with cells where the polymer provides the initial mechanical support to the engineered tissue and later, as it degrades, it is replaced by a protein matrix secreted by the cells. [57] Collagen scaffolds constructed from decellularized porcine aorta present a suitable scaffold of choice for cardiovascular tissue engineering. They retain their natural biological composition and three-dimensional architecture suitable for cell adhesion and proliferation. In vivo results indicated that these types of scaffolds are controllable and reveal adequate mechanical characteristics, porosity, biodegradability and biocompatibility. Furthermore, their surfaces and compositions efficiently promoted cell adhesion, proliferation and infiltration into the deep layers of the tissue constructs. [58]

Jux et al. [59] used an intestinal collagen layer (ICL), a purified bioengineered Type-I collagen derived from porcine submucosa, as septaloccluder in percutaneous transcatheter closure of interventionally created atrial septal defects in lambs. They compared them to implants with the commercially available occluders (CardioSeal, NMT Medical Inc., Boston, MA, US), which were considered the control group. They followed up the implants with histology and pathomorphological analysis after 2, 4, and 12 weeks. After 2 weeks, the devices were already covered completely by neo-endothelium. Compared with the conventional synthetic scaffold, ICL showed a quicker endothelialization, decreased thrombogenicity, and superior biocompatibility with no significant cellular infiltration observed in the histology of explants with ICL fabrics. After 3 months in vivo, the collagen layer remained mechanically intact but began to show the first histological signs of mild disintegration, gradual reabsorption, and remodeling. It was concluded that using bioengineered collagen matrix as an occluder tissue scaffold provide an acceptable approach with superior biocompatibility and overall results. [59] Hudon et al. [60] developed an impressive model of endothelialized reconstructed dermis that promotes the spontaneous formation of a human capillary-like network. The endothelialized dermis was prepared by co-culturing two human cell types, dermal fibroblasts and umbilical vein endothelial cells, in a collagen sponge biomaterial. They studied quantitatively and qualitatively the influence of angiogenic and angiostatic drugs on the capillary-like tube formation in vitro in the model. The confocal microscopy results showed that the endothelial structures were not cord-like but rather capillary-like tubes with well-defined lumina. Moreover, these tubes were organized in a complex network of branching structures. When angiogenic factors (vascular endothelial growth factor or basic fibroblast growth factor) were added to the model, 1.8 and 1.4 times more capillaries were observed, respectively, whereas the addition of progesterone reduced the number of tubes compared to the control by 2.4 times.

CONCLUSION

The use of collagen-based scaffolds in tissue engineering applications has evolved during the past two decades. It is well established that the type of the scaffold and its components are crucial for controlling the behavior of the cells and for the success of the therapy. This chapter has highlighted the benefits and limitations of collagen-based scaffolds for tissue engineering purposes. It is worth mentioning that to hasten the bench to bedside clinical application of novel tissue engineering based therapies, it still remain crucial that the intimate team contain stem cell biologists, material scientists and engineers, as well as basic and clinical biomedical investigators.

ACKNOWLEDGMENT

The authors are thankful to Mr. Mark A. Dirlam at Indiana University School of Dentistry for helping with illustrations presented in Figures 1 and 2.

REFERENCES

[1] Freed, L., Guilak, F., Guo, X., Gray, M., Tranquillo, R., Holmes, J., Radisic, M., Sefton, M., Kaplan, D., Vunjak-Novakovic, G. Advanced tools for tissue engineering: scaffolds, bioreactors, and signaling. *Tissue Engineering* 2006; 12: 3285-3305.

[2] Patrick, C. W., Mikos, A. G., McIntire, L. V., McIntire, L. V., editor. *Frontiers in Tissue Engineering*. 1998 Pergamon: Oxford.

[3] Ma, P. Scaffolds for tissue fabrication. *Materials today* 2004; 5: 30-40.

[4] Allen, K. D., Athanasious, K. A. Tissue engineering of the TMJ disc: a review. *Tissue Eng*. 2006; 12:1183-1196.

[5] Vats, A., Tolley, N., Polak, J., Gough, J. scaffolds and biomaterials for tissue engineering: a review of clinical applications. *Clin. Otolaryngol*. 2003; 28: 165-172.

[6] Stock, U., Vacanti, J. Tissue engineering: current state and prospects. *Annu. Rev. Med.* 2001; 52: 443-451.

[7] Hutmacher, D., Schantz, T., Zein, I., Ng, K., Teoh, S., Tan, K. Mechanical properties and cell cultural response of polycaprolactone scaffolds designed and fabricated via fused deposition modeling. *J. Biomed. Mater. Res.* 2001; 55: 203-216.

[8] Sachlos, E., Czernuszka, J. Making tissue engineering scaffolds work. Review: the application of solid freeform fabrication technology to the production of tissue engineering scaffolds. *Eur. Cell Mater*. 2003; 30:29-39.

[9] Yang, S., Leong, K., Du, Z., Chua, C. The design of scaffolds for use in tissue engineering. Part I. Traditional factors. *Tissue Eng*. 2001; 7: 679-89.

[10] Glowacki, J., Mizuno, S. *Biomaterials in cartilage and bone tissue engineering* 2004; 15: 347-354.

[11] Glowacki, J., Mizuno, S. Collagen scaffolds for tissue engineering. *Biopolymers* 2007; 89: 338-344.

[12] Lee, C., Singla, A., Lee, Y. Biomedical applications of collagen. *International Journal of Pharmaceutics* 2001; 221:1-22.

[13] Lee, K., Yuk, S. Polymeric protein delivery systems. Progress in Plymer *Science* 2007; 32: 669-697.

[14] Desai, T. Micro- and nano-scale structures for tissue engineering constructs. *Med. Eng. Phys*. 2000; 22: 595.

[15] Mo, X., Iwata, H., Matsuda, S., Ikada, Y. Soft tissue adhesive composed of modified gelatin and polysaccharides. *J. Biomater. Sci. Polym*. 2000; 11, 341.

[16] Murugan, R., Ramakrishna, S. Nano-featured scaffolds for tissue engineering: A review of spinning methodologies. *Tissue Engineering* 2006; 12: 435-447.

[17] Fratzl, P. *Collagen: structure and mechanics*, Springer, New York, NY, US, 2008.

[18] Jensen, L., Host, N. Collagen: scaffold for repair or execution. *Cardiovascular Research* 1997; 33: 535-539.

[19] Silver, F., Yannas, I., Salzman, E. In vitro blood compatibility of glycosaminoglycan-precipitated collagens. *J. Biomed. Mater. Res*. 1979;13: 701-16.

[20] Charulatha, V., Rajaram, A. Influence of different crosslinking treatments on the physical properties of collagen membranes. *Biomaterials* 2003; 24: 759-767

[21] Daminik, L., Dijkstra, M., Van Luyn, M., Van Wachem, P., Nieuwenhuis, P., Feijen, J. Glutaraldehyde as a crosslinking agent for collagen-based biomaterials. *Journal of Materials Science* 1995; 6: 460-472.

[22] Nimni, M., Cheung, D., Strates, B., Kodama, M., Sheikh, K. Chemically modified collagen: a natural biomaterial for tissue replacement. *J. Biomed. Mater. Res.* 1987;21:741-71.

[23] Xu, B., Chow, M. J., Zhang, Y. Experimental and modeling study of collagen scaffolds with the effects of crosslinking and fiber alignment. *International Journal of Biomaterials* 2011; doi:10.1155/2011/172389.

[24] O'Brien, F. Biomaterials and scaffolds for tissue engineering. *Materials today* 2011; 14:88-95.

[25] Karring, T., Nyman, S., Gottlow, J., Laurell, L. Development of the biological concept of guided tissue regeneration--animal and human studies. *Periodontol.* 2000 1993;1:26-35

[26] Chen, F., Zhang, J., Zhang, M., An, Y., Chen, F., Wu, Z. A review on endogenous regenerative technology in periodontal regenerative medicine. *Biomaterials* 2010;31:7892

[27] Giannobile, W., Somerman, M. J. Growth and amelogenin-like factors in periodontal wound healing. A systematic review. *Annals of Periodontology* 2003; 8: 193-204

[28] Sculean, A., Nikolidakis, D., Schwarz, F. Regeneration of periodontal tissues: combinations of barrier membranes and grafting materials – biological foundation and preclinical evidence: a systematic review. *Journal of Clinical Periodontology* 2008; 35: 106–116

[29] Wang, H. L., Greenwell, H., Fiorellini, J., Giannobile, W., Offenbacher, S., Salkin, L., Townsend, C., Sheridan, P., Genco, R. J. Periodontal regeneration. *Journal of Periodontology* 2005; 76, 1601–1622

[30] Felipe, M., Andrade, P., Grisi, M., Souza, S., Taba, M., Palioto, D. Comparison of two surgical procedures for use of the acellular dermal matrix graft in the treatment of gingival recession: a randomized controlled clinical study. *Journal of Periodontology* 2007;78:1209.

[31] Santos, A., Goumenos, G., Pascual, A. Management of gingival recession by the use of an acellular dermal graft material: a 12-case series. *Journal of Periodontology* 2005;76: 1982.

[32] Behring, J., Junker, R., Walboomers, X. F., Chessnut, B., Jansen, J.A. Toward guided tissue and bone regeneration: morphology, attachment, proliferation, and migration of cells cultured on collagen barrier membranes. A systematic review. *Odontology* 2008;96:1.

[33] Bottino, M. C., Jose, M. V., Thomas, V., Dean, D. R., Janowski, G. M. Freeze-dried acellular dermal matrix graft: effects of rehydration on physical, chemical, and mechanical properties. *Dental Materials* 2009;25:1109.

[34] Bottino, M. C., Thomas, V., Jose, M. V., Dean, D. R., Janowski, G. M. Acellular dermal matrix graft: synergistic effect of rehydration and natural crosslinking on mechanical properties. *Journal of Biomedical Materials Research Part B: Applied Biomaterials* 2010;95:276

[35] Gouk, S. S., Lim, T. M., Teoh, S. H., Sun, W. Q. Alterations of human acellular tissue matrix by gamma irradiation: histology, biomechanical property, stability, in vitro cell repopulation, and remodeling. *Journal of Biomedical Materials Research Part B: Applied Biomaterials* 2008;84:205.

[36] Livesey, S. A., Herndon, D. N., Hollyoak, M. A., Atkinson, Y. H., Nag, A. Transplanted acellular allograft dermal matrix—potential as a template for the reconstruction of viable dermis. *Transplantation* 1995;60:1.

[37] Ma, L., Gao, C., Mao, Z., Zhou, J., Shen, J., Hu, X., Han, C. Collagen/chitosan porous scaffolds with improved biostability for skin tissue engineering. *Biomaterials* 2003; 24: 4833-4841.

[38] Yannas, I., Burke, J., Orgill, D., Skrabut, E. Wound tissue can utilize a polymeric template to synthesize a functional extension of skin. *Science* 1981; 215:174.

[39] Yannas, I., Orgill, D. Artificial skin: A fifth route to organ repair and replacement. In: Piskin, E. and Hoffman, A Eds. *Polymeric Biomaterials*, 1986, Dordrecht: MartinusNijhoff

[40] Silver, F., Pins, G. Cell growth on collagen: A review of tissue engineering using scaffolds containing extracellular matrix. *Journal of Long-Term Effects of Medical Implants* 1992; 2:67-80.

[41] Carter, D., Lin, A., Varghese, M., Caldwell, D., Pratt, L. Eisinger M. Treatment of junctionalepidermolysisbullosa with epidermal autografts. *J. Am. Acad. Dermatol.* 1997; 17: 246-250.

[42] Bell, E., Ehrlich, P., Buttle, D., Nakatsuji, T. Living tissue formed in vitro and accepted as skin equivalent tissue of full thickness. *Science* 1981; 211:1052- 1054.

[43] Bell, E., Ehrlich, P., Sher, S., Merrill, C., Saber, R., Hull, B., Nakatsuji, T., Buttle, D. Development and use of a living skin substitute. *Plast. Reconstr. Surg.* 1981; 67:386-92.

[44] Guerret, S., Govignon, E., Hartmann, D. J., Ronfard, V. Long-term remodeling of a bilayered living human skin equivalent (Apligraf) grafted onto nude mice: Immunolocalization of human cells and characterization of extracellular matrix. *Wound Repair Regen.* 2003; 11:35–45.

[45] Langer, R., Vacanti, J. Tissue engineering. *Science* 1993;260: 920-6.

[46] Hutmacher, D. Scaffolds in tissue engineering bone and cartilage. *Biomaterials* 2000;21:2529-2543.

[47] Wakitani, S., Goto, T., Pineda, S., Young, R., Mansour, J., Caplan, A., Goldberg, V. Mesenchymal cell-based repair of large, full-thickness defects of articular cartilage. *J. Bone Joint Surg.* 1994; 76:579–592.

[48] Sellers, R., Zhang, S., Glasson, H., Kim, D., Peluso, D., Beckwith, K., Morris, E. Repair of articular cartilage defects one year after treatment with recombinant human bone morphogenetic protein-2 (rhBMP-2). *J. Bone Joint Surg.* 2000; 82:151–160.

[49] Frenkel, S., Toolan, B., Menche, D., Pitman, M., Pachence, J. Chondrocyte transplantation using a collagen bilayer matrix for cartilage repair. *J. Bone Joint Surg.* 1997; 79:831– 836.

[50] Byrne, E., Farrell, E., McMahon, L., Haugh, M., O'Brien, F., Campbell, V., Prendergast, P., O'Connell, B. Gene expression by marrow stromal cells in a porous collagen-glycosaminoglycan scaffold is affected by pore size and mechanical stimulation. *J. Mater. Sci. Mater. Med.* 2008;19:3455-63.

[51] Alhag, M., Farrell, E., Toner, M., Lee, T. C., O'Brien, F. J., Claffey, N. Evaluation of the ability of collagen-glycosaminoglycan scaffolds with or without mesenchymal stem cells to heal bone defects in Wistar rats. *Oral Maxillofac. Surg.* 2012;16:47-55.

[52] O'Brien, F. A collagen/hydroxyapatite composite scaffold, and process for the production thereof. WO2008096334, (2008).

[53] Gleeson, J., Plunkett, N., O'Brien, F. Addition of hydroxyapatite improves stiffness, interconnectivity and osteogenic potential of a highly porous collagen-based scaffold for bone tissue regeneration. *Eur. Cell Mater.* 2010;20: 218-30.

[54] Gentleman, E., Lay, A., Dickerson, D., Nauman, E., Livesay, G., Dee, K. Mechanical characterization of collagen fibres and scaffolds for tissue engineering. *Biomaterials* 2003; 24: 3805-3813.

[55] Bellincampi, L., Closkey, R., Prasad, R., Zawadsky, J., Dunn, M. Viability of fibroblast-seeded ligament analogs after autogenous implantation. *J. Orthod. Res.* 1998; 16: 414-20.

[56] Stegemann, J., Kaszuba, S., Rowe, S. Review: Advances in vascular tissue engineering using protein-based biomaterials. *Tissue Engineering* 2007; 13: 2601-2613.

[57] Mendelson, K., Schoen, F. Heart valve tissue engineering: concepts, approaches, progress, and challenges. *Annals of Biomedical Engineering* 2006; 34:1799–1819

[58] Lu, Q., Ganesan, K., Simionescu, D., Vyavahare, N. Novel porous aortic elastin and collagen scaffolds for tissue engineering. *Biomaterials* 2004; 25: 5227-5237.

[59] Jux, C., Wohlsein, P., Bruegmann, M., Zutz, M., Franzbach, B., Bertram, H. A new biological matrix for septal occlusion. *J. Intv. Cardiol.* 2003; 16: 149-152.

[60] Hudon, V., Berthod, F., Black, A., Damour, O., Germain, L., Auger, F. A tissue engineered endothelialized dermis to study the modulation of angiogenic and angiostatic molecules on capillary-like tube formation in vitro. *Br. J. Dermatol.* 2003; 148:1094-1104.

In: Type I Collagen
Editors: Maria Eduarda Henriques and Marcio Pinto
ISBN: 978-1-62257-625-8

Chapter VII

BIOMEDICAL IMPLICATIONS OF TYPE I COLLAGEN: A MARINE PERSPECTIVE

Ramjee Pallela[1,*], Venkateswara Rao Janapala[2], Yoon-Bo Shim[1] and Se-Kwon Kim[3]

[1]Institute of Biophysio Sensor Technology, Department of Chemistry, Pusan National University, Busan, South Korea
[2]Toxicology Unit, Biology Division, Indian Institute of Chemical Technology, Hyderabad, India
[3]Department of Chemistry and Marine Bioprocess Research Center, Pukyong National University, Busan, South Korea

ABSTRACT

Among all the collagens, Type I collagen plays an important role in the extracellular matrix (ECM) of skin, bone and other tissues. This protein is involved in many human and animal diseases, including fibrosis, osteoporosis, cancer, atherosclerosis etc. In spite of or because of the fact that it is widely distributed in the body, the different parts (degradation products) of type I collagen molecule are frequently utilized to monitor physiological changes in tissues as well as being used as diagnostic tools in various pathophysiological conditions. Collagens from marine sources are proved to be suitable for human applications as is metabolically compatible, non-toxic, low inflammatory and less immunogenic, however, type I collagen from marine sources has not yet been made available for extensive commercial medical uses. Hence, in the current book chapter, for the first time, we provide comprehensive information on the past explorations of type I collagens exclusively from marine sources; isolation and characterization, biomedical applications basing on our previous experiences. Further, the future prospects and perspectives are well covered in the present manuscript in order to bring the wide-ranging viewpoints that are useful for the next generation ECM researchers as well as marine medical biologists.

Keywords: Type I collagen, marine sources, biomaterial, tissue engineering

---

* Corresponding author: Phone: +8210-2056-4148; Email: rpallela@gmail.com.

INTRODUCTION

Collagen plays a crucial role in maintaining structural integrity as well as a regulating role in developing tissues there by serving as a structural backbone or scaffolding of animals (Prockop 1998). It is the common protein (about 30% of the human body) that provides texture, resiliency and shape; and found in most of the animal connective tissues *viz.*, dermis, bones, tendons, cartilage (hyaline), ligaments, blood vessels, teeth, cornea, intervertebral discs, vitreous bodies, placenta (fetal), etc. The use of collagen as a biomaterial has generated a great deal of interest during the past few decades in food, medical, pharmaceutical, cosmeceutical applications (Friess 1998; Lee et al. 2001; Rao et al. 2011). Although ruminant-derived collagens are prominently exploited in various human applications, apparent health complications like Bovine Spongiform Encephalopathy (BSE) and Transmissive Spongiform Encephalopathy (TSE) becoming potential threat nowadays (Pallela et al. 2011; Pallela et al. 2012; Swatschek et al. 2002a). As an alternative to these sources, collagens from other vertebrate and invertebrate sources are considered, however, the problem is still obvious and the collagens from marine sources have been evolved to use in food, biomedical and cosmetic applications. Very few investigations are performed on the ultrastructural and biochemical properties of sponge collagens towards their similarity and compatibility with the vertebrate collagens (Heinemann et al. 2007).

Traditionally speaking of collagen, it usually means type I collagen, the most common of the collagens in vertebrates and comprises up to 90% of the mammalian skeleton. Among all the collagens, type I collagen became the superior for exploring and exploiting it in various *in vitro* and *in vivo* evaluations. The presence of type I collagen is widespread in the animal kingdom, from invertebrates to vertebrates (Exposito et al. 2002). Moreover, the invertebrate species from marine origin are getting attracted towards the extraction of these collagens because of the safety reasons as well as due to the notion that 'life originated from marine'. However, research on type I collagen from marine animals is still at the budding stage. In the current chapter, we elucidated brief information on the structural and functional properties of type I collagen along with the biomedical implications of this most valuable protein derived from marine origin.

STRUCTURAL AND FUNCTIONAL ASPECTS OF TYPE I COLLAGEN

Type I collagen is widespread in the human body as in addition to bones; it exists in skin, tendons, ligaments, cornea, intervertebral disks, dentine, arteries and granulation tissues as the main locations. Although cartilage mainly contains of type II collagen, it is reported to contain type I collagen additionally (Wardale and Duance 1993).

Along with types II, III, V, and XI; type I collagen belongs to the group of classical fibril-forming collagens (Fibril Associated Collagens with Interrupted Triple helices, FACIT) (Rossert and De Crombrugghe 2002). Structurally, type I collagen is characterized as a highly orientated supramolecular aggregate with a characteristic suprastructure, with a typical quarter-staggered fibril-array of diameters ranging from 25 and 400 nm. The fibrils of type I collagen are defined by a characteristic banding pattern (electron microscope and atomic microscope), with a periodicity of about 70 nm (called the D-period) based on a staggered arrangement of individual collagen monomers (Gelse et al. 2003). Each molecule of type I collagen composed of two α1 chains and one α2 chain [$\alpha 1(1)_2$-$\alpha 2(1)$] coiled around each other in a characteristic triple helix. Both the α1 and α2 chains consist of a long helical domain preceded by a short N-terminal peptide and followed by a short C-terminal peptide (van der Rest and Garrone 1991). The mechanism of formation of type I collagen molecules by the stoichiometric control is still not well understood. It is evident that a number of type I collagen molecules can be formed by three α1 chains [$\alpha 1(1)_3$] and the homotrimeric type I collagen isotype contains three pro α1(1) collagen chains, a major isotype, whose role is not defined well. It is also observed from the previous studies that homotypic/homomeric and heterotypic/heteromeric collagens are noticed in the animal kingdom (Bairati and Gioria 2004; Pallela et al. 2011). However, it is very difficult to differentiate these types in case of invertebrate collagens due to the re-arrangements that occur between the collagen chains, resulting a different molecular pattern than the mammalian collagens.

Functionally, these triple helical molecules are, *in vivo*, mostly incorporated into a composite matrix either with type III collagen (in skin and reticular fibres) or with type V collagen (in bone, tendon, cornea). In most organs and notably in tendons and fascia, type I collagen provides tensile stiffness. Particularly in bone, type I collagen defines considerable biomechanical properties concerning the load bearing, tensile strength, and torsional stiffness especially after calcification (Gelse et al. 2003). Because of the fact that type I collagen is widely distributed in the body as degradation products or of intact form; these molecules are frequently utilized to monitor physiological changes in tissues as well as being used for diagnostic tools in various pathological conditions.

BIOMEDICAL APPLICATIONS OF TYPE I COLLAGEN

Type I collagen is currently the gold standard in the field of tissue-engineering because of its highest biocompatible characteristics than other collagens (Parenteau-Bareil et al. 2010). Immune response reaction against collagen mainly involves the epitopes in the telopeptide region at each end of the tropocollagen molecule. The difference of immunogenicity between polymerized collagen and their smaller counterpart lies on the accessibility of the antigenic determinants that decrease during the polymerization process. However, type I collagen is a suitable material for any tissue implantation because, only a small amount of people possess humoral immunity against it and a simple serologic test can verify if a patient is susceptible to an allergic reaction in response to this collagen-based biomaterial. Although type I collagen can be used in broad range of applications, forms, or medical products, e.g., medical devices, tissue engineered medical products (TEMPs) or cell, drug, or DNA delivery devices for implantation; its uses in a practical application should be based on the other factors, on the biocompatibility and on the available physical test data (Kaplan 2004).

Type I collagen is an important molecule used in several aspects e.g., it is used in the gelatin industry and in many biomaterial based industries. In the fact, leather is for instance, composed extremely of type I collagen molecules. In spite of several industrial applications, type I collagen has been used in noticeable biomedical and pharmacological applications (Meena et al. 1999). Several biodegradable collagen-based matrices either in sponge or sheet conformation, incorporated with carrier compounds e.g., fibronectin, laminin, hyaluronate, antibiotic, etc. have been developed by the use of type I, II, III collagens. These matrices were generated by mixing them with liquid medium containing a dispersing agent in order to make it feasible for freeze drying. Crosslinking agents like carbodimer or a succinimidyl can be added either prior to or after freeze drying procedures. These freeze-dried atherocollagens cure the wounds by accelerating the rate of wound healing. Since collagen is a material exhibiting excellent adhesive and proliferative properties towards fibroblasts, these dressings likewise exhibits vital adhesion and therapeutic effect for the wounds (Komatsuzaki et al. 1994).

Several collagen based medical, pharmacological as well as cosmetic products have been came forward for meeting the health demands of human beings e. g., Collasate® (a hydrolyzate of type I collagen for the management of postoperative and trauma sites). This hydrolyzate possessing the qualities of fast-acting healing gel for postoperative and trauma sites, first and second degree burns, skin lesions, dental extractions and oral surgery, pressure ulcers, venous stasis ulcers, ulcers resulting from arterial insufficiency, spay and neutering, de-clawing, foot pad injuries, hot spots, diabetic ulcers, lick granulomas, ocular wounds and general dermatologic wounds (PRN Pharmacal).

Marine Derived Type I Collagen and Its Biomedical Significance

As a first stage study of unexploited resources, several marine animals and their byproducts have been used for the preparation and characterization of collagens. However, very little information is available on the bio-medically important collagen from marine resources. Because of the difficulties in isolating marine collagen, there are very few animals are explored for collagens e.g., sponges (Garrone et al. 1975; Heinemann et al. 2007; Pallela et al. 2011b; Rao et al. 2011; Swatschek et al. 2002a), jellyfish (Addad et al. 2011; Nagai et al. 1999), cuttlefish (Nagai et al. 2001), starfish (Kimura et al. 1993), sea urchin (Omura et al. 1996), fish (Sikorski and Borderias 1994) etc.

Research on biomedical applications of marine sponge collagen is at the budding stage; however, few researchers are succeeded to isolate sponge collagens towards their biomedical and cosmetic applications e.g., skin parameters, enteric coatings, dermal delivery of all-*trans* retinol etc. (Nicklas et al. 2009; Swatschek et al. 2002a; Swatschek et al. 2002b). The novel enteric coating of the marine sponge collagen (using 12.9 mg/cm^2 coating material) complied with the requirements of European Pharmacopoeia (Ph. Eur.) for gastroresistant tablets. In addition, this coating material also meets the regulatory requirements for dietary supplements. Studies on type I collagens from marine sponge are at the verge of understanding the structural and functional roles to use them as effective biomedical materials (Heinemann et al. 2007). Our previous studies assessed that the sponge (*Ircinia fusca*) collagens that contain type I collagen in combination with chitosan and hydroxyapatite can also be used for bone tissue engineering applications based on the biophysicochemical and cyto-compatibility properties (Pallela et al. 2012). The main objective of bone tissue engineering is to mimic the natural process of bone formation by delivering a source of cells and/or growth factors through a scaffold matrix which can induce cellular attachment, migration, proliferation and osteoblastic differentiation. Although the selection of a suitable scaffold matrix is critical for cell-based bone tissue engineering applications, poriferans are aimed to identify and characterize natural marine sponges (*Callyspongiidae*) as potential bioscaffolds for osteogenesis (Lin et al. 2011).

On the other hand, jellyfish are also gaining much importance for isolation, characterization and application of collagens. The resilience, transparent and softness of coelenterate body is an indicative to the easy isolation of pure form of collagens which is in contrast to marine sponges that are highly contaminated with sediment particles etc. It is recently proved that broad harmlessness of jellyfish (*Aurelia aurita*, *Cotylorhiza tuberculata*, *Pelagia noctiluca*, and *Rhizostoma pulmo*) collagens and their biological effects on human cells are similar to that of mammalian type I collagen. Based on the bioavailability and biophysicochemical properties of jellyfish collagen, this marine biomaterial thus can be a good candidate for replacing terrestrial originated collagens in selected biomedical applications (Addad et al. 2011).

Although fish are the major resources for collagens from marine environment, the research on their biomedical implications is not well explored (Ikoma et al. 2003). In regard of investigating through the more effective use of under-utilized resources, type I collagen can be prepared from skin, bone and fins of marine fish and fish wastes. Marine fish collagens have been proposed to use in tissue engineering applications (Hayashi et al. 2011). Type I collagens derived from lower marine vertebrates such as bony fishes and lamprey were found to exhibit a high degree of structural similarity between their α1 α2 and skin related α3 chains compared with type I collagen from calf (Hayashi et al. 2011; Kimura 1992). Numerous attempts have been recently made to use type I collagen for biomedical applications by making them to assemble with other biomedical molecules through chemical and physical measures towards the bio-stability and effectiveness of working as a biomaterial. Type I collagen from marine fish (*Oncorhynchus keta* and *Theragra chalcogramma*) acts as an adequate culture substrate, in either serum-supplemented or serum-free conditions, to support the adhesion and proliferation of cells depending on the culturing conditions (Kaneko et al. 1995). Just recently, drug delivering potential of type I collagen isolated from eel fish *Evenchelys macrura* has been reported (Veeruraj et al. 2012). The eel collagen was successfully tested for its drug delivering capacity through standard drugs embedded in gels and films of the eel extracted acid soluble and pepsin soluble collagens (ASC and PSC, respectively). In an independent study by Noitup (2005), ASC and PSC of albacore tuna (*Thunnus alalunga*) and silver-line grunt (*Pomadasys kaakan*), as skin by-products from frozen fish fillet industry) had been extracted, purified and characterized. Analysis of these collagens by SDS-PAGE indicated the absence of a disulfide bond, which is a characteristic of type I collagen that contain different subunits, α, β and γ (Noitup et al. 2005).

The notion of utilizing these marine based type I collagens is still in the emergent stage and there is a need of understanding the physiofunctional aspects of these collagens for the application in suitable biomedical studies. Moreover, diverging approaches are put forward to use type I collagen as a 2D or 3D matrix for cellular growth and proliferation towards the development of stable *in vitro* and *in vivo* biosensors (Ju et al. 2009). The current chapter could provide proper scientific trend to the young researchers for choosing appropriate source of collagens and the biomedical approach towards the development of novel collagen based biomedical materials.

CONCLUSION

Biomedicine is an emerging field of science that implies the principles of natural sciences, more importantly biology, to investigate the problems in clinical medicine. Natural and synthetic materials can be characterized for their biocompatibility to use them *in vitro* and *in vivo* for providing a platform for the end user applications. One such pioneering biological macromolecule is collagen, which has been put forward for various biomedical applications from several decades. Although marine collagen extraction procedures are very limited, the biomedical results of these marine derived collagens are proved to be promising. Among the marine derived collagens, type I collagen became the superior contributor of biomedical applications *viz*., tissue engineering scaffolds, gels, plasters etc. Although it is challenging, advanced strategies to be followed properly for the extraction of type I collagen and there is a further need of focusing these biomolecules towards their implications in biomedical fields.

REFERENCES

Addad, S., Exposito, J. Y., Faye, C., Ricard-Blum, S., Lethias, C. (2011). Isolation, characterization and biological evaluation of jellyfish collagen for use in biomedical applications. *Marine Drugs* 9(6), 967-983.

Bairati, A., Gioria, M. (2004). Collagen fibrils of an invertebrate (*Sepia officinalis*) are heterotypic: immunocytochemical demonstration. *Journal of Structural Biology* 147(2), 159-165.

Exposito, J., Cluzel, C., Garrone, R., Lethias, C. (2002). Evolution of collagens. *The Anatomical Record* 268(3), 302-316.

Friess, W. (1998). Collagen – biomaterial for drug delivery. *European Journal of Pharmaceutics and Biopharmaceutics* 45(2), 113-136.

Garrone, R., Huc, A., Junqua, S. (1975). Fine structure and physicochemical studies on the collagen of the marine sponge Chondrosia reniformis Nardo. *Journal of Ultrastructure Research* 52(2), 261-275.

Gelse, K., Pöschl, E., Aigner, T. (2003). Collagens--structure, function, and biosynthesis. *Advanced Drug Delivery Reviews* 55(12), 1531-1546.

Hayashi, Y., Yamada, S., Ikeda, T., Yanagiguchi, K. (2011). Fish Collagen and Tissue Repair. In: Kim. S. K., (Ed.) *Marine cosmeceuticals: trends and prospects*, CRC-Taylor and Francis: Boca Rotan, pp. 133-142.

Heinemann, S., Ehrlich, H., Douglas, T., Heinemann, C., Worch, H., Schatton, W., Hanke, T. (2007). Ultrastructural studies on the collagen of the marine sponge *Chondrosia reniformis* nardo. *Biomacromolecules* 8(11), 3452-3457.

Ikoma, T., Kobayashi, H., Tanaka, J., Walsh, D., Mann, S. (2003). Physical properties of type I collagen extracted from fish scales of *Pagrus major* and *Oreochromis niloticas*. *International Journal of Biological Macromolecules* 32(3–5), 199-204.

Ju, Y.M., Yu, B., West, L., Moussy, Y., Moussy, F. (2010). A novel porous collagen scaffold around an implantable biosensor for improving biocompatibility. II. Long-term *in vitro/in vivo* sensitivity characteristics of sensors with NDGA- or GA-crosslinked collagen scaffolds. *Journal of Biomedical Materials Research* Part A 92(2), 650-6588.

Kaneko, Y., Igarashi, M., Iwashita, M., Suzuki, K., Kojima, H., Kimura, S., Hasobe, M. (1995). Effects of fish and calf type I collagens as culture substrate in the adhesion and spreading process of established fish cells. In *Vitro Cellular & Developmental Biology - Animal* 31(3), 178-182.

Kaplan, D. S. (2004). Development of standards for the characterization of natural materials used in tissue engineered medical products (TEMPs). *Tissue Engineered Medical Products* (1452), 172.

Kimura, S. (1992). Wide distribution of the skin type I collagen α3 chain in bony fish. Comparative Biochemistry and Physiology Part B: *Comparative Biochemistry* 102(2), 255-260.

Kimura, S., Omura, Y., Ishida, M., Shirai, H., 1993. Molecular characterization of fibrillar collagen from the body wall of starfish Asterias amurensis. Comparative Biochemistry and Physiology Part B: *Comparative Biochemistry* 104(4), 663-668.

Komatsuzaki, S., Hirayama, T., Toyokawa, T. (1994). *Wound dressing and method of manufacturing the same*. EP Patent 0407943.

Lee, C. H., Singla, A., Lee, Y. (2001). Biomedical applications of collagen. *International Journal of Pharmaceutics* 221(1), 1-22.

Lin, Z., Solomon, K. L., Zhang, X., Pavlos, N. J., Abel, T., Willers, C., Dai, K., Xu, J., Zheng, Q., Zheng, M. (2011). *In vitro* evaluation of natural marine sponge collagen as a scaffold for bone tissue engineering. *International Journal of Biological Sciences* 7(7), 968-977.

Meena, C., Mengi, S., Deshpande, S. (1999). Biomedical and industrial applications of collagen. *Journal of Chemical Sciences* 111(2), 319-329.

Nagai, T., Ogawa, T., Nakamura, T., Ito, T., Nakagawa, H., Fujiki, K., Nakao, M., Yano, T. (1999). Collagen of edible jellyfish exumbrella. *Journal of the Science of Food and Agriculture* 79(6), 855-858.

Nagai, T., Yamashita, E., Taniguchi, K., Kanamori, N., Suzuki, N. (2001). Isolation and characterisation of collagen from the outer skin waste material of cuttlefish (*Sepia lycidas*). *Food Chemistry* 72(4), 425-429.

Nicklas, M., Schatton, W., Heinemann, S., Hanke, T., Kreuter, J. (2009). Enteric coating derived from marine sponge collagen. *Drug Development and Industrial Pharmacy* 35(11), 1384-1388.

Noitup, P., Garnjanagoonchorn, W., Morrissey, M.T. (2005). Fish skin type I collagen: Characteristic comparison of albacore tuna (*Thunnus alalunga*) and silver-line grunt (*Pomadasys kaakan*). *Journal of Aquatic Food Product Technology* 14(1), 17-28.

Omura, Y., Urano, N., Kimura, S. (1996). Occurrence of fibrillar collagen with structure of $(\alpha1)_2\alpha_2$ in the test of sea urchin *Asthenosoma ijimai*. Comparative Biochemistry and Physiology Part B: *Biochemistry and Molecular Biology* 115(1), 63-68.

Pallela, R., Bojja, S., Janapala, V. R. (2011). Biochemical and biophysical characterization of collagens of marine sponge, *Ircinia fusca* (Porifera: Demospongiae: Irciniidae). *International Journal of Biological Macromolecules* 49(1), 85-92.

Pallela, R., Venkatesan, J., Janapala, V. R., Kim, S. K. (2012). Biophysicochemical evaluation of chitosan-hydroxyapatite-marine sponge collagen composite for bone tissue engineering. *Journal of Biomedical Materials Research* Part A 100A(2), 486-495.

Parenteau-Bareil, R., Gauvin, R., Berthod, F. (2010). Collagen-based biomaterials for tissue engineering applications. *Materials* 3(3), 1863-1887.

PRN Pharmacal: http://www.prnpharmacal.com/collasate/index.php.

Prockop, D. J. (1998). What holds us together? Why do some of us fall apart? What can we do about it? *Matrix Biology* 16(9), 519-528.

Rao, J. V., Pallela, R., Prakash, G.V.S.B. (2011). Prospects of marine sponge collagen and its applications in cosmetology. In: Kim. S.K., (Ed.) *Marine cosmeceuticals:Trends and prospects*, CRC-Taylor and Francis: Boca Rotan, pp. 77-103.

Rossert, J., De Crombrugghe, B. (2002). Type I collagen: structure, synthesis, and regulation. In: Bilezikian, J. P.; Raisz, L. G.; Rodan, G. A. (Eds.) *Principles of bone biology*, Academic Press: New York, pp.189-210.

Sikorski, Z. E., Borderias, J. A. (1994). Collagen in the muscles and skins of marine animals. In: Sikorski, Z.E., Pan, B.S., Shahidi, F. (Eds.) *Seafood Proteins*, Chapman and Hall: New York, pp.58-70.

Swatschek, D., Schatton, W., Kellermann, J., Müller, W.E.G., Kreuter, J. (2002a). Marine sponge collagen: isolation, characterization and effects on the skin parameters surface-pH, moisture and sebum. *European Journal of Pharmaceutics and Biopharmaceutics* 53(1), 107-113.

Swatschek, D., Schatton, W., Müller, W. E. G., Kreuter, J. (2002b). Microparticles derived from marine sponge collagen (SCMPs): preparation, characterization and suitability for dermal delivery of all-trans retinol. *European Journal of Pharmaceutics and Biopharmaceutics* 54(2), 125-133.

van der Rest, M., Garrone, R. (1991). Collagen family of proteins. *The FASEB journal* 5(13), 2814-2823.

Veeruraj, A., Arumugam, M., Ajithkumar, T., Balasubramanian, T. (2012). Isolation and characterization of drug delivering potential of type-I collagen from eel fish *Evenchelys macrura*. *Journal of Materials Science: Materials in Medicine*, 1-10.

Wardale, R. J., Duance, V. C. (1993). Quantification and immunolocalisation of porcine articular and growth plate cartilage collagens. *Journal of Cell Science* 105(4), 975.

Reviewed by:

1. Dr. A. Veeruraj, Professor,

Centre of Advanced Study in Marine Biology, Faculty of Marine Sciences, Annamalai Univeristy, Parangipettai-608502, TamilNadu, India, Email: anguveeruraj@gmail.com.

2. Dr. Narsinh L. Thakur, Senior scientist,

Bio-organic Chemistry Group, Chemical Oceanography Division, National Institute of Oceanography, Dona Paula, Goa-403004, India. Email: thakurn@nio.org.

3. R. Jayakumar, Professor,

Amrita Institute of Medical Sciences & Research Center, Amrita Lane, AIMS Ponekkara P.O; Kochi-682041. Kerala, India. Email: rjayakumar@aims.amrita.edu.

In: Type I Collagen
Editors: Maria Eduarda Henriques and Marcio Pinto
ISBN: 978-1-62257-625-8

Chapter VIII

Role of Extracellular Matrix in the Wound Repair Process

Simona Martinotti, Bruno Burlando and Elia Ranzato*
Dipartimento di Scienze e Innovazione Tecnologica, DiSIT,
University of Piemonte Orientale "Amedeo Avogadro," Italy

Abstract

The extracellular matrix (ECM) serves as scaffolding to hold tissues together, its form and its composition help to determine tissue characteristics. Wound repair processes heal by progressing through distinct but overlapping phases: haemostasis, inflammation, proliferation and remodeling. Throughout these phases, components of the ECM play an important role in regulating and integrating many key processes of healing mechanisms. The components of the ECM provide strength, elasticity and compressibility in normal skin. In acute wounds the provisional wound matrix, containing fibrin and fibronectin, plays several key roles, including providing a scaffold to direct cells into the injury as well as stimulating them to proliferate, differentiate and synthesize new ECM. It has also been proposed that the prolonged inflammatory phase causes increased levels of proteases such as MMPs, elastase, plasmin and thrombin, which destroy components of the ECM, damaging the growth factors and their receptors that are essential for healing. This article reviews the multifaceted molecular roles of ECM in normal and abnormal wound-healing process, and touches on potential therapies based on recent acquisitions of tissue biology.

The Extracellular Matrix

The process of wound repair involves the timed and balanced activity of inflammatory, vascular, connective tissue and epithelial cells. All of these components need an extracellular matrix (ECM) to facilitate the healing process [1]. Skin is composed of thin and high cellular epidermis and relatively acellular dermis of collagen-rich ECM. The few cellular constituents

* E-mail: ranzato@unipmn.it

of dermis, mainly fibroblasts, are responsible for the exact anatomical and physiological reproduction of both epidermis and dermis during the normal tissue turnover process. This replacement occurs every several weeks for epidermis and every several months for dermis [2]. Research over the past 20 years has increased our understanding of the ECM composition, identifying distinct families of matrix structures. These ECM elements interact closely with each other, thereby constructing large networks with structural and non-structural components [3]. The components of ECM include proteins, complex carbohydrates and a combination of the two. Collagen is the most prominent protein of ECM, representing a group of diverse protein subfamilies containing at least 28 different collagen types, which are encoded by more than 42 genes. All members share a common element, represented by the presence of at least one triple helical domain. Collagen type I makes up 96% of the dermal collagen, and collagen type II most of the remaining collagen. Collagen type IV is present in the basement membrane and plays a significant role in epithelial cell adherence to the ECM and subsequent migration. Collagens not only provide structure or scaffold, but also critical signaling for cell proliferation, and migration into the wound [4, 5].

Elastin represents another important element of elastic tissues, such as connective tissue and vessel walls. Elastin fibers are not detected in the granulation tissue during the early phase of wound repair, suggesting that a certain differentiated status of fibroblasts is required to produce elastic tissue [6]. Proteoglycans are a combination of protein and sugars, consisting of a "core protein" with one or more covalently attached glycosaminoglycan (GAG) chains. These large molecules are highly hydrophilic, and confer viscoelasticity and compression resistance to tissue. Proteoglycans are involved in the scaffolding for new granulation tissue, and also provide a conduit for cell and nutrient movement in the wound [7]. Hyaluronic acid is a main glycosaminoglycan that maintains matrix hydration and directs the healing process. High molecular-weight molecules help to modulate inflammation, protecting the new granulation tissue, while small molecular-weight molecules, often deriving from fragmentation of larger molecules, activate angiogenesis and granulation tissue formation [8]. One of the best characterized glycoprotein of the ECM is fibronectin, a major product of dermal fibroblasts and myofibroblasts. Fibronectin is a large adhesive glycoprotein with a huge number of functions. Besides its structural role, fibronectin is the main cell adhesion molecule, modulating many cellular activities. In humans, alternative splicing generates 20 fibronectin variants with different functions [9]. After injury, fibronectin is rapidly deposited from blood plasma, playing an important role in platelet adhesion, activation and growth factors release [10].

Laminin represents a family of 16 members of large trimeric ECM glycoproteins consisting of three different polypeptide chains [11]. These factors control cell migration, proliferation and differentiation, in particular re-epithelialization and vascularization [12]. More recently a group of proteins named matricellular proteins has been identified. In this group, there are thrombospondins, a family of five members of proteins, specifically expressed during different phases of wound processes [13]. The family of tenascin proteins comprises four members in mammals. Tenascins are large glycoproteins with structural similarity to fibronectin [14]. Secreted protein acidic and rich in cysteine (SPARC), a matricellular glycoprotein, was initially identified in bone where it binds collagen and Ca^{2+}, initiating nucleation during bone mineralization [15]. However, SPARC is also secreted by non-epithelial cells in non-ossifying tissues, during both development and tissue repair, where it mediates ECM remodeling and turn-over, and cell-ECM interactions [16].

The wound healing process is, in large part, regulated by the ordered production of cytokines that control gene activation responsible for cellular migration, proliferation, and synthetic activities [17]. Platelets and macrophages are the key sources of cytokines. The control of cytokine release is regulated by other cytokines and, in part, by the tissue milieu [18]. The healing of wounds follows a predictable chain of events that occurs in a reproducible fashion. Five overlapped phases have been described: hemostasis, inflammation, cellular migration and proliferation, wound contraction and matrix remodeling [19]. During inflammation, immediately after injury, platelets aggregate and induce the formation of the fibrin clot. This clot is important not only for stopping bleeding, but also as a reservoir of ECM proteins and growth factors, providing a first suitable milieu for initiating the wound repair process [20]. After this first step, re-epithelialization begins to protect the wound bed from excessive water loss and exposure to bacterial infections. This period is characterized by endothelial cell and fibroblast proliferation and ECM production, replacing the losses imposed by wound injury. The subsequent phases of healing, including remodeling can be identified by characteristic patterns of cellular infiltrates and compositional changes of the ECM. Fibroblasts migrating into the wound, especially at the wound edges, begin to produce an early form of ECM, termed provisional matrix [21]. This early matrix is composed mainly of fibrin, fibronectin and hyaluronic acid. These components allow the adherence of cells to the ECM for subsequent cell migration into the wound. A temporary scaffold is also created by these components to direct cell movement. These phenomena induce the proliferation of fibroblasts, the formation of granulation tissue and the migration and proliferation of keratinocytes to close the wound [22, 23]. When the natural healing process is dysregulated as a consequence of vascular disease, diabetes and/or microbial infection, wounds may heal slowly and sometimes become chronic.

CELL–MATRIX INTERACTIONS

The functioning of cells is dependent on their interaction with the surrounding ECM, mediated by specific cellular receptors, which binds to ECM components [24]. Integrins are the largest family of receptors mediating the interaction of cells with the ECM [25]. These receptors have a relatively restricted, cell type-specific and context-dependent expression, with defined substrate specificity. Integrins are transmembrane heterodimers glycoproteins comprising 18 different α and 8 different β subunits. The combination of α and β subunits determines binding specificity for the ligands. The cytoplasmatic domain of integrins is anchored to the actin cytoskeleton through cytoskeletal linkage proteins such as vinculin and paxillin [26]. The cytoplasmic domain of integrins may function as a tyrosine kinase receptor with respect to cross-talk and induction of signaling [27]. Usually, integrins are expressed at the cell surface in an inactive form. Signals arising from the cytoskeleton activate integrins by modulating their conformation, resulting in increased affinity for ECM molecules and clustering to focal adhesions [28, 29]. Several ECM proteins, such as fibronectin, fibrinogen, osteopontin, tenascin, and vitronectin contain an arginine-glycine-aspartate (RGD) cell-binding domain that is recognized by specific integrins. The RGD sequence on many proteins is cryptic, i.e. it becomes exposed only upon proteolytic cleavage, thus allowing a regulatory mechanism of the RGD site function [30]. The degree of cell attachment and spreading, determined by ECM substrate, controls anchorage-dependent gene expression, cell growth, differentiation and cell survival [31]. Thus, integrins in absence of their cognate ligand may trigger apoptosis [32].

ADVANCED WOUND HEALING THERAPIES

The extracellular matrix plays an important regulatory role in the biological behavior of epidermal cells. These latter are induced to migrate from wound edges by contacts established with early matrix containing fibronectin, fibrin and collagen. These migrating cells move toward the center of wound by traveling along fibrin, fibronectin and collagen strands [33]. The ongoing signaling between cells and ECM direct the migration of the single epithelial sheet, and thereafter activatescell proliferation to build a multilayered epidermis. A bulk of studies has demonstrated the benefits of ECM or its components in the healing process, especially with diabetic and venous ulcers. A better understanding of the ECM role in tissue repair and regeneration can give new opportunities for wound treatment and management. Part of these efforts has been directed to correct conditions of matrix deficiency, thereby changing the biology of scar surface [26]. The first strategy is to decrease the continuous ECM degradation induced by inflammation. Such an approach would require the control of chronic inflammationin the wound bed through the inhibition of pro-inflammatory cytokine and metalloproteinase release. Unfortunately, no cytokine modifiers or MMP inhibitors are clinically available yet [34].

Another interesting strategy is to increase the local ECM production, so inducing dormant fibroblasts to produce ECM components. A number of products suitable to this aim are commercially available and many others are in development [35]. Examples of skin substitutes are cellular products with/without matrix, including epithelial cell sheets and dermal replacements. Acellular products are also available, containing ECM components based on natural or synthetic materials [36]. Collagen, in the form of synthetic matrices, is a commonly used topical product. With the exception of few products, which contain a natural collagen matrix architectures composed of native collagen, these products consist more frequently of synthetic collagen-like sponges obtained from denatured collagen. The advantage of this kind of device is to provide a matrix scaffold for cell proliferation and migration [37]. Fibronectin is another ECM element, which could be utilized as a topical agent. Fibroblasts exposed to fibronectin proliferate and produce a much greater amount of ECM than those exposed to collagen. There is currently no clinical use of topical fibronectin for stimulating the healing process [38].

Hyaluronic acid, a known wound stimulant, is available in several topical products but its reparative properties in poor-healing wounds has not been well established [39]. Another currently used approach is the topical application of growth factors, an ECM component known to be deficient in slowly healing wounds [40]. A number of growth factors have been shown to increase ECM production by fibroblasts and stimulate various wound healing steps. Platelet lysate (PL), a platelet-enriched fraction purified from whole blood by platelet apheresis, has been shown to increase the healing rate in *in vitro* studies [41, 42] and *in vivo* applications [43, 44]. PL promotes keratinocyte epithelialization and regulates fibroblast matrix deposition through modulation of modulates MMP-9 collagenase, collagen and syndecan-4 expression [45]. These data explain the ability of this platelet derivative to heal severe and problematic wounds without leading to heavy scarring and keloid formation [46].

Conclusions and Perspectives

Tightly controlled ECM homeostasis is crucial for regulating essential cellular processes, allowing for a correct development of the organism as well as tissue repair and regeneration [3]. When this homeostasis is perturbed, aberrant ECM contributes to pathological conditions, including fibrotic disease, tumor progression and metastasis. Diseases involving ECM alterations are responsible for millions of deaths worldwide, and represent a challenging obstacle with respect to clinical treatment [36].

Investigating processes underlying ECM perturbation, and the resulting altered cell-ECM interactions will allow us to identify therapeutic targets for clinical benefits. Gene therapy has already been used to repair a Laminin-332 (Laminin-5) defect in a patient with *epidermolysis bullosa* [47]. Furthermore, a potential alternative to gene therapy is to use extracellular matrix biomaterials for skin repair [48]. Tissue scaffolds have been used for wound dressing or skin tissue engineering in a variety of wound conditions. These implantations can not only cover the wound and provide a physical barrier, but also stimulate re-epithelialization and formation of granulation tissue. A variety of scaffolds fabricated based on naturally occurring materials or manufactured synthetically have been studied [1]. However, there are still many challenges faced by bioengineers, cell biologists and clinicians, and further developments in this area will require ongoing interactions and collaborations [1, 49].

References

[1] Zhong SP, Zhang YZ, Lim CT. Tissue scaffolds for skin wound healing and dermal reconstruction. *Wiley Interdiscip. Rev. Nanomed. Nanobiotechnol.* 2010;2(5):510-25.

[2] Keller KE, Aga M, Bradley JM, Kelley MJ, Acott TS. Extracellular matrix turnover and outflow resistance. *Exp Eye Res* 2009;88(4):676-82.

[3] Eckes B, Nischt R, Krieg T. Cell-matrix interactions in dermal repair and scarring. *Fibrogenesis Tissue Repair* 2010;3:4.

[4] Heino J, Tunyan K, Calvetti D, Somersalo E. Bayesian flux balance analysis applied to a skeletal muscle metabolic model. *J. Theor. Biol.* 2007;248(1):91-110.

[5] Abreu-Velez AM, Howard MS. Collagen IV in Normal Skin and in Pathological Processes. *N Am J Med Sci* 2012;4(1):1-8.

[6] Zhou Z, Wang J, Cao R, Morita H, Soininen R, Chan KM, et al. Impaired angiogenesis, delayed wound healing and retarded tumor growth in perlecan heparan sulfate-deficient mice. *Cancer Res.* 2004;64(14):4699-702.

[7] Hynes RO, Naba A. Overview of the matrisome--an inventory of extracellular matrix constituents and functions. *Cold Spring Harb. Perspect. Biol.* 2012;4(1):a004903.

[8] Bansal J, Kedige SD, Anand S. Hyaluronic acid: a promising mediator for periodontal regeneration. *Indian J. Dent. Res.* 2010;21(4):575-8.

[9] Kosmehl H, Berndt A, Katenkamp D. Molecular variants of fibronectin and laminin: structure, physiological occurrence and histopathological aspects. *Virchows. Arch.* 1996;429(6):311-22.

[10] Clark RA. Fibronectin matrix deposition and fibronectin receptor expression in healing and normal skin. *J. Invest. Dermatol.* 1990;94(6 Suppl):128S-34S.

[11] Aumailley M, Bruckner-Tuderman L, Carter WG, Deutzmann R, Edgar D, Ekblom P, et al. A simplified laminin nomenclature. *Matrix Biol.* 2005;24(5):326-32.

[12] Hallmann R, Horn N, Selg M, Wendler O, Pausch F, Sorokin LM. Expression and function of laminins in the embryonic and mature vasculature. *Physiol. Rev.* 2005;85(3):979-1000.

[13] Armstrong LC, Bornstein P. Thrombospondins 1 and 2 function as inhibitors of angiogenesis. *Matrix Biol.* 2003;22(1):63-71.

[14] Chiquet-Ehrismann R, Chiquet M. Tenascins: regulation and putative functions during pathological stress. *J. Pathol.* 2003;200(4):488-99.

[15] Murphy-Ullrich JE, Lane TF, Pallero MA, Sage EH. SPARC mediates focal adhesion disassembly in endothelial cells through a follistatin-like region and the Ca(2+)-binding EF-hand. *J. Cell Biochem.* 1995;57(2):341-50.

[16] Chlenski A, Guerrero LJ, Peddinti R, Spitz JA, Leonhardt PT, Yang Q, et al. Anti-angiogenic SPARC peptides inhibit progression of neuroblastoma tumors. *Mol. Cancer* 2010;9:138.

[17] Ranzato E, Burlando B. Signaling pathways in wound repair. In: Middleton J, editor. *Wound healing: process, phases and promoting.* Hauppauge, New York: Nova Publishers Inc, 2011:123-35.

[18] Circolo A, Welgus HG, Pierce GF, Kramer J, Strunk RC. Differential regulation of the expression of proteinases/antiproteinases in fibroblasts. Effects of interleukin-1 and platelet-derived growth factor. *J. Biol. Chem.* 1991;266(19):12283-8.

[19] Monaco JL, Lawrence WT. Acute wound healing an overview. *Clin. Plast. Surg.* 2003;30(1):1-12.

[20] Nurden AT, Nurden P, Sanchez M, Andia I, Anitua E. Platelets and wound healing. *Front Biosci.* 2008;13:3532-48.

[21] Greiling D, Clark RA. Fibronectin provides a conduit for fibroblast transmigration from collagenous stroma into fibrin clot provisional matrix. *J. Cell Sci.* 1997;110 (Pt 7): 861-70.

[22] Wood F. Tissue engineering of skin. *Clin Plast Surg* 2012;39(1):21-32.

[23] Reish RG, Eriksson E. Scar treatments: preclinical and clinical studies. *J. Am. Coll Surg.* 2008;206(4):719-30.

[24] Tran KT, Griffith L, Wells A. Extracellular matrix signaling through growth factor receptors during wound healing. *Wound Repair Regen.* 2004;12(3):262-8.

[25] Widgerow AD. Chronic wounds - is cellular 'reception' at fault? Examining integrins and intracellular signalling. *Int. Wound J.* 2012.

[26] Watt FM, Fujiwara H. Cell-extracellular matrix interactions in normal and diseased skin. *Cold Spring Harb. Perspect. Biol.* 2011;3(4).

[27] Blystone SD. Integrating an integrin: a direct route to actin. *Biochim. Biophys. Acta.* 2004;1692(2-3):47-54.

[28] Hynes RO. Integrins: bidirectional, allosteric signaling machines. *Cell* 2002; 110(6):673-87.

[29] Calderwood DA. Integrin activation. *J. Cell Sci.* 2004;117(Pt 5):657-66.
[30] Davis GE, Bayless KJ, Davis MJ, Meininger GA. Regulation of tissue injury responses by the exposure of matricryptic sites within extracellular matrix molecules. *Am. J. Pathol.* 2000;156(5):1489-98.
[31] Stupack DG. Integrins as a distinct subtype of dependence receptors. *Cell Death Differ* 2005;12(8):1021-30.
[32] Chen CS, Mrksich M, Huang S, Whitesides GM, Ingber DE. Geometric control of cell life and death. *Science* 1997;276(5317):1425-8.
[33] Ruszczak Z. Effect of collagen matrices on dermal wound healing. *Adv. Drug Deliv. Rev.* 2003;55(12):1595-611.
[34] Arwert EN, Mentink RA, Driskell RR, Hoste E, Goldie SJ, Quist S, et al. Upregulation of CD26 expression in epithelial cells and stromal cells during wound-induced skin tumour formation. *Oncogene.* 2012;31(8):992-1000.
[35] Rizzi SC, Upton Z, Bott K, Dargaville TR. Recent advances in dermal wound healing: biomedical device approaches. *Expert Rev. Med. Devices* 2010;7(1):143-54.
[36] Cox TR, Erler JT. Remodeling and homeostasis of the extracellular matrix: implications for fibrotic diseases and cancer. *Dis. Model Mech.* 2011;4(2):165-78.
[37] Purna SK, Babu M. Collagen based dressings--a review. *Burns* 2000;26(1):54-62.
[38] Midwood KS, Mao Y, Hsia HC, Valenick LV, Schwarzbauer JE. Modulation of cell-fibronectin matrix interactions during tissue repair. *J. Investig. Dermatol. Symp. Proc.* 2006;11(1):73-8.
[39] Chen WY, Abatangelo G. Functions of hyaluronan in wound repair. *Wound Repair Regen.* 1999;7(2):79-89.
[40] Fitzpatrick RE. Endogenous growth factors as cosmeceuticals. *Dermatol Surg* 2005;31(7 Pt 2):827-31; discussion 31.
[41] Ranzato E, Mazzucco L, Patrone M, Burlando B. Platelet lysate promotes in vitro wound scratch closure of human dermal fibroblasts: different roles of cell calcium, P38, ERK and PI3K/AKT. *J. Cell Mol. Med.* 2009;13(8B):2030-8.
[42] Ranzato E, Boccafoschi F, Mazzucco L, Patrone M, Burlando B. Role of ERK1/2 in platelet lysate-driven endothelial cell repair. *J. Cell Biochem.* 2010;110(3):783-93.
[43] Mazzucco L, Medici D, Serra M, Panizza R, Rivara G, Orecchia S, et al. The use of autologous platelet gel to treat difficult-to-heal wounds: a pilot study. *Transfusion* 2004;44(7):1013-8.
[44] Greppi N, Mazzucco L, Galetti G, Bona F, Petrillo E, Smacchia C, et al. Treatment of recalcitrant ulcers with allogeneic platelet gel from pooled platelets in aged hypomobile patients. *Biologicals* 2011;39(2):73-80.
[45] Ranzato E, Martinotti S, Volante A, Mazzucco L, Burlando B. Platelet lysate modulates MMP-2 and MMP-9 expression, matrix deposition and cell-to-matrix adhesion in keratinocytes and fibroblasts. *Exp. Dermatol.* 2011;20(4):308-13.
[46] Ranzato E, Mazzucco L, Burlando B. Platelet Derivatives: A New Horizon in Regenerative Medicine. In: Berhardt LV, editor. *Advances in Medicine and Biology.* Hauppauge, New York: Nova Publishers Inc, 2010:245-54.
[47] Mavilio F, Pellegrini G, Ferrari S, Di Nunzio F, Di Iorio E, Recchia A, et al. Correction of junctional epidermolysis bullosa by transplantation of genetically modified epidermal stem cells. *Nat. Med.* 2006;12(12):1397-402.

[48] Wolf K, Alexander S, Schacht V, Coussens LM, von Andrian UH, van Rheenen J, et al. Collagen-based cell migration models in vitro and in vivo. *Semin Cell Dev. Biol.* 2009;20(8):931-41.
[49] Griffith LG, Naughton G. Tissue engineering--current challenges and expanding opportunities. *Science* 2002;295(5557):1009-14.

INDEX

A

D

E

F

G

H

N

O

P

Q

R

S

T

U

V

W

X

Y

Z